A Practical Approach to the Care of Adolescents and Young Adults with Cancer

Julia Chisholm • Rachael Hough
Louise Soanes
Editors

A Practical Approach to the Care of Adolescents and Young Adults with Cancer

Springer

Editors
Julia Chisholm
Royal Marsden Hospital
Sutton, Surrey, UK

Rachael Hough
University College Hospital
London, UK

Louise Soanes
University College Hospital
London, UK

ISBN 978-3-030-09762-2 ISBN 978-3-319-66173-5 (eBook)
https://doi.org/10.1007/978-3-319-66173-5

Printed on acid-free paper

This Springer imprint is published by Springer Nature
The registered company is Springer International Publishing AG
The registered company address is: Gewerbestrasse 11, 6330 Cham, Switzerland

Foreword

It is only very recently that an increasing number of countries have begun to recognise the special needs of adolescents and young adults (AYA) compared with those of younger children and especially those with life-threatening illnesses like cancer. At this age (around 13–25 years) young people are going through significant physical, emotional, hormonal and psychological development and seeking progressive, greater independence from their parents. No matter where or how the doctors, nurses and other professionals who care for these young people have been trained in clinical aspects of care, they must also learn to recognise and help their patients with the more complex issues which face AYA patients receiving cancer treatment.

There is good evidence of greater delays in diagnosis amongst AYA patients especially with Hodgkin's Lymphoma, some brain tumours and bone tumours. Lack of awareness that young people can get cancer (it is rare) by the public and even more by doctors, decreasing parental advocacy, the patient not being believed when presenting with symptoms and young people not feeling empowered to insist on action have all been cited for such delays. Public and professional awareness is crucial through education. The tumours which AYAs acquire are different from younger children with only 10% being the 'tail' of childhood malignancies, 25–30% being adolescent peak tumours like Hodgkin's lymphoma, bone tumours especially osteosarcoma, and some germ cell tumours and 60–65% are early onset more 'adult type' diseases, including carcinomas. In a number of studies the longest symptom intervals (time from first symptoms/signs to diagnosis) have been seen in Hodgkin's lymphoma, osteosarcoma and some brain tumours. The consequences of delays are potential tumour progression and hence need for more intensive therapy, raised anxiety/anger/guilt, distrust of doctors and health care systems and subsequent greater risk of non-adherence to therapy and guidelines. Whether survival chances are decreased is difficult to verify. All those who care for teenagers and young adults need to be aware of these issues and help to educate the public and professionals about listening to patients and taking their histories seriously. They must also understand why such delays may make patients hostile to them initially.

There is also good evidence of decreased entry into clinical trials for this age group of patients. Where we do not know the optimal therapy for a specific tumour, a trial comparing the best current therapy against a new and potentially better drug or combination of drugs is the recognised best way to make progress. Low trial entry has been shown principally to be due to doctors not even considering entering patients on the false premise that young people will not adhere to treatment. Again this results from a failure to communicate well with patients and help them to understand what it is all about. Adherence can be attained not only we all 'tell it straight and honestly' about what we are doing and what our patients can expect but also what they must do to get through their treatment plus how we can help them.

Cancer treatment can have significant side effects but, with first class nursing, supportive care and relief of symptoms, most toxicity can be ameliorated to some degree. Like all aspects of care, adolescents and young adults are much better listeners than we give them credit for and they certainly recognise and respect truthfulness, sincerity and honesty in all discussions. So the nurses and doctors looking after young people must know what they are talking about, be well trained, be good listeners and show empathy.

This book is an excellent practical manual for all professionals working in this specialist field, covering different models of care, supportive, psychological and palliation, late effects and survivorship. Research has to be mentioned because we do not have all the answers as to why young people acquire cancer, how to optimally treat some tumours or actually prevent any of them.

Working in a team is crucial for the care of young people but it must be a truly well-co-ordinated one with the ability to give support to each other whilst working in often very emotional situations.

Finally we do have to realise that worldwide, in most low-middle income countries, childhood ceases at 13–14 years (just as it did in the UK in the 1970s) and patients over that age are treated as adults without usually any of the care which this manual is championing. There must be a very determined effort in the interests of young people worldwide to spread the messages which have been shown to help young people along their cancer pathway.

University of Manchester
Manchester, UK

Tim Eden

Contents

Overview of Adolescent and Young Adult Cancer

1

Martin G. McCabe

1.1 Adolescent and Young Adult Cancer: What Do We Mean?

The concept of Teenage and Young Adult (AYA) or Adolescent and Young Adult (AYA) cancer came to prominence in the 2000s with the recognition that progress in improving the outcomes of childhood and adult cancer patients had been the direct result of specific, coordinated, national and international initiatives designed around children and adults respectively [1, 2]. Little attention had been paid to the intervening age group, the 'lost tribe' of adolescents and young adults, for whom treatment was relatively poorly coordinated and largely divided between 'adult' and 'paediatric' practice [3, 4]. Professional concerns were crystallised by several national initiatives that developed in parallel in different countries and were built around a combination of clinical service provision and clinical research agendas. In the United States (US), a National Institutes of Health Progress Review Group suggested five key recommendations (Table 1.1) [5] followed soon afterwards by

Table 1.1 Recommendations of the NIH Report of the Adolescent and Young Adult Oncology Progress Review Group 2006 [5]

1	Identify the characteristics that distinguish the unique cancer burden in the AYA oncology patient
2	Provide education, training and communication to improve awareness, prevention, access and quality cancer care for AYAs
3	Create the tools to study the AYA cancer problem
4	Ensure excellence in service delivery across the cancer control continuum (i.e., prevention, screening, diagnosis, treatment, survivorship and end of life)
5	Strengthen and promote advocacy and support of the AYA cancer patient

M.G. McCabe
Christie Hospital, Manchester, UK
e-mail: martin.mccabe@manchester.ac.uk

J. Chisholm et al. (eds.), *A Practical Approach to the Care of Adolescents and Young Adults with Cancer*, https://doi.org/10.1007/978-3-319-66173-5_1

Bleyer et al.'s treatise on cancer in those aged between 15 and 29 years of age at diagnosis [6]. In the United Kingdom (UK), professional concern and lobbying by patient and charity representatives resulted in a clear government strategy to actively support AYA cancer, embodied initially in the National Institute of Clinical Excellence's 2005 publication 'Improving Outcomes in Children and Young People with Cancer' and its key recommendations (Table 1.2) [7], and more recently in the formation of a national Clinical Reference Group for the commissioning of childhood and young adult specialist cancer care in England, and equivalent initiatives in devolved UK nations. Similar professional and governmental initiatives have taken place elsewhere in Europe, North America and Australia [5, 8, 9]. In each case, the drive to improve AYA cancer care has been centred around a small number of core principles: that AYA cancer survival outcomes need to improve in absolute terms; that improvements in survival outcomes should occur at a similar pace to improvements in younger children and older adults; that AYA patients should have access to appropriate clinical trials to drive improvement in outcomes.

So what are the features that characterise a competent, clinical service for AYA cancer patients? Inevitably, some are designed with the above aims in mind: medical, nursing and allied health professional staff with knowledge and expertise relevant to the cancers that affect young people; adequate clinical trial infrastructure at local, national and international levels to develop and deliver the clinical trials needed to drive the required improvements; effective multidisciplinary teams built with patients at their centre to deliver holistic patient care; and effective survivorship care to manage late toxicities of treatment. However, adolescence and early adulthood are periods of life characterised by several major physiological and societal life events: completion of pubertal development, completion of mandatory education, entrance into higher education and/or paid employment, the beginning of independent living, for some parenthood and for some the responsibility of caring for infirm and ageing relatives. These form a constantly fluctuating backdrop of physical, emotional and social change for young people in their late second, third

Table 1.2 Recommendations of the UK National Institute of Health and Clinical Excellence [3]

1	Care should be coordinated across the whole of the NHS and be available as close to the patient's home as possible
2	Cancer networks should ensure that they meet the needs of children and young people with cancer
3	Multidisciplinary teams should provide cancer care
4	Each child or young person with cancer should have a key worker
5	Care should be appropriate to the child's or young person's age and type of cancer
6	Time in the operating theatre and a children's anaesthetist should be available when needed
7	Children and young people with cancer should be offered the chance to take part in research trials
8	Treatment should be based on agreed protocols
9	A register of all cancers in people aged 15–24 should be urgently considered
10	Cancer networks should ensure there are sufficient specialist staff

and fourth decades. Cancer occurs against this complex backdrop and cannot be successfully managed unless these other factors are recognised. Therefore, in addition to medical and surgical management of the cancer, AYA services must also take account of the non-disease-related factors that are critical to young people at this stage of their lives such as education, activity, childcare, employment and social care. Moreover, young people temporarily removed from their lives by a diagnosis of cancer can easily become isolated from and left behind by their peers, and exhibit high levels of distress and post-traumatic stress symptom during and after treatment [10, 11]. Psychological and peer support are therefore also key features of successful AYA cancer services. Thus, AYA cancer services have evolved as a conflation of multiple sources of input that converge around the needs of patients diagnosed with cancer during the decades that follow early childhood and precede middle age.

Necessarily, defining precise age criteria that mark the upper and lower age limits of the 'adolescent and young adult' period is an artificial exercise, but one that is nonetheless necessary to plan and deliver clinical services. Countries and professional groups have approached this differently. The initial publications in the US defined the AYA period as 15–29 years of age [4]. In the UK, clinical service provision is based on patients aged 15–24 years [7], but the national AYA research agenda takes a broader age range of 15–39 years. The latter is also the age range applied to an on-going collaboration between the European Society of Medical Oncology (ESMO) and the International Society of Paediatric Oncology: Europe (SIOPE) [12], and the age range favoured in recent publications from the US National Cancer Institute.

The multitude of professional, charitable, consumer and government groups now involved in AYA cancer care in many developed countries undoubtedly bring a richness of holistic expertise to the multi-faceted challenges faced by young cancer patients; each party contributes something different to the overall whole. However, despite advances in almost every aspect of AYA cancer care during the last two decades, the major issues that stimulated the professional community's original concerns about AYA cancers still hold true: AYA cancer patients are less likely to enter clinical trials and, in general, have worse outcomes than children with the same diseases; improvements in cancer survival in some countries lag behind those of children and older adults; cancer is rare in this age group, frequently presents initially with poorly predictive, non-specific features [13] and the diagnostic process is generally more prolonged involving more healthcare visits prior to referral than in older adults [14], and is frequently associated with advanced disease at presentation; many AYA patients remain isolated during treatment with little or no support from peers with similar diseases.

Much of the remainder of this chapter will present data on the changing patterns of incidence, survival and mortality in the AYA age group over recent years to describe the extent of the 'problem' of AYA cancer and to show where improvements have been made and where they are still very much needed. Much of the data is not directly comparable between countries due to discrepancies in the age ranges and types of data recorded and reported by different national groups.

1.2 Epidemiological Considerations

To facilitate descriptive epidemiological study of the spectrum of tumours that occur during adolescence and early adulthood an appropriate tumour classification is needed that allocates similar tumours into functionally meaningful groups. The International Classification of Diseases for Oncology (ICD-O) encodes tumours based on their anatomical site (topography), morphology and behaviour and forms the basis for the International Classification of Childhood Cancer, currently at version 3 (ICCC3) [15]. The ICCC3 is ideally suited to the classification of childhood cancer with its particular spectrum of tumour types, and particularly the prominence of embryonal tumours, characteristic of early childhood. However, these embryonal tumours are increasingly uncommon with advancing age and some occur only very rarely during adolescence and adulthood. In contrast, carcinomas and melanomas become increasingly common such that by the end of the third decade almost 50% of tumours are poorly classified by the ICCC3 [16]. An alternative classification system more suited to the tumours typical of the AYA age spectrum has been proposed [17] and modified [16] and is the classification that should be used in publications dealing specifically with AYA cancer epidemiology (Table 1.3). Not all groups have reported epidemiological data according to the same criteria, resulting in some important differences between groups and over time that should be borne in mind when interpreting reported data. For instance, UK reports on AYA cancer in recent years have described incidence and survival in young people aged 15–24 at diagnosis, in line with UK clinical service provision for AYA patients; other national reports include data from patients aged 15–29 or 15–39 at diagnosis. Some reports include amalgamated data from regional registries, others include nearly complete population data. In the case of data from the US National Cancer Institute's Surveillance, Epidemiology and End Results (SEER) database, cases are collated from nine, or more recently 13, states and metropolitan areas which together represent approximately 13% of the US population. Tumour classification systems vary between reports: those not designed for AYA cancer cannot adequately classify all AYA tumour groups. Importantly, the inclusion of some tumour types such as low-grade brain tumours, borderline malignancies and in situ tumours, varies between analyses, or their inclusion is unclear, and may result in apparent discrepancies in incidence, survival and mortality rates between countries.

1.2.1 Incidence

The data presented here are derived principally from statistics published by Cancer Research UK relating to cancers diagnosed in young people in the UK [18]. Additional data are described in the text.

Cancers in 15–24-year-olds account for less than 1% of all cancers in the UK, in 15–29-year olds they account for 1.4% and in 15–39-year-olds for 3.8% of all cancers. After an initial fall in incidence rates from infants to early school age children, cancer incidence increases steadily with age until the end of the seventh decade. Cancer incidence therefore rises steadily during the AYA years up to a maximum of approximately 800/million males per year and 1600/million females per year towards the end of the

Table 1.3 Classification scheme for AYA tumours, according to Birch and Barr [16]

1	Leukemias
1.1	Acute lymphoid leukemia
1.2	Acute myeloid leukemia
1.3	Chronic myeloid leukemia
1.4	Other and unspecified leukemias
1.4.1	Other lymphoid leukemia and lymphoid leukaemia, NOS
1.4.2	Other myeloid leukemia and myeloid leukaemia, NOS
1.4.3	Other specified leukemias
1.4.4	Unspecified leukemias
2.1	Lymphomas
2.1.1	NHL, specified subtype
2.1.2	Unspecified NHL
2.2	Hodgkin disease:
2.2.1	Hodgkin disease, specified subtype
2.2.2	Hodgkin disease, NOS
3	CNS and other intracranial and intraspinal neoplasms (tumors with any behavior code were included)
3.1	Astrocytoma
3.1.1	Specified low-grade astrocytic tumors
3.1.2	Glioblastoma and anaplastic astrocytoma
3.1.3	Astrocytoma, NOS
3.2	Other glioma
3.3	Ependymoma
3.4	Medulloblastoma and other PNET
3.4.1	Medulloblastoma
3.4.2	Supratentorial PNET
3.5	Other specified intracranial and intraspinal neoplasms
3.6	Unspecified intracranial and intraspinal neoplasms
3.6.1	Unspecified malignant intracranial and intraspinal neoplasms (behavior code of 3 or more)
3.6.2	Unspecified benign and borderline intracranial and intraspinal neoplasms (behavior code of less than 3)
4	Osseous and chondromatous neoplasms, Ewing tumor, and other neoplasms of bone
4.1	Osteosarcoma
4.2	Chondrosarcoma
4.3	Ewing tumor
4.4	Other specified and unspecified bone tumors
4.4.1	Other specified bone tumors
4.4.2	Unspecified bone tumors
5	Soft tissue sarcomas
5.1	Fibromatous neoplasms
5.2	Rhabdomyosarcoma
5.3	Other specified soft tissue sarcoma:
5.3.1	Specified
5.3.2	Unspecified

(continued)

Table 1.3 (continued)

6	Germ cell and trophoblastic neoplasms
6.1	Germ cell and trophoblastic neoplasms of gonads.
6.2	Germ cell and trophoblastic neoplasms of nongonadal sites
6.2.1	Intracranial (tumors with any behavior code are included)
6.2.2	Other nongonadal sites
7	Melanoma and skin carcinomas
7.1	Melanoma
7.2	Skin carcinomas
8	Carcinomas
8.1	Thyroid carcinoma
8.2	Other carcinoma of head and neck
8.2.1	Nasopharyngeal carcinoma
8.2.2	Other sites in lip, oral cavity and pharynx.
8.2.3	Nasal cavity, middle ear, sinuses, larynx, and other and ill-defined head and neck
8.3	Carcinoma of trachea, bronchus, and lung
8.4	Carcinoma of breast
8.5	Carcinoma of genitourinary tract:
8.5.1	Carcinoma of kidney
8.5.2	Carcinoma of bladder
8.5.3	Carcinoma of gonads
8.5.4	Carcinoma of cervix and uterus
8.5.5	Carcinoma of other and ill-defined sites in genitourinary tract
8.6	Carcinoma of gastrointestinal tract
8.6.1	Carcinoma of colon and rectum
8.6.2	Carcinoma of stomach
8.6.3	Carcinoma of liver and intrahepatic bile ducts
8.6.4	Carcinoma of pancreas
8.6.5	Carcinoma of other and ill-defined sites in gastrointestinal tract
8.7	Carcinoma of other and ill-defined sites, NEC
8.7.1	Adrenocortical carcinoma
8.7.2	Carcinoma of other and ill-defined sites, NEC
9	Miscellaneous specified neoplasms, NEC
9.1	Other pediatric and embryonal tumors, NEC:
9.1.1	Wilms tumor
9.1.2	Neuroblastoma
9.1.3	Other pediatric and embryonal tumors, NEC
9.2	Other specified neoplasms, NEC
9.2.1	Paraganglioma and glomus tumors
9.2.2	Other specified gonadal tumors
9.2.3	Myeloma, mast cell tumors, and miscellaneous lymphoreticular neoplasms, NEC
9.2.4	Other specified neoplasms, NEC
10	Unspecified malignant neoplasms, NEC

NOS not otherwise specified, *NHL* non-Hodgkin lymphoma, *CNS* central nervous system, *PNET* primitive neuroectodermal tumor, *NEC* not elsewhere classified fourth decade (Fig. 1.1). Until the mid-twenties, there is very little difference in the incidence of cancer between males and females. From the mid twenties female cases progressively outnumber male cases to the extent that by the end of the fourth decade the incidence in females is almost double that in males (Fig. 1.2).

The most common cancer types in the 15–24-year-old age group according to the Birch AYA cancer classification are lymphomas, early onset carcinomas and germ cell tumours (Fig. 1.3). However, the cancer spectrum changes significantly with

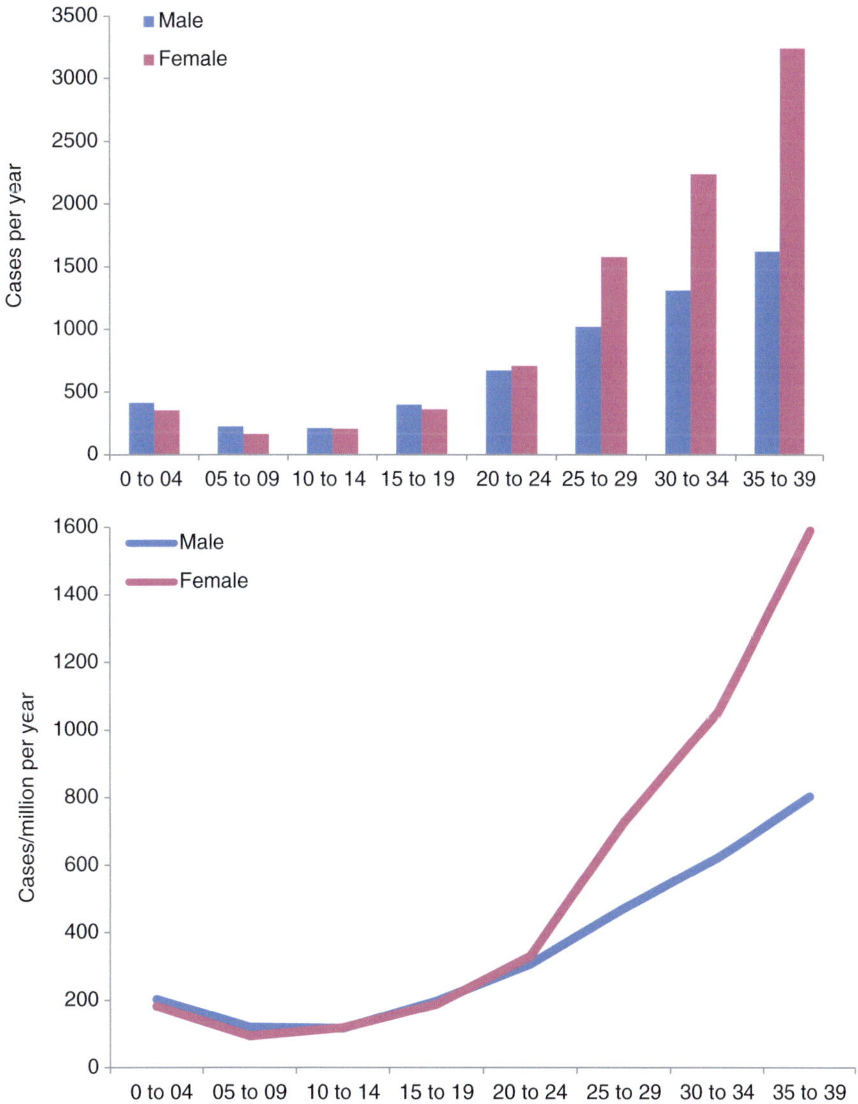

Fig. 1.1 Incidence of AYA cancers in males and females, UK, 2011–2013. Data extracted from [18]

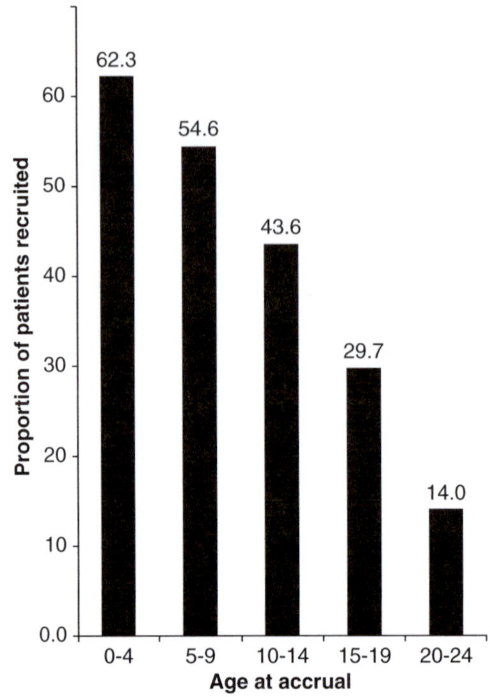

Fig. 1.2 Female: male ratio of cancer incidence, UK, 2011–2013. Data extracted from [18]

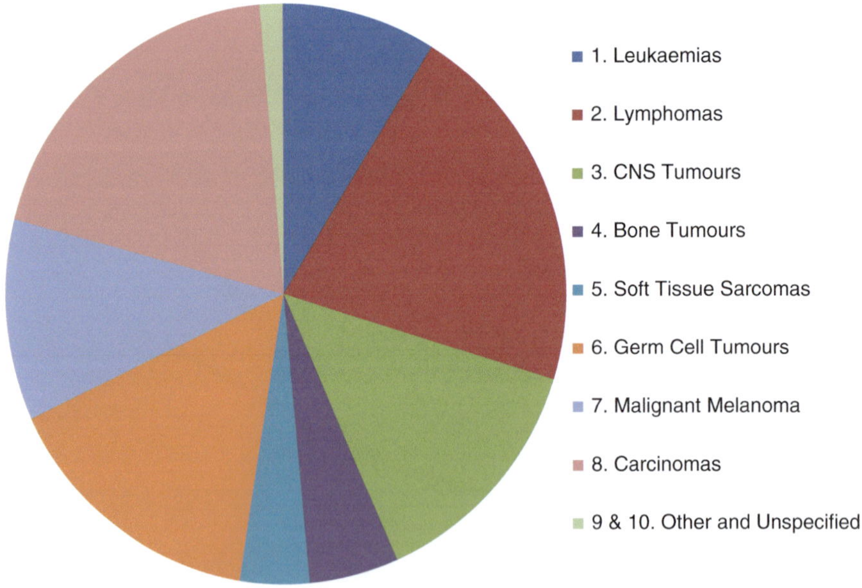

Fig. 1.3 Proportion of tumours in UK patients aged 15–24 at diagnosis arranged by AYA diagnostic classification. Data extracted from [18]

age. At the beginning of the period Hodgkin disease predominates in males and females. During the ensuing decade, female early onset carcinomas, particularly carcinomas of the breast, ovary, cervix and thyroid, and male testicular germ cell tumours become significantly more common. Malignant melanomas also become more common in both sexes. By the end of the AYA age range these cancers together outnumber haematological malignancies. The changing incidence patterns in the UK of these cancers are shown in Figs. 1.4 and 1.5. Similar changing incidence patterns have been reported across multiple countries including the Netherlands, US, Canada and France [4, 16, 19, 20]. The continued rise in female predominance with increasing age is largely explained by a progressive increase in the incidence of carcinomas of the breast, ovary and cervix, and of malignant melanoma. The bone and soft tissue sarcomas characteristic of adolescence occur less frequently, while non-rhabdomyosarcoma soft tissue sarcomas become more common, particularly beyond the age of 25.

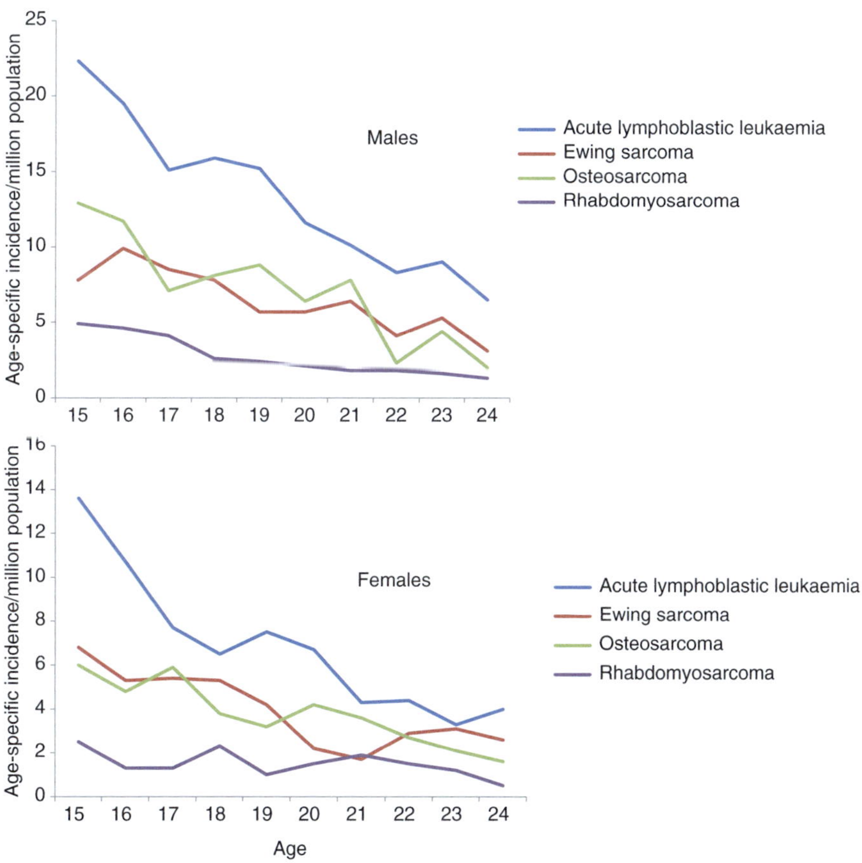

Fig. 1.4 Age-specific incidence, UK, 2000–2009. Tumour types whose incidence falls with increasing age. Data extracted from [18]

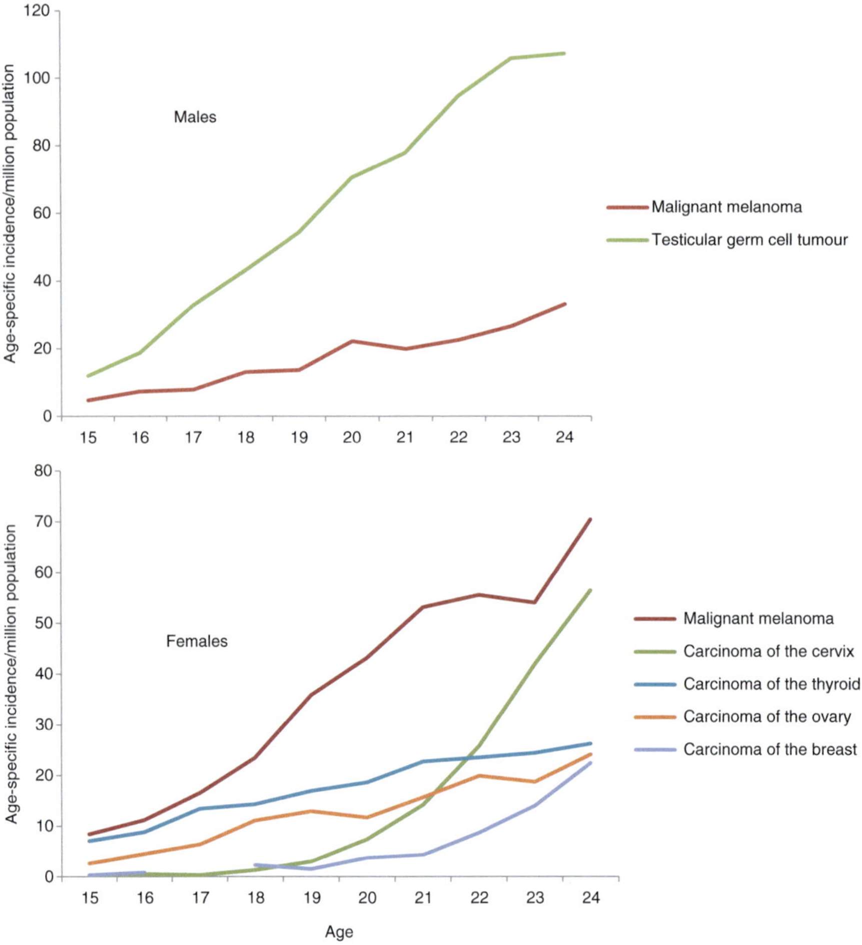

Fig. 1.5 Age-specific incidence, UK, 2000–2009. Tumour types whose incidence rises with increasing age. Data extracted from [18]

The incidence rates of AYA cancer have increased since the 1970s and are still continuing to rise (Fig. 1.6). Increases are apparent across most AYA cancer types (Fig. 1.7). The rise is not fully understood and is likely due to a combination of real changes in the incidence of some cancers, better recording of other cancers and changes in how some malignancies are registered, particularly for the subset of cancers whose behaviour codes have changed with successive versions of ICD-O between 'benign,' 'borderline' or 'uncertain' and 'malignant.' At least for some cancers there are plausible behavioural changes that may explain the observed variations in incidence. For instance, malignant melanoma has become more common in some Western populations, including the UK and the white population of the US, whilst in Australia melanoma incidence in the AYA population is falling in line with changing sun exposure practices and public health campaigns advocating skin

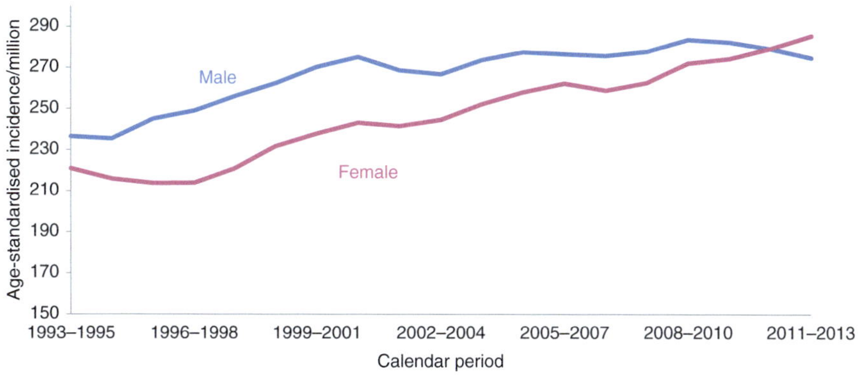

Fig. 1.6 European age-standardised incidence rates, ages 15–24, Great Britain, 1993–2014. Data extracted from [18]

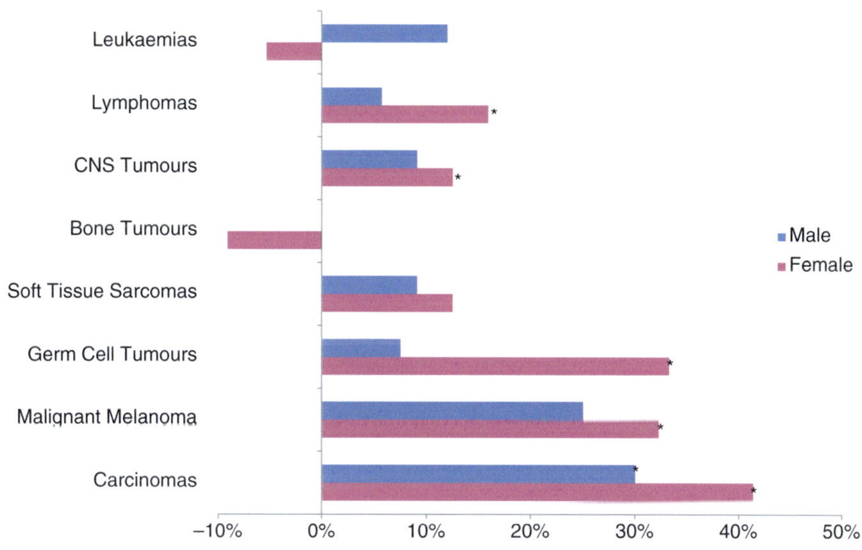

Fig. 1.7 Percentage change in European age-standardised 5 year average incidence rates per million population, UK, 1995–2009. *$p < 0.05$. Data extracted from [18]

protection [21, 22]. The incidence of cervical cancer in England has fallen overall since the early 1980s. However, its incidence in the AYA population has increased, and there is significant geographical variation [23]. Its changing demographics have been suggested to be related to younger age at first intercourse, higher rates of sexually transmitted infections in young people and younger age of cigarette smoking in the most recent AYA population cohorts studied compared to earlier cohorts, together with an effect from the introduction of active screening for cervical cancer. However, much of the observed increase in incidence across multiple cancers—leukaemias, lymphomas, CNS tumours, bone sarcomas, germ cell tumours and certain carcinomas—is unexplained, yet consistent, across age, sex and geographical region and presumed to be a real phenomenon [24]. In the US, additional significant increases were observed in recent decades in Kaposi sarcoma and non-Hodgkin lymphomas, particularly in young adult males, that were consistent with an effect of the Human Immunodeficiency Virus epidemic [4].

The 2006 SEER monograph has reported the most complete data so far on variations in AYA cancer incidence by racial/ethnic origin. Across the AYA age range the non-Hispanic white population had the highest cancer incidence and American Indians the lowest. The incidence rate in African Americans rose progressively with age and by the early 40s was higher than that in the white population. UK data from the Yorkshire Specialist Register of Cancer in Children and Young People diagnosed between 1990 and 2005 [25] did not find a difference in incidence between South Asian and non-South Asian populations, although there was a sustained rise in incidence in South Asians during the study period.

1.2.2 Survival

Overall, AYA cancer survival has steadily improved through successive eras in most reported series, to the extent that recent cohorts of European and American AYA patients diagnosed since 2000 have 5-year survival in excess of 80% [4, 19, 20, 26, 27]. Some diseases have seen very marked improvements in outcome within the last two decades, particularly the haematological malignancies (Fig. 1.8); in the UK, between 1992 and 2006, 5-year survival of patients aged 15–24 at diagnosis with acute lymphoblastic and acute myeloid leukaemia both rose by 17%, and non-Hodgkin lymphomas rose by 12% [27]. Similar improvements in survival across multiple cancer types have been reported in the AYA populations of other countries [19, 20, 28]. However, this overall very positive picture of improving long-term survival masks the outcomes of some cancers for which there has been very little improvement in population-level survival for many years despite widespread collaboration between cooperative trial groups and centralisation of treatment. High grade gliomas and some bone and soft tissue sarcomas fall into the latter group.

AYA outcomes have historically lagged behind improvements in the survival of both younger children and older adults. Indeed, the 2006 SEER monograph on AYA cancer [4] identified an age cohort of male cancer patients between 25 and 35 at diagnosis for whom there had been no measurable survival improvement in 22 years of SEER data collection. A recent update of that analysis [28] reported significant improvements in 5-year survival for 14 AYA cancers. However, survival improved less in AYA than in children for acute myeloid leukaemia and medulloblastoma and less in AYA than in adults for 14 cancers, including acute myeloid and acute lymphoblastic leukaemias, low and high grade astrocytomas, Hodgkin disease and carcinomas of the liver, pancreas, stomach, oropharynx and ovary.

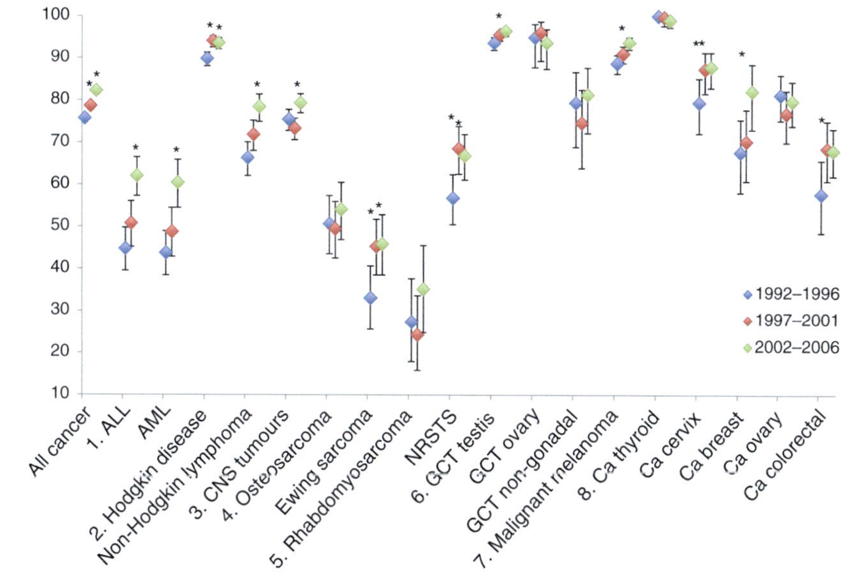

Fig. 1.8 Trends in 5-year survival, UK, 1992–2006. Arranged by AYA diagnostic group. *ALL* acute lymphoblastic leukaemia, *AML* acute myeloid leukaemia, *CNS* central nervous system, *NRSTS* non-rhabdomyosarcoma soft tissue sarcoma, *GCT* germ cell tumour, *Ca* carcinoma. *$p < 0.05$ for the change in survival compared to survival in 1992-1996. Data extracted from [27]

In contrast, EUROCARE 5 recently reported the results of an analysis of cancer outcomes in 56,505 children, 312,483 AYAs, and 3,567,383 adults diagnosed between 2000 and 2007 in Europe [29]. For the first time, survival improvements occurred in parallel in children and AYAs. Indeed, European AYAs generally had better outcomes than children in the cohort, largely due to the preponderance of good prognosis cancers such as Hodgkin and non-Hodgkin lymphomas, melanoma, thyroid carcinoma and germ cell tumours in the AYA population that were less common in the childhood population. Females in general had better survival than males throughout the AYA age range. In part that was related to their increased likelihood of developing thyroid carcinoma and melanomas, both of which have good prognosis, but there were also significant gender differences across a range of good and poor prognosis cancers, a phenomenon that has been reported previously in the UK AYA population [27]. Variations in cancer outcomes by country of origin were reported under the EUROCARE-4 programme for patients aged 15–24 and diagnosed between 1995 and 2002 [30] but have not yet been updated for the expanded age group of 15–39 included in the EUROCARE-5 cohort.

Notwithstanding the parallel improvements in outcomes across children and AYAs in the most recent EUROCARE cohort, outcomes for AYAs remain worse than for children in UK, US and European patients with some of the worst prognosis malignancies to affect this age group: acute leukaemias, low and high grade astrocytomas and bone and soft tissue sarcomas. The survival of AYAs with bone and soft tissue sarcomas is also worse than in older adults. Thus, the data would appear to suggest that some of the cancers with worst outcome in AYAs—bone and soft tissue sarcomas—are at the nadir of their survival distribution during the age when their incidence reaches its peak. However, it is likely that in part these observations are due to age-related variations in the histological entities prevalent across the age spectrum; with advancing age the AYA sarcomas with worst outcomes—alveolar rhabdomyosarcoma, osteosarcoma and Ewing sarcoma—are replaced with better prognosis sarcoma histotypes. Nevertheless, it is clear that there are age-related discrepancies in survival outcomes from childhood to mid-adulthood that remain to be explained. In contrast to the sarcoma age-outcome distribution, AYAs have either equivalent or better outcome than older adults for acute leukaemias, Hodgkin's disease, CNS tumours, melanomas and for most carcinomas.

Given the recently reported findings of EUROCARE-5 it is not now clear whether the absence of improvement in the survival of AYA patients previously reported by Bleyer and colleagues from the US has been addressed, or alternatively may be an issue of relevance to the US healthcare system but not to Europe. There are many reasons why AYA patients may not experience the survival improvements witnessed in younger and older age groups. Critically, these include potentially remediable factors related to differences in service delivery, clinical trial accrual and diagnostic pathways. The patient and professional communities involved in managing AYA cancer have recognised these issues for at least a decade. None are yet optimally managed for young people, although national and international initiatives are attempting to improve the situation [31]. Indeed, it is efforts to abolish these avoidable factors that have largely driven the evolution of specific services for AYAs with cancer across much of the world.

1.2.3 Mortality

There have been few reports of mortality rates across the AYA age spectrum. In general, mortality rates rise in line with incidence rates: as cancer incidence rises with increasing age, so does mortality. In the SEER data from 1975 to 2000 there was a male preponderance in AYA deaths under the age of 30 and a female preponderance over 30 [4]. However, when the SEER incidence and mortality rates are compared there is an excess of male deaths at all ages from 15 to 39. Moreover, while cancer is most common in the white population throughout the AYA age range, deaths are most common in the African American/black population at all ages from 15 to 39, and the preponderance of non-white deaths increases with increasing age. Across the study period from 1975 to 2000 there were reductions in observed mortality rates at all ages and in all ethnic groups. The smallest observed reductions in mortality during the study period were in patients aged in their early 30s at diagnosis. Both sexes were affected but the finding was more prominent in males. When ethnic origin was examined, the smallest reduction in mortality was in the African American/black population aged 15–25.

Australian mortality data have been reported from a cohort of Western Australian AYA cancer patients aged 15–39 and diagnosed between 1980 and 2005 [32]. Reductions in mortality rates were observed through the study period in males and females and across most major AYA cancer groups. In the Australian cohort too the reduction in mortality with time was more marked in females than males and was not evenly distributed across cancer types.

Early mortality data have also been reported from a cohort of patients diagnosed between 2005 and 2009 in England and aged 15–24 at diagnosis (Fig. 1.9) [33]. Deaths at 30 days, 90 days and 1 year after diagnosis were reported. Overall, 6.9% of patients died within 1 year of diagnosis. The patterns of death varied significantly by tumour type to a maximum of 23% mortality 1 year after diagnosis in patients with acute myeloid leukaemia. Some cancer types, particularly haematological malignancies were more likely to be associated with very early mortality, within 30 days of diagnosis.

1.3 The Future of AYA Cancer Across Geographical and Professional Boundaries

It is undoubtedly true that outcomes for AYAs with cancer have improved significantly during the last two decades. Apportioning the cause for this success is challenging for the reasons outlined in the discussion above: most AYA patients are not

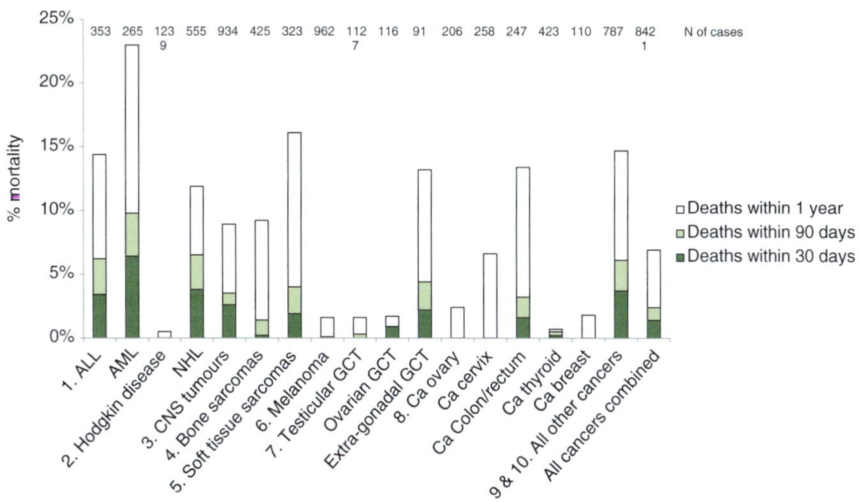

Fig. 1.9 Early cancer mortality, UK, aged 15–24, 2005–2009 by time from diagnosis. Arranged by AYA diagnostic group. *ALL* acute lymphoblastic leukaemia, *AML* acute myeloid leukaemia, *NHL* Non-Hodgkin lymphoma, *CNS* central nervous system, *GCT* germ cell tumour, *Ca* carcinoma. Data extracted from [33]

recruited to clinical trials, many are not treated in high-volume centres with AYA expertise or disease expertise, some are diagnosed via referral pathways that take far too long or are inappropriate. Referral of AYA patients to 'centres of excellence' for diagnosis and treatment is espoused as a desirable outcome by some professional and governmental bodies. In the UK, clinical service guidance published by the National Institute for Health and Clinical Excellence in 2005 mandated referral of all patients aged 15–24 with cancer to a regional AYA principal treatment or AYA designated hospitals [7]. The guidance has not been universally followed: in the years 2009–2010 approximately 43% of patients were referred [34] and in 2011–2013 the proportion rose to just over 50% [35]. One reason for maintenance of poor referral rates to principal treatment or AYA designated centres is that they have not yet been comprehensively evaluated as a component of treatment. The Brightlight study [36] is attempting to do that for the UK population and is expected to report its findings within the coming years. Data from the UK National Cancer Patient Experience Survey (NCPES) gives some insight into the impact on patient experience of principal treatment centres [37]. The NCPES randomly surveys a cohort of cancer patients across the adult age spectrum who are undergoing treatment and allows a useful comparison between the experiences of AYA patients compared to older adults. Approximately a decade after the introduction of the clinical service guidance, patients aged 16–24 were more likely to have prolonged diagnostic pathways and multiple healthcare attendances prior to diagnosis and more likely to feel excluded from conversations and decisions about their healthcare than older patients. On the other hand, they were seen more urgently once cancer was suspected, and were more likely to feel satisfied about the quality and quantity of explanation given about treatment and side effects than older patients. Importantly, AYA patients reported being invited to take part in clinical research more frequently than older patients. There were some significant differences between patients in defined centres of AYA cancer expertise compared to other centres: those treated in AYA centres had fewer problems understanding information given by healthcare staff, were more likely to feel involved in discussions about treatment, took a greater part in decision making, and felt more enabled to express their fears, concerns and opinions to healthcare staff.

In light of the progress that has been made to date, what does the future hold for AYA cancer and AYA cancer services? There have been some significant changes in professional practice around AYA patients during recent years designed to contribute to better working between the multiple different professional groups responsible for the care of AYA patients and better outcomes for AYA patients:

- A recognition that clinical trial age eligibility criteria either directly or indirectly exclude groups of AYA patients without a valid rationale
- The development of increasingly comprehensive AYA cancer services in many countries resulting from better communication and closer cooperation between paediatric and adult services locally, nationally and internationally
- Increasing focus on AYAs with cancer from professional groups, governmental health bodies, research funders, clinical research collaboratives and patient charities leading to improvements in the clinical services experienced by AYA patients and the burgeoning of a profusion of AYA-related cancer research.

These are all positive steps that should lead to a better understanding of AYA cancer, its causes, treatment and effects and ultimately to better treatment outcomes for AYA patients. There remain, however, some significant barriers: slow progress in influencing the events that take place prior to a cancer diagnosis, low availability of appropriate clinical trials to recruit patients to, variable patient access and accrual to the clinical trials that are available, incomplete understanding of the contribution of individual biology to patient outcomes, variations in how patients are managed that are not based on clinical evidence, generally under-developed services and an under-developed clinical evidence base for cancer survivors. If the outcomes of AYA cancer patients are to improve, these barriers will need to be managed and/or eliminated. Is there likely to come a time when AYA cancer is no longer needed as a concept to bring professionals together to work towards better outcomes for AYA cancer patients? Not in the foreseeable future!

References

1. Benowitz S. Children's oncology group looks to increase efficiency, numbers in clinical trials. J Natl Cancer Inst. 2000;92:1876–8.
2. Cancer Progress Report. National Cancer Institute, National Institutes of Health, US Department of Health and Human Services. 2001.
3. Bleyer A. Older adolescents with cancer in North America deficits in outcome and research. Pediatr Clin North Am. 2002;49:1027–42.
4. Bleyer A, O'Leary M, et al. Cancer epidemiology in older adolescents and young adults 15 to 29 years of age, including SEER incidence and survival: 1975–2000. National Cancer Institute: Bethesda; 2006.
5. Albritton K, Caligiuri M, et al. Closing the gap: research and care imperatives for adolescents and young adults with cancer: report of TEH adolescent and young adult oncology progress review group. National Cancer Institute Lance Armstrong Foundation. 2006.
6. Bleyer WA, Barr RD. Cancer in adolescents and young adults. 1st ed. Berlin: Springer; 2007.
7. NICE: Improving outcomes in children and young people with cancer. NH Service London, 2005.
8. National service delivery framework for adolescents and young adults with cancer, Commonwealth of Australia. 2008.
9. van Gaal JC, Bastiaannet E, et al. Cancer in adolescents and young adults in north Netherlands (1989–2003): increased incidence, stable survival and high incidence of second primary tumours. Ann Oncol. 2009;20:365–73.
10. Clerici CA, Massimino M, et al. Psychological referral and consultation for adolescents and young adults with cancer treated at pediatric oncology unit. Pediatr Blood Cancer. 2008;51:105–9.
11. Seitz DC, Besier T, et al. Posttraumatic stress, depression and anxiety among adult long-term survivors of cancer in adolescence. Eur J Cancer. 2010;46:1596–606.
12. ESMO/SIOPE Adolescents and Young Adults Working Group, ESMO. 2016.
13. Dommett RM, Redaniel MT, et al. Features of cancer in teenagers and young adults in primary care: a population-based nested case-control study. Br J Cancer. 2013;108:2329–33.
14. Lyratzopoulos G, Neal RD, et al. Variation in number of general practitioner consultations before hospital referral for cancer: findings from the 2010 National Cancer Patient Experience Survey in England. Lancet Oncol. 2012;13:353–65.
15. Steliarova-Foucher E, Stiller C, et al. International classification of childhood cancer, third edition. Cancer. 2005;103:1457–67.
16. Barr RD, Holowaty EJ, et al. Classification schemes for tumors diagnosed in adolescents and young adults. Cancer. 2006;106:1425–30.

17. Birch JM, Alston RD, et al. Classification and incidence of cancers in adolescents and young adults in England 1979–1997. Br J Cancer. 2002;87:1267–74.
18. Cancer Research UK. Teenagers' and young adults' cancers incidence statistics. 2016.
19. Aben KK, van Gaal C, et al. Cancer in adolescents and young adults (15–29 years): a population-based study in the Netherlands 1989–2009. Acta Oncol. 2012;51:922–33.
20. Desandes E, Lacour B, et al. Cancer incidence and survival in adolescents and young adults in France, 2000–2008. Pediatr Hematol Oncol. 2013;30:291–306.
21. Wallingford SC, Iannacone MR, et al. Comparison of melanoma incidence and trends among youth under 25 years in Australia and England, 1990–2010. Int J Cancer. 2015;137:2227–33.
22. Whiteman DC, Green AC, et al. The growing burden of invasive melanoma: projections of incidence rates and numbers of new cases in six susceptible populations through 2031. J Invest Dermatol. 2016;136:1161–71.
23. Foley G, Alston R, et al. Increasing rates of cervical cancer in young women in England: an analysis of national data 1982–2006. Br J Cancer. 2011;105:177–84.
24. Alston RD, Geraci M, et al. Changes in cancer incidence in teenagers and young adults (ages 13 to 24 years) in England 1979–2003. Cancer. 2008;113:2807–15.
25. van Laar M, McKinney PA, et al. Cancer incidence among the south Asian and non-south Asian population under 30 years of age in Yorkshire, UK. Br J Cancer. 2010;103:1448–52.
26. Furlong W, Rae C, et al. Surveillance and survival among adolescents and young adults with cancer in Ontario, Canada. Int J Cancer. 2012;131:2660–7.
27. O'Hara C, Moran A, et al. Trends in survival for teenagers and young adults with cancer in the UK 1992–2006. Eur J Cancer. 2015;51:2039–48.
28. Keegan THM, Ries LAG, et al. Comparison of cancer survival trends in the united states of adolescents and young adults with those in children and older adults. Cancer. 2016;122:1009–16.
29. Trama A, Botta L, et al. Survival of European adolescents and young adults diagnosed with cancer in 2000–07: population-based data from EUROCARE-5. Lancet Oncol. 2016;17:896–906.
30. Gatta G, Zigon G, et al. Survival of European children and young adults with cancer diagnosed 1995–2002. Eur J Cancer. 2009;45:992–1005.
31. Stark D, Bielack S, et al. Teenagers and young adults with cancer in Europe: from national programmes to a European integrated coordinated project. Eur J Cancer Care (Engl). 2016;25:419–27.
32. Haggar FA, Preen DB, et al. Cancer incidence and mortality trends in Australian adolescents and young adults, 1982–2007. BMC Cancer. 2012;12:151.
33. Moran T, Purkayastha D, et al. Pattern of deaths in the year following diagnosis in cancer patients aged 15–24 years in England, National Cancer Intelligence Network; 2013.
34. O'Hara C, Khan M, et al. Notifications of teenagers and young adults with cancer to a Principal Treatment Centre 2009–2010, National Cancer Intelligence Network; 2013.
35. Khan M, Moran A, et al. TYAC Notification System Report 2009–2013, vC: Teenagers and Young Adults with Cancer. 2015.
36. Taylor RM, Fern LA, et al. Development and validation of the BRIGHTLIGHT Survey, a patient-reported experience measure for young people with cancer. Health Qual Life Outcomes. 2015;13:107.
37. Furness CL, Smith L, et al. Cancer patient experience in the teenage young adult population-key issues and trends over time: an analysis of the United Kingdom National Cancer Patient Experience Surveys 2010–2014. J Adolesc Young Adult Oncol. 2017. [Epub ahead of print].

Cancer Research and AYA

2

Lorna A. Fern and Jeremy Whelan

2.1 Young People and Research

2.1.1 Introduction

The significant advances made in cancer survival are due in part to successive generations of clinical trials and research, identifying and testing new agents and new combinations of older agents to confer a survival advantage, reduction in toxicity and/or improved quality-of-life for patients [1]. Research may be defined as an activity '*to advance scientific knowledge directly or indirectly, leading to improvement in the prevention and treatment of disease*' [2]. Consequently, participation to high quality research, particularly clinical trials, is advocated as the gold standard of care in many health care systems [3–5].

Adolescents and young adults (AYA) are less likely to be entered into cancer clinical trials compared to children and some older adults [5–10]. This pattern of lower inclusion rates is reported internationally regardless of healthcare system and is proposed to link to consequent suboptimal improvements in survival and outcomes for this group [11–15]. Unique cancer biology [16, 17], complex pathways to diagnosis [18], differences in treatment protocols [19] and place of care may also contribute. As such, many national and local AYA healthcare policies and initiatives have improving inclusion to cancer clinical trials as a 'key recommendation' or 'action' for young people [4, 20].

The reasons behind lesser inclusion of young people in cancer clinical trials are multifaceted and complex [5, 9, 21, 22]. Many of them are entrenched in traditional

L.A. Fern, Ph.D. (✉) • J. Whelan
University College London Hospitals NHS Foundation Trust, 250 Euston Road, London NW1 2PG, UK
e-mail: Lorna.Fern@nhs.net; Jeremy.whelan@nhs.net

J. Chisholm et al. (eds.), *A Practical Approach to the Care of Adolescents and Young Adults with Cancer*, https://doi.org/10.1007/978-3-319-66173-5_2

structural and organisational configurations of our health services which are conveniently and neatly divided into 'paediatric' and 'adult' services, neither of which satisfactorily meet the needs of young people with cancer [13, 23]. In addition, we are also beginning to understand more about the perspectives of young people around entry into research, where there can be conflicting views of the '*right to know about and have access to all available research*' versus feeling '*overwhelmed with too much information*' and an individual's view may fluctuate between these two opinions during their cancer timeline [21, 24].

With this in mind, this chapter will describe some of the evidence around lower involvement in clinical trials, why trials are important and how young people and parents can be included in the research process to maximise recruitment opportunities for young people.

2.1.2 Where is the Evidence for Lower Involvement in Cancer Research?

Inequalities in access to research are well described, in particular affecting ethnic minority groups, those of lower socioeconomic status, elderly patients and those who flank adult and paediatric care boundaries, namely teenagers and young adults, which refers to those broadly aged 13–24 years [22]. Age related inequalities for young people and the elderly are well documented [22], however the reasons behind exclusion of these two patient populations are likely to be different. Older patients are more likely to be excluded due to the presence of age related co-morbidities which are largely absent in young people. Data pertaining to the lack of enrolment in cancer clinical trials compared to children first emerged from the United States by Archie Bleyer and colleagues [6]. This was subsequently followed by reports from Australia [11], France [13], the United Kingdom (UK) [8], Italy [25] and more recently Canada [26]. Despite variation in methodology the results are consistent across countries and healthcare systems, in that, compared to children and some older adults, young people were less likely to be included in cancer clinical trials. Bleyer and colleagues later correlated the association of lower involvement in trials with lesser improvement in survival compared to children and older adults [12, 15]. Figure 2.1 shows recruitment to cancer trials in common cancer types in young people in Scotland, England and Wales during 2005–2014.

2.1.3 Why Do We Need Clinical Trials?

Entry into a clinical trial is viewed as a measure of a high standard of care in many healthcare systems. The planning, running and the reporting of clinical trials is not a straight forward process and is fraught with many challenges including securing funding, regulatory hurdles and often difficulties relating to recruiting anticipated numbers of patients on time. Despite this, developing trials and research studies is considered a worthwhile pursuit and remains the only reliable way to generate level

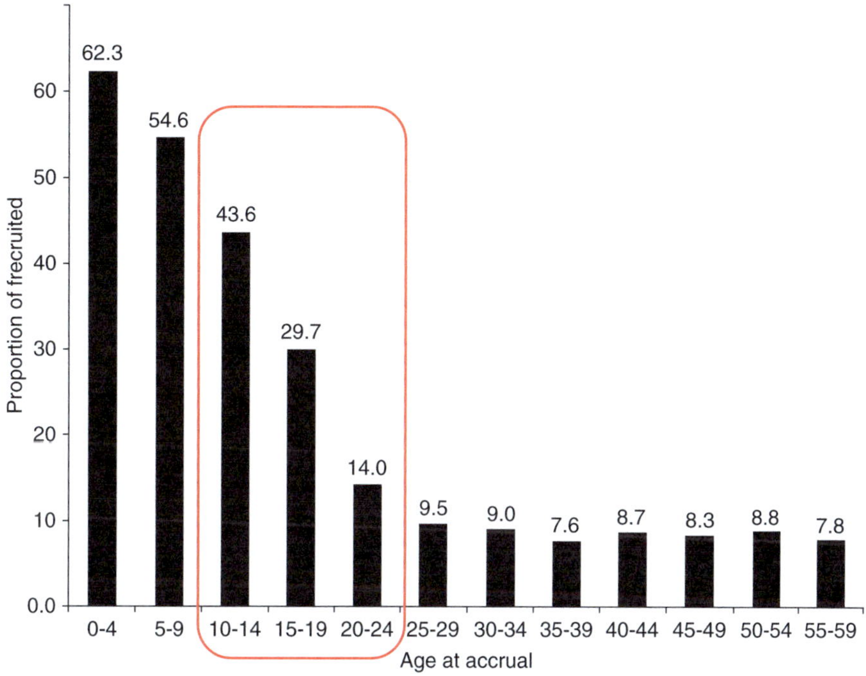

Fig. 2.1 Recruitment to cancer trials in common cancer types in young people in Scotland, England and Wales during 2005–2010

three evidence of the effectiveness of new therapies or combinations of therapies compared to current standards of care.

2.1.3.1 Improvements in Outcomes

Successive generations of cancer clinical trials have now resulted in five year survival rates in excess of 90% for certain cancer types, including some cancers found in young people such as male germ cell tumours and Hodgkin's disease [1]. The benefits of participation in clinical trials are not thought to be restricted to the specific medications used within the trial but extend to a higher standard of care including access to a wider multidisciplinary team, enhanced safety and care that is protocol-driven [15]. Patients may also benefit from a sense of altruism or 'giving back', particularly true of young people [21, 27].

2.1.3.2 Allows Legitimate Comparison between Treatments

Clinical trials allow systematic evaluation of new, more effective therapies or less toxic therapies. Their structure minimises 'selection bias' whereby the treating physician may consciously or subconsciously offer different treatments to patients who have a better performance status, may be more compliant or the physician just 'thinks' may do better. By randomly allocating patients between different treatments arms one can be sure patient demographics (age, gender, cancer type, stage, prognostic indicators, and performance status) are well matched between treatment groups. Additionally, adherence to drug doses, schedules and supportive care within the parameter of a trial also ensures that groups can be fairly compared.

2.1.3.3 Adequate Recording of Disease Response and Toxicities

The rigorous documentation required of trial conduct mandates precise and accurate recording of dosages, effectiveness and side effects in a standardised manner [28]. This allows toxicities as well as tumour response to be accurately recorded in a standardised manner allowing inter-patient and centre comparison. Again this facilitates fair comparisons between new therapies and current standards of care.

2.1.3.4 Collection of Biological Material

Collection of biological material within the context of a trial allows molecular targets, prognostic indicators and drivers of malignant growth to be identified and correlated with prospectively collected clinical outcome data. This is beneficial within the trial as it may indicate subgroups of patients who may be particularly responsive to the drug and/or be more prone to toxicities. Storage of biological samples with clinical data provides a rich source of knowledge from which we can expect to decipher the molecular and cellular drivers of malignant growth and transformation therefore allowing us to develop more precise therapies in the future.

We give an example of the importance of clinical trials in Sect. 2.4, case study 1.

2.1.4 Optimising Recruitment Opportunities for Young People with Cancer

The efforts of many international investigators have allowed us to understand better some of the reasons for under-representation of young people in clinical trials. In this section we will briefly summarise some of the key findings.

2.1.5 Availability of Trials

The availability of open clinical trials and other study types is a key determinant of inclusion in research. This presents a specific challenge for young people because of the relative rarity of cancer in this population, accounting for around 1% of all newly diagnosed cases [29], and the associated problems of developing trials for small populations. In the UK, there are approximately 2400 incidence cases (the number of new cases per year) and 14,000 across Europe [30]. Approximately three quarters of young people will present with leukaemia (primarily acute lymphoblastic leukaemia), lymphoma (mainly Hodgkin's disease), brain and central nervous system (CNS) tumours, bone and soft tissue sarcomas and germ cell tumours (gonadal and CNS) [29]. Within each of these cancer types are histological subgroups which further segment this group. In comparison approximately 80% of all new cancers in older adults are carcinomas and around half of these will be carcinomas of the breast, prostate, colon and lung [31]. Consequently, many cancer services and research activities are centred on these latter diseases types due to the numbers of newly diagnosed patients per year. The attractiveness of developing drugs for rare cancers is less for the pharmaceutical industry with high costs and attrition rates (the number of drugs which do not make it from Phase I to the clinic) and limited returns on drugs for small patient populations, despite incentives such as 'orphan drug status' which confer privileges including extended patents for drugs approved for rare or niche indications. Therefore, for many young people there may not be trials available for their cancer types/subtype.

2.1.6 Accessible

Even when a trial has been established and activated, the inclusion of a young person can still be prevented by a lack of accessibility to the study. This can be influenced by structural/organisation barriers and also professional attitudinal barriers. As discussed earlier young people are more likely to present with rare cancers compared to the general population [29]. If a trial is available it may not be open in all hospitals where young people are treated. Young people may be referred to either a paediatric centre, adult oncology centre or a specialist AYA centre depending on local practice and service configuration. For young people presenting with late onset paediatric cancers and who are referred to an adult centre it is less likely that paediatric studies will be open in the adult centre, or that the adult physicians will be aware of ongoing paediatric studies in a neighbouring institute or department. If the physicians are aware of local paediatric studies then referral of that young person into a paediatric centre to access the trial may be prohibited by age restrictions applying in the paediatric unit [23]. The lengthy regulatory procedures and unfamiliarity with paediatric protocols may prohibit opening of paediatric studies in adult centres.

In the adult unit the range of studies available is likely to reflect the dominant adult cancer types such as breast, colorectal, prostate and lung which are rare in young people and if found are likely to have different cancer biology to older adults which may preclude young people from these studies. Additionally, unfamiliarity in communicating research with young people may inhibit healthcare professionals discussing studies when they are trained and most familiar with discussing research with an older population.

Referral of young people into a specialist AYA centre presents an ideal scenario where young people should have access to age appropriate facilities, staff and a complement of trials/studies appropriate for young people. Healthcare professionals play a key role in maximising opportunities for including young people in clinical trials, bridging the gap between clinical care and research [24]. Recently, the dependence on this role has become apparent in a nationwide study in England, BRIGHTLIGHT (see case study 2) where a main contributing factor to lower than anticipated accrual was that young people were not being approached to be offered information about the study despite fulfilling the eligibility criteria [24]. The concept of professional gate keeping is not new, reflecting the beliefs of healthcare professionals in their role as protectors of some ill-defined "vulnerable" groups for whom judgements are made that research is too burdensome [22]. However, young people have expressed their 'right to be informed' about all available research relevant to them and provided with opportunities to make their own informed choices about all aspects of their care including research [24]. The delivery of information is also key to the acceptance of uptake whereby if healthcare professionals do not convey the value of the study young people are unlikely to respond [24]. This is discussed in more detail in the Sect. 2.1.9.

2.1.7 Appropriate

The 'appropriateness' of a study in this context principally refers to the eligibility criteria which define the patient population to be enrolled in the study. Eligibility criteria are predominately based on clinical characteristics identifying which patients are most likely to respond to the drug in question. However, restrictive eligibility criteria have come under criticism recently mainly with reference to the effect on the generalisability of study results to non-trial populations with the same disease [32].

It is common for eligibility criteria to cite lower and upper ages for trial inclusion and common for these to have little scientific or clinical rationale [9]. Despite international documents cautioning about the use of age as criterion for inclusion in research, the application of inappropriate age eligibility criteria on studies persists [9, 28, 33–36].

Appropriate age eligibility criteria are those that are suitably matched to an age range predicted by the biology of the disease(s) and the expected toxicity profile of the agent(s) being studied. Figure 2.2 shows appropriate age eligibility criteria applied to the EURAMOS-1 trial which was open to patients with osteosarcoma up to the age of 40 years [37]. This matched the incidence rates for osteosarcoma—which peak between the age of 15–20 years [38]. The application of an upper age cut-off at 40 years was clinically based in that beyond this age the clinical and biological features of osteosarcoma tend to be different and the treatment included not tolerated by older patients. Also shown in Fig. 2.2 is the age eligibility criteria of the Phase 3 RATHL trial (Response-adapted therapy for advanced Hodgkin lymphoma) which was a study aimed to identify patients who may be spared side effects of treatment [39]. The study recruited patients over the age of 18 years, however, as can been seen the peak incidence of Hodgkin's Disease begins at 16 years, and so a population of patients who could have benefited from inclusion in this study were excluded based on age rather than clinical or biological criteria. RATHL opened in 2008 and closed in 2012 and presents perhaps a historical picture of Hodgkin's lymphoma trials in the UK with the next HD trial which is due to open having an upper age eligibility of 25 years. However, it serves as an example of how giving attention to studies with an inappropriate age eligibility criterion can drive change. Currently, the National Cancer Research Institutes Lymphoma Clinical Studies Group has agreed that all 'adult' Hodgkin's disease studies generated by the Group should have as minimum criteria 16 years as a lower age eligibility criteria. Further to this, a major funder of cancer research in the UK has mandated that all new

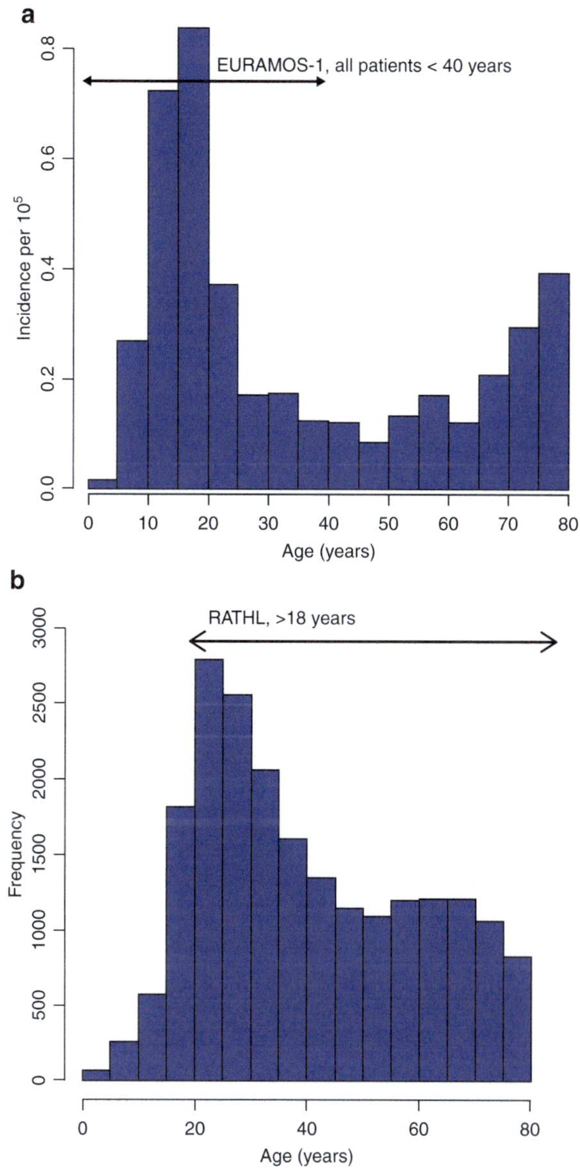

Fig. 2.2 The use of age as an inclusion and exclusion criterion. (**a**) Appropriate age eligibility criteria. (**b**) Inappropriate age eligibility criteria

investigators must give scientific justification for the use of age as inclusion or exclusion criteria on all new funding applications [9]. A model which could be used by other funders in other countries:

> 'Is age to be included as an inclusion/exclusion criterion?
>
> *If yes, please provide specific justification for both upper and lower age limits. Please note that if a lower age limit for studies involving adults is deemed essential it should normally be set at 16 rather than 18 years. Low incidence of patients aged 16 and 17 is not sufficient reason for selecting a lower age criterion of 18 years'* This is a great move forward for cancer research in the UK. However, industry sponsored studies continue to have a lower age eligibility criteria on studies in AYA relevant diseases.

2.1.8 Aware

Broad awareness of clinical trials and the importance of offering entry to research for young people amongst professionals and public is critical to improve inclusion of young people in studies. Healthcare professionals may not be aware of studies available either within their own institution if there are separate adult and children's jurisdictions or neighbouring sites to which patients may be referred. Young people themselves may not realise the importance of entering a research study and may be reliant on healthcare professionals to inform them of studies rather than proactively asking if there are studies available.

2.1.9 Acceptability

Another essential contributor to successful recruitment to a research study is the acceptability of study design to the treatment team, the young person and often, their family, partners or carers [9, 15, 21]. If the research question is deemed unsuitable or lacking clinical relevance by the physician or treating team they are less likely to offer participation in the study to young people. Similarly, if the question and/or outcomes are not important to the young person then they may not see the relevance of suggested participation. Central to participation is the study design, particularly for young people whose focus may be more inclined to prioritise being able to continue their normal activities as far as possible and therefore study designs which interfere with this may prove to be unattractive.

To lessen the risk of study question and study design having low acceptability, early engagement is recommended from the research team with young people. This is ideally done at the concept stage and during protocol development, prior to securing funding for a study. While researchers are familiar with creating multidisciplinary, multi-centre collaborative teams for study design, they may be less comfortable in involving young people early on in study design. The term 'user involvement', 'consumer involvement' and 'patient representative' has become common place within many healthcare and social care systems over the past decade.

2.2 Involving Young People in Research

2.2.1 What is User Involvement?

'User involvement' refers to 'research being carried out '**with**' or '**by**' members of the public rather than '**to**', '**about**' or '**for**' them' [40]. The premise that people who have had first-hand experience of a disease and its related treatment, clinical and psychosocial side-effects are well placed, and in some instances, best placed to contribute to the design and conduct of research, clinical and social services is now generally accepted across most disciplines. As such, evidence of user involvement in research funding submissions is often a prerequisite for funding, certainly within the UK.

2.2.2 Why User Involvement?

User involvement has become common place over the past decade due to perceived benefits conferred to the research study, participants, professionals and also those involved in 'user involvement.' However, rigorous evaluation of the extent of benefit produced by user involvement is challenging [41].

Traditionally, most user involvement activity has been confined to the design and content of study materials such as patient information sheets. However, there are multiple ways young people can contribute to research and they can, with some thought and careful consideration, be involved throughout the research pathway from formulating the research question, through data collection, analysis and dissemination [24, 27, 42–45]. Table 2.1 illustrates how young people can be involved. Introducing and maintaining effective user involvement can be resource intensive, requiring considerable advance planning and organisation. We have offered some practical considerations when approaching user involvement and the associated resources alongside a case study of how we have sucessfully involved young poeple in a longtudinal cohort study, see Sect. 2.4.3.

2.2.2.1 Funding

Funding to support user involvement activity is essential but is often limited, particularly if not considered early enough in study budgeting and funding applications. It is crucial to be clear from the outset with young people whether or not they will be remunerated for their time but payment of travel and sustenance during the meeting should be considered a minimum criterion for involvement. Costs can be minimised by choice of meeting rooms and utilising online platforms such as Facebook (closed groups) and emails.

The UK National Institute of Health Research (NIHR) advocates that during the costing of a research proposal (the process prior to submission where the exact research budget it calculated), researchers should allocate specific costs for user involvement. In this context, as well as adequate travel and sustenance allowance for user involvement, it is typical to budget for remuneration of time spent contributing to the project. In the UK, the national organisation, INVOLVE, suggests a daily rate,

Table 2.1 Research cycle and how young people can contribute

Part of research cycle	Young person contribution/questions to consider
Study concept	Is this area of research relevant to young people?
	Does the question reflect current experience?
Study design	Is the outcome measure relevant to young people?
	Is the study design acceptable to young people?
	Is the method of approach acceptable to young people (timing, person recruiting)?
	Are study materials acceptable to young people (content, length, depth of relevant information)?
	Are data collection methods acceptable to young people (questionnaire, survey, focus groups, digital versus on line, face to face, telephone, multiple mode)?
Study conduct	Can recruitment rates be optimised?
	Are current retention strategies optimal?
Analysis	Can young people add additional insight into analysis?
	Validation of results by young people, is interpretation of the results a valid and accurate reflection of young people's experiences?
Dissemination	Are the results presented in a way which is understandable to young people?
	Young people can disseminate findings back to other young people which can add impact?
	Can young people contribute to conference proceedings and publications?

of £150/day [46]. It should be noted that payments may affect social support/benefits and young people should be made aware of this prior to accepting payment. It is common for some research groups to offer vouchers instead of cash payment which are less likely to negatively impact social support payments. An online tool to assist with calculating costs can be found on the INVOLVE website [47].

2.2.2.2 Time

Effective user involvement requires adequate time to plan the involvement. Young people need sufficient time to consider meeting materials prior to meetings and it is useful to have a key person who can be responsible for translating/converting complex documents into easily understandable formats. Young people may also need assistance in booking and/or paying for travel and overnight accommodation in advance.

It is important to clearly define what is expected from young people prior to their engagement in terms of number of meetings, amount of pre-reading material prior to meetings, email and telephone/teleconference participation. Many young people are keen to engage however, in reality, may not have the capacity to fully participate and may be better suited to other engagement events such as focus groups.

Ensuring that young people are aware of the anticipated length of the project and how long their involvement is likely to be for will mitigate any disappointment or feelings of rejection when the project finishes.

2.2.2.3 Venues and Activities

The choice of venue and activities will be influenced by how much time and money is available for user involvement. In feasibility phases and during grant preparation, when resources are most likely to be scarce then utilising local hospital rooms may be the only viable option. However, ideally rooms are hired away from the clinical area where young people may feel more relaxed about discussing their care and cancer experience. Another thing to consider when choosing a venue is accessibility for those with limited mobility and sight.

A number of resources exist to creatively involve young people and are worth pursuing for ideas on how to best capture different types of experience [48] [49]. It also worth looking around at how other industries conduct their user involvement and applying modifications for your group [27].

2.3 Gaining Other Public Advocacy Support

Widening the partners in a clinical research project beyond the traditional restraints of funder- researcher- research subject can, as has been described above, improve the overall quality of a research project whether qualitative study or clinical trial. Creating partnerships with appropriate stakeholders has been achieved from different directions, driven either by research organisations, patient and public organisations or through individual research projects.

In the UK, opportunities for patients/parents or advocacy groups to engage researchers has been supported in the clinical research infrastructure. Maintenance of dynamic national clinical trials portfolios are the responsibility of individual tumour-specific expert clinical study groups (CSGs), membership of which is mandated to include patient/parent representatives thus giving an effective additional voice to contribute both to strategy and direction as well as work on detail of individual projects. Early consideration of the potential acceptability to patients of trial designs and questions can avoid extensive development of ideas which have a low chance of being successfully completed while assistance with the production of patient-centred information sheets has proved beneficial both from faster processing through ethical review to better uptake of trial participation.

These structural approaches to widen involvement are matched by patient organisations reaching out to researchers at local, national and international level.

2.4 Case Studies

2.4.1 Evidence of the Importance of Clinical Trials

In the following 'case study' we have used Acute Lymphoblastic Leukaemia as an example to illustrate the value of clinical trials to young people's cancer care.

2.4.2 Case Study 1: Acute Lymphoblastic Leukaemia

2.4.2.1 Improvements in Outcomes: Acute Lymphoblastic Leukaemia

Substantial improvements in survival for children with acute lymphoblastic leukaemia (ALL) have been observed over the last three decades and treatment for ALL is considered to be one of the most significant success stories of modern childhood cancer treatment [50]. Advances in treatment have resulted in five-year survival for children with ALL increasing from 47% in 1974 to approximately 90% for those diagnosed today [1, 50]. However, comparable advances in survival were not observed in teenagers and young adults with increasing age being recorded as an adverse prognostic indicator.

2.4.2.2 Allows Legitimate Comparison between Treatments: Paediatric Versus Adult

From 2005 a growing body of evidence from a number of groups including the UK began to emerge indicating significant improvements in outcomes for AYAs with ALL when treated on a paediatric protocol, compared to those treated on the more myelosuppressive and transplant focused adult protocols [19, 51]. As the majority of these observations were made from clinical trial data it was possible to make some comparisons between the studies, albeit there was no randomisation between paediatric and adult protocols in the same study [19, 51].

2.4.2.3 Improving the Appropriateness of Trial Design

A consequence of these observations was collaboration between adult haematologists and paediatric haematologists so that a national ALL trial, UKALL2003, amended its upper age eligibility criterion to include patients up to 24 years. Patients recruited to this study have survival rates not dissimilar to their paediatric counter parts with five year overall survival in the region of 76% [52].

2.4.2.4 Conferring Survival Advantage to Individuals in a Study: UKALL2003 Experience

There has been little evidence to demonstrate that participation in a clinical trial by itself is associated with a survival advantage for an individual. However, recent data published by the National Cancer Intelligence Network has shown that young people in the UKALL2003 trial had significantly better survival at 1 and 2 years compared to those who were not on trial [53]. One year survival for those on trial was 90.8% compared to 81.9% for those not on trial and at 2-years this difference had become more marked with 85.4% survival for those on trial versus 67.5% for those not on trial [53]. Furthermore, young people not in trial were more likely to die within 3 months of diagnosis (8%) than those on trial (2.5%) [53].

2.4.2.5 Adequate Recording of Disease Response and Toxicities

The move from adult to paediatric protocols for young people with ALL has conferred significant survival advantages. However, an increase in serious adverse events exists for those patients over ten years old with a pattern of age specific treatment related toxicities being reported [52]. The increased toxicities associated with this protocol suggest that it may be best delivered in a specialist AYA centre.

2.4.3 Case study 2

2.4.3.1 Contribution of Young People to the BRIGHTLIGHT Study

BRIGHTLIGHT [54], a national evaluation of specialist cancer services for young people in England is unique in many ways, not least the contribution young people made to study design, management and dissemination. BRIGHTLIGHT is funded by national NIHR funding in England (NIHR RP-PG-1209-10013). Prior to BRIGHTLIGHT, the 'Core Consumer Group'(CCG), five young people with a previous cancer diagnosis, worked with the study team as co-researchers on a feasibility study for the main programme, 'Essence of Care', collecting data from other young people in the form of peer-to-peer interviews, identifying priorities for a specialist AYA unit, data analysis, dissemination and consultation with a wider group of young people on acceptability of study design and choice of a primary end point for BRIGHTLIGHT [24, 27, 42–45, 55]. Critically, during study set-up the CCG suggested the proposed name for the study 'The 2012 Cancer Cohort Study' or 'Essence of AYA Care' was not an appropriate engaging name for young people. Young people were subsequently engaged in a branding naming process adapted from healthcare advertisement to re-name and brand the study as BRIGHTLIGHT [27].

2.4.3.2 Measuring Impact: Study Uptake and Retention

This level of user involvement, where young people are involved in data collection, analysis and dissemination is resource intensive. However, the benefits conferred to study in terms of acceptably of study design and research materials are indicated by an uptake of 80% for those young people who were offered entry into BRIGHTLIGHT compared to an anticipated 60% which was calculated based on other cohort studies in young people [24, 44].

Young people have continued to be involved in BRIGHTLIGHT and have been invaluable in assisting the study team with advice on recruitment, retention and dissemination [44]. The BRIGHTLIGHT Young Advisory Panel (YAP) is a group of around 20 young people who advise on all aspects of BRIGHTLIGHT. Their contributions to recruitment have included modifications to the approaches used for both timing and patient information materials, inviting the wider treatment team (social workers and youth support workers) to be involved in recruitment and advocating that all young people who are eligible for any research study should be made aware of all opportunities in order to make an informed choice about their care [24]. In this context their impact on improving recruitment rates was difficult to measure as it was not possible to randomise young people to receiving YAP influenced materials versus healthcare professional influenced materials only. Additionally, the majority of recruitment difficulties were around young people not being approached by healthcare professionals about the study.

Uptake for BRIGHTLIGHT, for those patients who were offered the study as was an impressive 80% and retention at Wave 2 also higher than anticipated at 69%

which may be related to the study being designed for young people by young people [45]. The BRIGHTLIGHT YAP was invited to contribute to the existing retention strategy acknowledging that retention rates were not aligned with what was anticipated given uptake and retention at Wave 2. A number of modifications were made based on the YAP recommendations and retention at Wave 3 increased from 30% to 59%[45].

2.4.3.3 Measuring Impact: Is User Involvement Beneficial to Young People?

The benefits to young people being involved with research are numerous. Practical benefits include learning new skills such as data collection, analysis, writing and presenting which can help with securing employment or entry to higher education and provide evidence of constructive use of time during periods of recovery. Personal attributes can include increased confidence and learning about communication with peers, healthcare professionals and the public. Additionally, young people have expressed a therapeutic value of involvement. The full impact of this warrants further exploration.

Conclusions

Cancer research rightly has a high public profile. For AYA, the demonstration of differences in participation rates in clinical trials compared with children and older adults has triggered efforts both to understand this phenomenon and identify interventions which might re-balance it. In the UK, taking part in clinical trials has been given a high priority within the delivery of AYA cancer care, setting considerable challenges for researchers to ensure there is a successful portfolio of research. Including young people themselves in the research process has been demonstrated to be both feasible and effective, thus making it a pre-requisite for future clinical research affecting young people.

Acknowledgements We would like to thank members of the Core Consumer Group and the BRIGHTLIGHT Young Advisory for their contribution to research studies under the aegis of the National Cancer Research Institutes Teenage and Young Adult Clinical Studies Group and BRIGHTLIGHT. The case study presents independent research funded by the National Institute for Health Research (NIHR) under its Programme Grants for Applied Research Programme (Grant Reference Number RP-PG-1209-10013). The views expressed are those of the author(s) and not necessarily those of the NHS, the NIHR or the Department of Health. Lorna Fern is funded by Teenage Cancer Trust.

References

1. Smith MA, Seibel NL, Altekruse SF, Ries LA, Melbert DL, O'Leary M, et al. Outcomes for children and adolescents with cancer: challenges for the twenty-first century. J Clin Oncol. 2010;28(15):2625–34.
2. Hayes A, et al. Clinical trials. In: Bleyer A, Barr R, Whelan J, Ferrari A, Ries L, editors. Cancer in adolescent and young adults. Cham: Springer; 2016. p. 549.

3. Bleyer A, Morgan S, Barr R. Proceedings of a workshop: bridging the gap in care and addressing participation in clinical trials. Cancer. 2006;107(7 Suppl):1656–8.
4. National Institute for Clinical Excellencec. Improving outcomes guidance for children and young people. London: Crown Publishers; 2005.
5. Freyer D, Seibel N. The clinical trials gap for adolescents and young adults with cancer: recent progress and conceptual framework for continued research. Curr Peadiatr Rep. 2015;3(2):137–45.
6. Bleyer WA, Tejeda H, Murphy SB, Robison LL, Ross JA, Pollock BH, et al. National cancer clinical trials: children have equal access; adolescents do not. J Adolesc Health. 1997;21(6):366–73.
7. Bleyer A, Budd T, Montello M. Lack of participation of older adolescents and young adults with cancer in clinical trials: impact in the USA. 2nd ed: Cancer Adolescent, Blackwell publishing; 2005. p. 32–45.
8. Fern L, Davies S, Eden T, Feltbower R, Grant R, Hawkins M, et al. Rates of inclusion of teenagers and young adults in England into National Cancer Research Network clinical trials: report from the National Cancer Research Institute (NCRI) Teenage and Young Adult Clinical Studies Development Group. Br J Cancer. 2008;99(12):1967–74.
9. Fern LA, Lewandowski JA, Coxon KM, Whelan J. Available, accessible, aware, appropriate, and acceptable: a strategy to improve participation of teenagers and young adults in cancer trials. Lancet Oncol. 2014;15(8):e341–50.
10. Ferrari A. Michael Montello Troy Budd Archie Bleyer. the challenges of clinical trials for adolescents and young adults with cancer. Pediatr Blood Cancer. 2008;50(S5):1101–4.
11. Mitchell AE, Scarcella DL, Rigutto GL, Thursfield VJ, Giles GG, Sexton M, et al. Cancer in adolescents and young adults: treatment and outcome in Victoria. Med J Aust. 2004;180(2):59–62.
12. Bleyer A, Montello M, Budd T, Saxman S. National survival trends of young adults with sarcoma - lack of progress is associated with lack of clinical trial participation. Cancer. 2005;103(9):1891–7.
13. Desandes E, Lacour B, Sommelet D, White-Koning M, Velten M, Tretarre B, et al. Cancer adolescent pathway in France between 1988 and 1997. Eur J Oncol Nurs. 2007;11(1):74–81.
14. Desandes E, Bonnay S, Berger C, Brugieres L, Demeocq F, Laurence V, Sommelet D, Tron I, Clavel J, Lacour B. Pathways of care for adolescents patients with cancer in France from 2006 to 2007. Peadiatr Blood Cancer. 2012;58:924–9.
15. Unger JM, Cook E, Tai E, Bleyer A. The role of clinical trial parctipation in cancer research: barriers, evidence, and strategies. Am Soc Clin Oncol Educ Book. 2016;35:185–98.
16. Bleyer A, Viny A, Barr R. Cancer in 15-to 29-year-olds by primary site. Oncologist. 2006;11(6):590–601.
17. Damenia AO, Turkevich EA, Semiglazov VF, Kochetova IA, Gurbanov SS, Bit-Sava EM, et al. Biological features of breast cancer in patients under 35. Vopr Onkologii. 2007;53(6):674–6.
18. Lethaby CD, Picton S, Kinsey SE, Phillips R, van Laar M, Feltbower RG. A systematic review of time to diagnosis in children and young adults with cancer. Arch Dis Child. 2013;98(5):349–55.
19. Boissel N, Auclerc MF, Lheritier V, Perel Y, Thomas X, Leblanc T, et al. Should adolescents with acute lymphoblastic leukemia be treated as old children or young adults? Comparison of the French FRALLE-93 and LALA-94 trials. J Clin Oncol. 2003;21(5):774–80.
20. Ferrari A. SIAMO: Italian pediatric oncologists and adult medical oncologists join forces for adolescents with cancer. Pediatr Hematol Oncol. 2014;31(6):574–5.
21. Pearce S, Brownsdon A, Fern L, Gibson F, Whelan J, Lavender V. The perceptions of teenagers, young adults and professionals in the participation of bone cancer clinical trials. Eur J Cancer Care (Engl). 2016.; [Epub ahead of print].
22. Ford JG, Howerton MW, Lai GY, Gary TL, Bolen S, Gibbons MC, et al. Barriers to recruiting underrepresented populations to cancer clinical trials: A systematic review. Cancer. 2008;112(2):228–42.

23. Ferrari A, Arico M, Dini G, Rondelli R, Porta F. Upper age limits for accessing pediatric oncology centers in Italy: a barrier preventing adolescents with cancer from entering national cooperative AIEOP trials. Pediatr Hematol Oncol. 2012;29(1):55–61.
24. Taylor RM, Solanki A, Aslam N, Whelan JS, Fern LA. A participatory study of teenagers and young adults views on access and participation in cancer research. Eur J Oncol Nurs. 2016;20:156–64.
25. Ferrari A, Bleyer A. Participation of adolescents with cancer in clinical trials. Cancer Treat Rev. 2007;33(7):603–8.
26. Hay AE, Rae C, Fraser GA, Meyer RM, Abbott LS, Bevan S, et al. Accrual of adolescents and young adults with cancer to clinical trials. Curr Oncol. 2016;23(2):e81–5.
27. Taylor RM, Mohain J, Gibson F, Solanki A, Whelan J, Fern LA. Novel participatory methods of involving patients in research: naming and branding a longitudinal cohort study, BRIGHTLIGHT. BMC Med Res Methodol. 2015;15:20.
28. Group IEW. Guideline for good clinical practice E6 (R1). International conference on harmonization. 1996.
29. Birch JM, Alston RD, Quinn M, Kelsey AM. Incidence of malignant disease by morphological type, in young persons aged 12–24 years in England, 1979–1997. Eur J Cancer. 2003;39(18):2622–31.
30. Stark D, Bielack S, Brugieres L, Dirksen U, Duarte X, Dunn S, et al. Teenagers and young adults with cancer in Europe: from national programmes to a European integrated coordinated project. Eur J Cancer Care (Engl). 2016;25(3):419–27.
31. Whelan J, Fern L. Cancer in adolescence: incidence and policy issues. In: Kelly D, Gibson F, editors. Cancer care for adolescents and young adults. Oxford: Blackwell Publishing Ltd.; 2008.
32. Aapro MS, Kohne CH, Cohen HJ, Extermann M. Never too old? Age should not be a barrier to enrollment in cancer clinical trials. Oncologist. 2005 Mar;10(3):198–204.
33. Association WM. Declaration of Helsinki- Ethical Principles for medical research involving human subjects. 2013.
34. Health Do. Cancer reform strategy, Chapter 6 Reducing cancer inequalities. London; 2007.
35. Administration FaD. Studies in support of special populations: geriatrics E7. Silver Spring; 1994.
36. Administration FaD. Clinical Investigation of medicinal products in the peadiatric population. Silver Spring; 2000.
37. Whelan JS, Bielack SS, Marina N, Smeland S, Jovic G, Hook JM, et al. EURAMOS-1, an international randomised study for osteosarcoma: results from pre-randomisation treatment. Ann Oncol. 2015;26(2):407–14.
38. Arora RS, Alston RD, Eden TO, Geraci M, Birch JM. The contrasting age-incidence patterns of bone tumours in teenagers and young adults: implications for aetiology. Int J Cancer. 2012;131(7):1678–85.
39. Johnson P, Federico M, Kirkwood A, Fossa A, Berkahn L, Carella A, et al. Adapted treatment guided by interim PET-CT scan in advanced Hodgkin's lymphoma. N Engl J Med. 2016;374(25):2419–29.
40. INVOLVE. 2017. http://www.invo.org.uk/find-out-more/what-is-public-involvement-in-research-2/.
41. Brett J, Staniszewska S, Mockford C, Herron-Marx S, Hughes J, Tysall C, et al. Mapping the impact of patient and public involvement on health and social care research: a systematic review. Health Expect. 2014;17(5):637–50.
42. Taylor RM, Fern L, Whelan J, Pearce S, Grew T, Millington H, et al. "Your place or mine?" Priorities for a specialist teenage and young adult (TYA) cancer unit: disparity between TYA and professional perceptions. J Adolesc Young Adult Oncol. 2011;1(3):145–51.
43. Fern LA, Taylor RM, Whelan J, Pearce S, Grew T, Brooman K, et al. The art of age-appropriate care: reflecting on a conceptual model of the cancer experience for teenagers and young adults. Cancer Nurs. 2013;36(5):E27–38.

44. Taylor RM, Fern LA, Solanki A, Hooker L, Carluccio A, Pye J, et al. Development and validation of the BRIGHTLIGHT Survey, a patient-reported experience measure for young people with cancer. Health Qual Life Outcomes. 2015;13:107.
45. Taylor RM. Optimising a retention strategy with young people: the BRIGHTLIGHT study. J Young Adult Adolesc Oncol. 2017 (in press).
46. INVOLVE. 2017. http://www.invo.org.uk/wp-content/uploads/2014/11/10002-INVOLVE-Budgeting-Tool-Publication-WEB.pdf.
47. INVOLVE. 2017. http://www.invo.org.uk/resource-centre/payment-and-recognition-for-public-involvement/involvement-cost-calculator/.
48. Children St. Participation—Spice it up!; 2003.
49. Shaw C, Brady LM, Davey C. Guidelines for research with children and young people. London: National Childrens Bureau Research Centre; 2011.
50. Rowe JM, Buck G, Burnett AK, Chopra R, Wiernik PH, Richards SM, et al. Induction therapy for adults with acute lymphoblastic leukemia: results of more than 1500 patients from the international ALL trial: MRC UKALL XII/ECOG E2993. Blood. 2005;106(12):3760–7.
51. Boissel N. Lymphoblastic leukaemia in adults. The European cancer congress 2015. Vienna; 2015.
52. Hough R, Rowntree C, Goulden N, Mitchell C, Moorman A, Wade R, et al. Efficacy and toxicity of a paediatric protocol in teenagers and young adults with Philadelphia chromosome negative acute lymphoblastic leukaemia: results from UKALL 2003. Br J Haematol. 2016;172(3):439–51.
53. Network NCI. Clinical trial participation and outcomes in teenagers and young adults in England with acute lymphoblastic leukaemia. 2015. http://www.ncin.org.uk/view?rid=2908.
54. Brightlight. 2017. www.brightlightstudy.com.
55. Gibson F, Fern L, Whelan J, Pearce S, Lewis IJ, Hobin D, et al. A scoping exercise of favourable characteristics of professionals working in teenage and young adult cancer care: 'thinking outside of the box'. Eur J Cancer Care (Engl). 2012;21(3):330–9.

3 Models of Delivery of Care for AYA

Dan Stark and Andrea Ferrari

To design services for AYA with cancer, it is a given that we need to understand the patterns of disease. However more importantly we need to respond to the specific clinical and organisational challenges inherent in this patient group.

Improving AYA cancer management involves bridging interfaces. The local nature of these interfaces determines the age-group considered as AYA. Specific skills are necessary in the clinical, the biological, and the psychosocial domains. Any specified age range should meet the local challenges in service provision. Geographical issues can require some specialisation, but models to minimise the down-side of that are known, described in detail and evaluate well. Local hospitals should work together with not-for-profit organisations that have public and business support, to deliver enhanced services to meet local needs, and to support local specialist places of care, such as wards or outpatient care environments.

AYA services need pragmatic support from policy as well as clinical and administrative health care professionals, which may have to be won by following a carefully considered and responsive strategy. National policy can help greatly, and is evolving in the UK, Australia, Canada and France and most recently in Italy.

D. Stark (✉)
St James Hospital, Leeds, UK
e-mail: D.P.Stark@leeds.ac.uk

A. Ferrari
Pediatric Oncology Unit, Fondazione IRCCS Istituto Nazionale Tumori, Milano, Italy
e-mail: andrea.ferrari@istitutotumori.mi.it

J. Chisholm et al. (eds.), *A Practical Approach to the Care of Adolescents and Young Adults with Cancer*, https://doi.org/10.1007/978-3-319-66173-5_3

Where these changes have been made, some outcomes have improved. Different parts of the world have taken similar but distinct approaches to this, which can be informative. This chapter discusses what forms of pragmatic health service design are meeting (or could in future meet) these devastating patterns of serious disease and, while doing that, also meet AYA patients' specific needs.

3.1 The Problem

In recent years evidence has increased to support the design of cancer services for adolescents and young adults (AYA) with cancer. The major considerations in these designs can be understood if we aim to meet the specific challenges that arise in the care of these patients, within the existing structures in healthcare. These are illustrated in Box 3.1.

Box 3.1: Some age-specific challenges facing specialist services for AYA with cancer

1. AYA with cancer are have *highly specific medical needs*;
   - Their symptom appraisal and pathway from symptoms to diagnosis are specific [1, 2]
   - Biologically their cancer types and treatments are specific [3]
   - They have distinct patterns of acute toxicity and late effects [4–6]
2. AYA with cancer bring *specific supportive care* challenges; [7]
   - Social context—balancing family, peer-group, and the individual context for the patient.
   - Personal development—where is this young person in their personal journey of developing biologically and personally, from early childhood to mature adulthood? [8–10]
   - Psychological needs are specific [11]
3. AYA cancer care involves *multiple different teams*;
   - Across cancer-site specific clinical teams (e.g., breast cancer, sarcoma, lymphoma) [9, 12]
   - Across administrative boundaries in health care systems (e.g., haematology and oncology, adult and pediatric) [13, 14].

These challenges all share a common feature–they are due to the 'interface' position of AYA. AYA is the interface group between childhood and adulthood in society, by definition [8, 9].

In the absence of specialist AYA services, AYA receive care either in pediatric or adult services. Both adult and pediatric care inform AYA care, but AYA care is AYA-specific (Box 3.1). The differences between the young adolescent and the emerging adult in social, psychological and physiological development have the potential to maintain misunderstandings between adult and pediatric services about optimal care [9]. Both seek to apply the supportive care and medical care paradigms they are familiar with, and may not therefore focus upon AYA issues. For example;

- They can be influenced by how the team would usually communicate, if this were a younger or an older patient.
- They can be influenced by how the team usually make decisions on chemotherapy dose reduction, by the more established principles laid down for childhood embryonal tumours and adult carcinomas respectively [15].
- Their experienced 'educated guesses' about how to resolve challenges in care can be influenced by their wider practices in older or younger patients.

Maintaining this interface doesn't serve the needs of patients, and delays the development of new improved treatment options, by delaying the study of the pros and cons of differing approaches in clinical trials. Bridging this clinical interface is key for AYA services and needs continually to be at the heart of the design of services.

As AYA age-based outcome data was previously divided between two specialty areas (at least) and not considered together, it can be marginal within professional and academic concerns. This means that, even 20 years after the first descriptions of these challenges [16, 17] and while progress is being made [18–20] it remains the case that

- Clinical outcomes are incompletely described,
- Biological specifics of AYA cancer, in tumour biology and the pharmacology, are incompletely described [21–29].

AYA with cancer themselves have a clear view on how care could be improved, and their view also supports bridging the interface; they reported that they were isolated from other young people [30]. This was because AYA were divided between many healthcare settings, rather than together - many did not know there were other young people being treated for cancer as well. Of course this is ironic, given the huge emphasis AYA place upon their own peer group in their usual lives [31]. Some professionals may feel this isolation is simply because AYA cancers are rare. Compared to adult carcinomas they are uncommon. However they are less rare than childhood cancer, and specialisation in childhood cancer care brought children and their families together many years ago [32]. The cross-cutting issues for AYA whatever cancer they have are certainly not rare within oncology. Therefore a successful AYA service needs to be designed to work across these interfaces, bring young people together for their cancer care, and bring professionals together who treat their cancer and care for them.

It is difficult to conceptualise a single, ideal "new" model of delivery of care for AYA. Neither the classic family-focused pediatric or the traditional patient-focused adult model of care are ideally suited to meet the needs of AYA patients. But to overcome these difficulties defining a specific model adapting the established systems may meet AYA's needs. To achieve we are *patient-focused*—using a multidisciplinary approach that implies the direct presence in the team of both pediatric oncologists and adult medical oncologists. We should involve young patients in the care process directly. We should promote their normalcy, including their being permitted to challenge authority. Moreover, an AYA program should adapt the overall model of care, to the local situation and variations in medical culture, as well as in resources. The different local issues have generated a great heterogeneity of solutions.

3.2 Practical Approaches to this Problem

3.2.1 Geography and Delivering AYA Care

AYA cancer is uncommon. If professionals are to be experts, with current experience and specific clinical skills to work with AYA, then they need regular and substantial exposure to the issues, and time to prioritise their professional education in this field. A centralisation of services (as seen in pediatric cancer) may be necessary to achieve this exposure [16, 19, 33]. This has disadvantages to weigh up; specifically in AYA, when compared to young children, a negative impact upon the young person's sensitive, local, fragile, personal and newly widening social, educational and vocational development. Cancer is diagnosed just when so often AYA are starting leave the support of a smaller family unit into a peer-group social network of friends and partner [34]. While a family travelling up to 60 miles repeatedly over many months for treatment is hugely disruptive, the key people supporting a young child (often parents) may be able to be present for many of the key events. For a 19-year old, embedded in a social group of a similar age, perhaps at a university or apprenticed in a company, sometimes with a newly starting intimate relationship, very little of the personal support their peers can provide can be maintained at high quality over longer distances. AYA may have to return to reliance upon family, or try to manage without support.

Some limited centralisation of services has taken place in some places, by policy and by some young people choosing to come to existing specialist services. In 2005 in England, the National Institute for Clinical Excellence (now the National Institute for Health and Care Excellence) published 'Improving Outcomes Guidance for cancer in children and young people' which has led to a network of AYA treatment centres [35, 36]. The guidance defines specific standards of care for people aged 15–24 years at their cancer diagnosis, which (although now uncertain in straightened financial times) are assessed through 'peer to peer' service reviews on a 2–3 yearly cycle. A semi-centralisation is part of this alongside other several key features:

- The definition of regional principal treatment centres where all care AYA might need, for rare or less rare cancers, for first line and relapsed disease and for severe complications, is available and of high quality. Moreover, an investment supports specific psychosocial care including a multi-professional team with specialist nurses, social work, rehabilitation, mental health care, educational and vocational experts and activity co-ordinators. This larger centre is allied in a network to local 'designated hospitals,' where some such elements of enhanced care are in place (but with a lesser investment in specialist staff) and active links with the principal centre.
- The definition of referral pathways to investigate symptoms. Which colleague or healthcare team a primary care physician should ask to investigate a symptom or sign, how to contact them and what timescales to expect are defined in publicly available network referral pathway documents in each region and inspected within a biennial peer review system.

- AYA aged 18 years or younger must *commence* their treatment in a principal centre. After that, if wished, local 'shared' care can be offered at a designated hospital.
- Older AYA aged 19–24 must be offered an informed choice of whether to go to the principal centre or chose care in a designated hospital, allowing them to trade off the risks and benefits. Defining how to explain that choice has been subject to a specialist national project (http://www.nhs.uk/young-cancer-care/pages/cancer-treatment-choices.aspx, accessed August 2016), but it remains unknown how this is done in practice.
- Non-designated hospitals within the NHS in England are not commissioned to provide treatment for cancer in AYA. Therefore if they provide treatment, they are not paid for that care by the NHS.
- Professionals including clinical and managerial groups across a region meet as a network and share their service enhancement and development.

In other nations, developments include varying degrees of centralisation of care and are described below, but the UK situation is (arguably) the best described in health service policy terms. The 'BRIGHTLIGHT' prospective evaluation of; the methodological aspects, nature in practice, impacts upon outcomes, costs and wider implications of this semi-specialisation are awaited [37, 38], as the less reliable but intriguing data widens internationally within site-specific patient cohorts [39]. It is important to note however that these systems of service specialisation are not immune to pressures to change. They are overseen by a clinically-led policy reference group in England, but most recently the pediatric and the AYA reference groups were merged, threatening some reduction in the place of AYA care within NHS policy.

Where young people chose not to travel to the principal treatment centre, peripatetic specialist AYA services can outreach to other hospitals. This has the potential to reduce geographical and social disruption for some patients and provide specialist support locally. Also however it maintains professional networks, and a pilot evaluation is complete and awaiting full dissemination [40].

3.2.2 What Age Range Should AYA Services Include?

There are very reasonable pressures to define the age which we mean by 'AYA.' It is a frequent criticism from peer reviewers of publications and those who may not support changes in structures of care that the age ranges used by different investigators are inconsistent. Defined age ranges promote clarity. For some these critics are seeking a decision by those in the field as to what their scope should be. For others the criticism is a simpler plea to retain a consistent structure in data about services, so that one analysis can be compared to another. However, in practice the age range should be made explicit and agreed at a local or individual project level, to solve a specific problem for the service or research project, because different purposes require their own age ranges (see Box 3.2). As AYA go from diagnosis, through treatment, to cancer survivorship (for over 80%) their personal development continues gradually, and their care and the study of their outcomes should develop with them [9]. A joint approach to care between children's and adult's services may support transition between healthcare providers, such as for late effects care. According to the findings of the 2013 ENCCA survey of AYA professionals AYA services should be flexible for patients with special needs, such as in educational or personal development [41].

Box 3.2: How age range for AYA studies may vary with the purpose of the study

To overcome the clinical interface challenge

- In the UK, AYA services cover an age of 13–24 years which crosses the problematic interface between adult and children's services.
- Considerable advantages may come from joint clinical care planning by pediatric and adult teams for patients in an age range which relatively equally encompasses the adolescent oncology patients at and after puberty (13–18) and the younger young adults (19–24). Both groups of professionals then actively share a responsibility for the patients aged 16–18, where the psychosocial and legal issues can be the most contentious [31]. Moreover this 13–24 age range leads to equity in multi-disciplinary clinical care discussions or clinic-pathological conferences; both what 'would be' pediatric cases and what 'would be' adult cases are discussed, jointly. We have found this is cohesive for a team, when compared to asking adult teams to come to a children's cancer meeting or *vice versa*.
- However this age interface is inconsistent internationally. Pediatric care ends at 14 or 15 years in some parts of southern Europe, but strictly at 18 years in Germany (Table 3.1).

To support young people in their personal development

- Including older patients is justified up to 39 years to provide this support. Erikson identified phases of young adolescence, older adolescence, very young adulthood and young adulthood [42]. Since this work in the 1970s society is very different—it includes older transitions, such as age of leaving education, or starting parenthood, or personal financial independence [43, 44, 45].

To study age-specific incidence and outcomes

Epidemiological data has been dominant in the process of determining age ranges, using their favoured 5-year groupings (e.g., 15–19 and 20–24). These 5-year age bands are ubiquitous. However modern computerised databases should make rigid grouping much less necessary, and prolonged registry processes and 'big-data' pooling should enable case numbers that allow analyses without groupings that are statistically driven [19, 31, 46].

Table 3.1 The age-groups, projects and selected challenges for AYA cancer services in selected European nations, to illustrate the variation in definitions and local needs.

	UK	France	Germany, Poland	Italy	Spain	The Netherlands	Denmark	Czech Republic
Age range	15–24 years in policy (13–24 in several departments)	15–25 years	Interface between pediatric and adult care at 18 years	19–24 years	14–30 years	18–35 years	Not defined	15–19
Local projects	25 AYA principal units and many designated hospitals, accredited and inspected	8 AYA programs, with 3 AYA units	Inter-disciplinary programs in 3 centers	2 AYA units, 1 regional project	1 AYA unit—local initiatives in pediatric centers	2 AYA centers	2 AYA units	Collaboration on Leukaemia trials
Next challenge	Maintain policy initiatives Increase research	Enhance medical oncology participation, prospective research	Extend the collaborative AYA infrastructure	Equitable access for all, through implementing national policy	National economic and political support	Prospective research; financial model	National policy	Financial support within health care systems

3.2.3 Environment of Care

Specific AYA medical 'units' generally arise from adaptation of existing services, followed by nomination of distinct spaces. Often this is not a policy change for many years after it begins, but instead a group of clinicians, with or without a policy change in their hospitals but with their practical support and consistently with strong support from young people as 'service user advocates,' have identified there is an unmet clinical need for suitable facilities, for shared models of care and to for peer group support between young people [32].

Often these begin by providing AYA out-patient environments, which is simpler than in-patient wards. A drop-in zone to support the clinic is an example, with charitable support for specific decor, facilities for electronic communication and the types of food that are popular for young people. When supported by staff who work well with young people, this environment can relax young people before a consultation, by enabling them to socialise with their peers while waiting for difficult news. These and in-patient specific environments are valuable to young people; undoubtedly décor and equipment can be contemporary in contrast to many healthcare environments [47, 48]. Young people when asked in detail however also value privacy, and most importantly the time with others of a similar age [49]. Internet based interactions are very important to young people (and others) and should be suitable for their needs, while bearing in mind the difficulties they may cause, such as for information governance [50]. The process of building a new AYA-specific place of care (as much as the work within it once completed) can prove a focus for joint collaborative working and mutual understanding across interfaces, provided that initial amicable inter-professional relationships are in place.

Within 6 European nations, as well as in Canada, USA, Australia, New Zealand, India, China, Morocco and Uruguay there are now specific AYA environments for oncology care. Prominent among the improvements that professionals want in an AYA service is a collaborative ethos [19, 51–53].

An environment of care for AYA may also change the culture of the hospital or clinic. AYA are born to challenge the *status quo* [12], including the design of health services. These challenges can be contentious sometimes, but extremely helpful to stimulate improvement if they remain constructive. This is why integrating AYA patients' voices into decisions is used widely in several international settings when designing and developing cancer care environments [54].

Environment of care may not in any sense be sufficient to achieve all outcomes professionals and young people would wish. A recent study from the European pediatric Soft tissue sarcoma Study Group (EpSSG) estimated the proportion of adolescents (defined as patients from 15 to 19 years old) enrolled in the EpSSG's protocols with the number of adolescent cases expected to occur, estimated from the incidence rates in population-based cancer registries. The study confirmed that adolescents were less represented in EpSSG protocols (the observed to expected ratio was 0.30 among patients 15–19 years old, as opposed to 0.64 for 0–14 years old), even though these trials were open to patients up to 21 years old. The UK despite specialist AYA services was among the lower trial inclusion proportion, lower for example, than

Italy and France [55]. AYA Patients and specialist AYA services still require close links with the available age-appropriate clinical trials even when they have an AYA-specific environment of care.

3.2.3.1 Services that promote prompt diagnosis of cancer in AYA

Consistently, specific studies report prolonged time periods between symptoms and treatment for AYA within healthcare systems [56–59]. What is less clear is whether this is an age-specific problem or relates to cancer in this age range being uncommon, and therefore from clinical use of 'prior probability' in making decisions whether or not to investigate symptoms. Problems for AYA include:

- Non-specific symptoms, not always specifically or classically described by a young person
- The frequency of non-cancer diagnoses that can explain many presenting symptoms
- Young people not having a clear understanding of their body's normal function, and not therefore seeking help for a problem (presuming the symptom to be a 'phase they are going through')
- AYA no longer (unlike small children) discussing any symptoms with older people with more experience of health issues
- Young people lacking the confidence, perceiving that they lack the free time, (or in some systems the financial means) to consult with a healthcare professional.
- In recent times is has also become less clear when a long period from first symptoms to cancer treatment can hinder prognosis and when it does not.

Skilled initial medical reassurance is often the logical approach at the initial presentation of a possible cancer symptom in a young person [60]. However multiple consultations are well documented. There is clear evidence that AYA do have an increased number of medical consultations with symptoms for some months before cancer is diagnosed [1, 61, 62]. The symptom interval is longer in AYA than children for both reasons related to the patients and the family's symptom appraisal (patient-delay) but also due to the interpretation that the doctors make of the symptoms and therefore whether to refer (doctor –delay) [59].

There are programmes designed which can improve young people's understanding of cancer symptoms [63]. A recent SIAMO project in Italy promoted a communication strategy (at various levels, i.e., community, family physicians, oncologists and institution). Two information campaigns dedicated to teenagers were launched to improve awareness that cancer can develop at their age, and also how to interpret symptoms they experience, with a view to reducing the time elapsing before they seek help, and thereby shortening the pathway to diagnosis [64, 65]. Danish studies in adult cancer care are beginning to define adjustments to care pathways that may speed a diagnosis for all [66–69], but will still need to be AYA-friendly.

AYA services might speed the processes of AYA cancer diagnosis and treatment once a young person is in the hospital also. In our local experience, rarer presentations are often discussed between clinical teams for some while, who are considering the illnesses they commonly see. Mediastinal masses may be seen by lymphoma and by germ cell teams, for example. Strong relationships built through routine case discussions between these teams may accelerate the correct diagnosis and management.

3.2.4 Providing Skilled Multi-professional Clinical Teams

The professional supportive care skills integral to delivering cancer care are multiple. Those specific to care for AYA extend beyond traditional oncology domains. An example might be working constructively using the various expressions of emotions from multiple generations within a family and extended carer network of peers, within a single consultation, to meet the distinct information preferences of all.

Currently, many health care professional training programs do not address AYA-specific issues routinely, such as communication, personal development or disease profiles [70, 71]. We have conducted professional opinion surveys within Europe, through the European Network for Cancer in Children and Adolescents ENCCA (www.encca.eu), which indicate a professional and service user consensus as to what expertise is most important [41, 72]. AYA services require a specific multi-professional team and acceptance of the training and competencies which define those roles, ideally with certification of completed training [73, 74]. Service managers also need to be willing to permit staff to work across traditional interfaces.

Training curricula are in place for cancer in AYA, each defining a similar body of knowledge, in the US, UK, Canada, Australasia and the EU [74–77]. However they vary substantially when going beyond knowledge, to the skills and attitudes which professionals require. They vary as to whether the interface between the pediatric and adult training schemes has been considered. Some, notably most recently in Canada, ask for advocacy, leadership, and service development knowledge skills and attitudes (A Gupta, personal communication 2014). Interestingly few emphasise collaborative skills.

At an international summit meeting hosted by ENCCA and the Teenage Cancer Trust in 2014, the consensus of experts in AYA cancer and medical education was:

- Accredited AYA-specific education is needed by cancer professionals. This must be collaborative between doctors and allied healthcare professionals and available to all who lead in AYA services
- There should be generic “working with AYA” training programmes for all health care professionals who work with young people with serious illness
- Detailed AYA training should be compulsory for all doctors leading in AYA cancer care, who should hold a validated qualification in AYA oncology
- Delivery of learning for training should be online, and the face-to-face work required should be delivered at key international congresses.
- This training should be accredited by Universities, in collaboration with professional societies

Delivering upon these aims is within on-going work.

3.3 AYA Cancer Care Services and Projects Across the World

UK services have been described in detail recently and are outlined above [35, 54].

3.3.1 In Continental Europe

AYA care in France has an integrated cooperative and cross-cutting program, joining pediatric and adult oncology/hematology. The last three successive national Cancer Plans since 2004 have included an AYA element, including regional pathways to care and increasing research. The Institut National du Cancer (INCa) has supported eight defined French AYA centres. Each must have

- A cross-cutting clinical team (at least one pediatric and one adult oncologist/hematologist, coordinating nurse)
- A specific psycho-social program including psychologists and social workers.

Groupe Onco-hematologie Adolescents et Jeunes Adultes (Go-AJA) is the national specialist group and charity, including patients, their representatives and professionals. This group with professional leadership has been the cornerstone of the coordinated national programme for AYA launched by INCa in May of 2016.

In Germany, cancer care for AYA has distinct infrastructures for pediatric and adult oncology, with a relatively unequivocal age barrier at 18 years. Inpatient treatment of adolescent cancer patients <18 years is not reimbursed unless it takes place within a German Society for Pediatric Oncology and Hematology (GPOH)-certified unit. Patients being managed both before and after their 18th birthday require specific action. Medical oncology national cooperative infrastructures are 'site-specific' (leukemia, lymphoma, germ cell tumours) but can support collaboration between pediatric and the adult national societies, while four centers have initiated AYA-specific interdisciplinary programs [78].

In Italy, two AYA units have developed, focussed upon cooperation between pediatric and adult medical oncologists [79]. The initial seed of an Italian national program arose in pediatric oncology, with the development of Committee on Adolescents of the pediatric cooperative group Associazione Italiana Ematologia Oncologia Pediatrica (AIEOP) established a, with the declared goal to assure adequate and equitable access to the best available care for Italian adolescents with cancer [79, 80].

SIAMO (Società scientifiche italiane Insieme per gli Adolescenti con Malattie Onco-ematologiche, Italian Scientific Societies Together for Adolescents with Oncohematological Diseases, www.progettosiamo.it) began in 2014 to develop a comprehensive national program, a national task-force with a cooperation between adult and pediatric groups [81]. More recently SIAMO has formal support from national health services (Andrea Ferrari, personal communication 2016). SIAMO aims to include a dedicated document in Italy's next National Oncology Plan, with the goal to identify the criteria and facilities that centers (be they pediatric or adult units) need to treat adolescents with cancer. New local programs are currently ready to be launched in different Italian centers under the auspicies of SIAMO. A recent update of the evaluation of the access of 15–19-year-old patients to AIEOP centers has showed a significant increase from the 0.10 observed to expected ratio of the 1989–2006 period to 0.28 for the 2007–2012 period, as a results of the various initiatives launched in the last years [82].

In the Netherlands, health professionals from regional centers started a national cooperative AYA project in 2013, initiated by medical oncology, and focussing upon 18–35 year-olds rather than more explicitly crossing the pediatric/adult care interface. There is an AYA (digital) community and research studies of fertility, preferences by age, acute and long term outcomes of treatment [83].

In Spain, in 2011 an Adolescents with Cancer Committee was established within Pediatric Haemato-oncology. Patients over 14 years are likely to be treated in adult oncology wards [84]. The charity AAA—'Spanish Association of Adolescents and Young Adult with Cancer' (www.aaacancer.org) is now raising awareness and maintains a community of patients including youth activities (www.adolescentesyjovenesconcancer.com/).

In Denmark, an AYA nurse-initiated project beginning in 2000 in Aarhus University Hospital [49] has been followed by developments in Copenhagen. The excellent complete and multi-faceted cancer registry data in Scandinavia and focussed researchers working within it have recently produced excellent epidemiological data about AYA-specific cancer survivorship outcomes and patient pathways [4, 5]. Policy is being considered by the Danish Cancer Society.

In other countries, across northern and western Europe (e.g., Belgium, Sweden, Norway), South Eastern Europe (Rumania, Bulgaria,) the Mediterranean (Greece, Slovenia) and central Europe (Lithuania, Poland, Czech Republic) there is no current national coordinated clinical project to improve outcomes for AYA with cancer, although there are some individual projects. For example leukaemia trials in Lithuania are now open collaboratively between adult and pediatric groups.

3.3.2 USA

An alliance between service users and the not-for-profit sector has picked up the gauntlet thrown down in unison by the poor outcomes described in; the Adolescent and Young Adult Oncology Progress Review Group report of 2006 [71, 85], and by the U.S. National Cancer Institute (NCI) monograph including survival data up to 2000 [86]. Work in AYA services has been in rapid evolution in the USA since then [87]. This has delivered biological [3] and psycho-social research programmes in AYA cancer [88, 89]. Meanwhile, embedding a collaboration between pediatric and adult oncology is central to the work of Teen Cancer America in identifying 10 partner centres, and is also central in work to provide certification of AYA Centres of Excellence, as long as those include clinical and multi-dimensional supportive care, research programmes and meet quality standards [90–92]. Improvements in outcomes are being seen in some but not all parts of the AYA field [93].

There is on-going work, with the organisation 'Critical Mass' linking academic, clinical, administrative and service user stakeholders. This includes work to identify and improve the extent to which AYA patients are referred to specialist AYA centres [94], are meeting the recommendations as to the quality of care [91], are working with not-for-profit organisations, are choosing optimal treatments [15], and are providing supportive care to manage the psychological, medical, financial and geographical needs of Americans aged 15–39 living with and after cancer [18]. These and other priorities are laid out as explicit priorities for on-going work in the field [95]. On-going concerns about access to care have remained, while challenges of under-insurance remain prevalent in young people [96, 97], with perhaps some moderation of that in some recent years in many states, notably through the Affordable Care Act and most significant for those aged under 26.

There is optimism that trial recruitment may be enhanced by collaborative working at the level of the hospital between pediatric and adult teams, and by the NCI Community Oncology Research Program [98, 99]. An influential change has been the restructuring of the US cooperative clinical trial groups to form the NCI Clinical Trials Network. This encourages (with administrative and financial incentives and collaborative trial design) hospitals with research infrastructure to enrol AYAs onto any suitable trials that may have originated in either pediatric or adult cooperative groups [100, 101]. This has either led to is or supporting the development of new trials as a result of collaborations across what were once adult and pediatric silos [102].

3.3.3 Canada

The response to the AYA disparities in care and outcomes in Canada has been led since 2008 by their Task Force on AYA with Cancer, working with the national Canadian Partnership against Cancer. Updates in 2011 and 2013 illustrated some distinct national priorities, such as their early recognition of palliative care issues, the need to consider 'virtual' specialist care (online), and their emphasis upon training future AYA leaders specifically in their leadership skills [103 105]. Extending col laboration and securing the necessary resources are challenging, as elsewhere [77].

Some of these challenges are pragmatically being addressed by international collaborations in research and clinical datasets [20, 106, 107]. Innovative and progressive individual programs within the overall national picture are pushing forward the boundaries in this field, with an increasing emphasis upon services that meet patient's needs after their cancer treatment [108, 109].

3.3.4 Australia

Across Australia, led nationally by the Youth Cancer Services team, each state has at least one specialist unit for AYA, aged 12–24 inclusive, living with cancer (http://youthcancer.com.au/Youth-Cancer-Services.aspx, accessed August 2016). They also include, within their policy, support for a young person with a parent, brother or sister, either having cancer or who has died from cancer. This initiative has been supported by two rounds of national governmental support, for management and care, as a result of inclusion in national policy since 2008. That support has been obtained, the centres are networked and the staff are trained with the support of the Canteen not-for-profit national service user support organisation (https://www.**canteen**.org.au/). Youth cancer Services were set up with young cancer patients at their heart in 2005 and are informed by four pragmatic advisory groups; strategy, research, data and involvement of young people.

Australia—idea of promoting centralisation of specialist care. The Australian model has focussed upon developing multidisciplinary AYA cancer teams, who are based in the Cancer Services in large regional hospitals but work with conventional oncology services.

Specific issues of particular interest in Australia include their use of telemedicine, specific needs of their indigenous young cancer population, their integration of health care professionals training alongside those treating AYA with other illnesses, and recently a focus upon psychological assessment and management of distress in AYA [110].

3.3.5 Elsewhere

Initiatives in this area are also underway in Morocco, India and China, although facing even greater challenges of resource and some very distinct challenges of public health culture [111].

Conclusions

Improving AYA cancer management requires us to bridge the interfaces that act to oppose excellence in care. Service designs should also do this, in the context of the specific local challenges, to create services with a specified age range, geographical coverage and skill-mix to diagnose promptly and provide excellent care in all domains. Professionals need to be accredited to show they are developing these skills and attitudes as well as their specific knowledge. The study and development of AYA services can reveal tensions, as differing approaches to the care and management of similar patients become apparent. This can be energising, decelerating, or frankly destructive depending upon the relationships that have been built.

This requires champions for these services, professionals and the public, to promote supportive relationships between existing clinical groups, built upon a supportive health service policy. Supranational groups such as ASCO, SIOPE and ESMO are continuing the process by constructive collaboration after the trailblazers led the way, and regional and national policy followed [112, 113].

Different European project have joined forces and aims in the European Network for Teenagers and Young Adults with Cancer (ENTYAC). ENTYAC was born as an offshoot of the European Network for Cancer in Children and Adolescents (ENCCA), a network of research institutes activated from 2011 to 2015 within the European Seventh Framework Programme for Research FP7. At the end of ENCCA in 2015, the ENCCA work package dedicated to "Improving

Outcomes for Teenagers and Young Adults with Cancer" evolved in the ENTYAC. The latter has become a nascent federation of the European national groups [19]. Evaluation of the models of care that exist are on-going [38, 88, 106] and for several data will be available in 2017–18, further informing the pragmatic design of high-quality, patient-centred and equitable services for AYA with cancer.

References

1. Dommett RM, et al. Features of cancer in teenagers and young adults in primary care: a population-based nested case-control study. Br J Cancer. 2013;108(11):2329–33.
2. Ferrari A, et al. The sooner the better? How symptom interval correlates with outcome in children and adolescents with solid tumors: regression tree analysis of the findings of a prospective study. Pediatr Blood Cancer. 2016;63(3):479–85.
3. Tricoli JV, et al. Biologic and clinical characteristics of adolescent and young adult cancers: acute lymphoblastic leukemia, colorectal cancer, breast cancer, melanoma, and sarcoma. Cancer. 2016;122(7):1017–28.
4. Rugbjerg K, et al. Cardiovascular disease in survivors of adolescent and young adult cancer: a Danish cohort study, 1943–2009. J Natl Cancer Inst. 2014;106(6):dju110.
5. Rugbjerg K, Olsen JH. Long-term risk of hospitalization for somatic diseases in survivors of adolescent or young adult cancer. JAMA Oncol. 2016;2(2):193–200.
6. Woodward E, et al. Late effects in survivors of teenage and young adult cancer: does age matter? Ann Oncol. 2011;22(12):2561–8.
7. Morgan S, et al. Sex, drugs, and rock 'n' roll: caring for adolescents and young adults with cancer. J Clin Oncol. 2010;28(32):4825–30.
8. World Health Organisation. Adolescent development. 2015. http://www.who.int/maternal_child_adolescent/topics/adolescence/dev/en/.
9. Arnett JJ. Emerging adulthood. A theory of development from the late teens through the twenties. Am Psychol. 2000;55(5):469–80.
10. Viner RM, et al. Life course epidemiology: recognising the importance of adolescence. J Epidemiol Community Health. 2015;69(8):719–20.
11. Whitaker KJ, et al. Adolescence is associated with genomically patterned consolidation of the hubs of the human brain connectome. Proc Natl Acad Sci USA. 2016;113(32):9105–10.
12. Erikson EH. Identity: youth and crisis. New York: Norton; 1968.
13. Abrams AN, Hazen EP, Penson RT. Psychosocial issues in adolescents with cancer. Cancer Treat Rev. 2007;33(7):622–30.
14. Barr RD, Holowaty EJ, Birch JM. Classification schemes for tumors diagnosed in adolescents and young adults. Cancer. 2006;106(7):1425–30.
15. Potosky AL, et al. Use of appropriate initial treatment among adolescents and young adults with cancer. J Natl Cancer Inst. 2014;106(11):dju300.
16. Leonard RC, et al. Strategy needed for adolescent patients with cancer. BMJ. 1995;311(7001):387.
17. Lewis IJ. Cancer in adolescence. Br Med Bull. 1996;52(4):887–97.
18. Nass SJ, et al. Identifying and addressing the needs of adolescents and young adults with cancer: summary of an Institute of Medicine workshop. Oncologist. 2015;20(2):186–95.
19. Stark D, et al. Teenagers and young adults with cancer in Europe: from national programmes to a European integrated coordinated project. Eur J Cancer Care (Engl). 2016;25(3):419–27.
20. Barr RD, et al. Cancer in adolescents and young adults: a narrative review of the current status and a view of the future. JAMA Pediatr. 2016;170(5):495–501.
21. Veal GJ, Hartford CM, Stewart CF. Clinical pharmacology in the adolescent oncology patient. J Clin Oncol. 2010;28(32):4790–9.

22. Gramatges MM, Rabin KR. The adolescent and young adult with cancer: state of the art—acute leukemias. Curr Oncol Rep. 2013;15(4):317–24.
23. Vriens MR, et al. Clinical and molecular features of papillary thyroid cancer in adolescents and young adults. Cancer. 2011;117(2):259–67.
24. Casanova M, et al. A prospective protocol for nasopharyngeal carcinoma in children and adolescents: the Italian Rare Tumors in Pediatric Age (TREP) project. Cancer. 2012;118(10):2718–25.
25. Daniotti M, et al. Cutaneous melanoma in childhood and adolescence shows frequent loss of INK4A and gain of KIT. J Invest Dermatol. 2009;129(7):1759–68.
26. Chan JK, et al. Ovarian cancer in younger vs older women: a population-based analysis. Br J Cancer. 2006;95(10):1314–20.
27. Tricoli JV, et al. Unique characteristics of adolescent and young adult acute lymphoblastic leukemia, breast cancer, and colon cancer. J Natl Cancer Inst. 2011;103(8):628–35.
28. Collinson K, et al. Age-related biological features of germ cell tumors. Genes Chromosomes Cancer. 2014;53(3):215–27.
29. Kohsaka S, et al. A recurrent neomorphic mutation in MYOD1 defines a clinically aggressive subset of embryonal rhabdomyosarcoma associated with PI3K-AKT pathway mutations. Nat Genet. 2014;46(6):595–600.
30. Kent EE, et al. Talking about cancer and meeting peer survivors: social information needs of adolescents and young adults diagnosed with cancer. J Adolesc Young Adult Oncol. 2013;2(2):44–52.
31. Hollis R, Morgan S. The adolescent with cancer—at the edge of no-man's land. Lancet Oncol. 2001;2(1):43–8.
32. Kelly D, Pearce S, Mulhall A. 'Being in the same boat': ethnographic insights into an adolescent cancer unit. Int J Nurs Stud. 2004;41(8):847–57.
33. Stark D, Lewis I. Improving outcomes for teenagers and young adults (TYA) with cancer. Klin Padiatr. 2013;225(6):331–4.
34. Clic-Sargent. A long way from home - the impact of travel on children and young people with cancer. London; 2010. p. 24.
35. Carr R, et al. Young adult cancer services in the UK: the journey to a national network. Clin Med. 2013;13(3):258–62.
36. NICE(UK). Improving outcomes in children and young people with cancer. Cancer service guidance: London; 2005.
37. Taylor RM, et al. Development and validation of the BRIGHTLIGHT Survey, a patient-reported experience measure for young people with cancer. Health Qual Life Outcomes. 2015;13(1):107.
38. Whelan J, Barber J, Feltbower R, Fern L, Gibson F, Hooker L, Lerner M, Millington H, Moran A, Morris S, O'Hara C, Pearce S, Raine R, Stark D, Taylor R. Do specialised services for TYA with cancer add value? London: NIHR (UK); 2012.
39. Wolfson J, et al. Impact of treatment site in adolescents and young adults with central nervous system tumors. J Natl Cancer Inst. 2014;106(8):dju166.
40. Coad J. Teenage Cancer Trust North West Pilot Evaluation. 2015. http://www.coventry.ac.uk/research/research-directories/current-projects/2015/teenage-cancer-trust-north-west-pilot-evaluation/.
41. Jones LJ, Pini SA, Morgan SJ, Birk GK, Stark DP. How Do Teenagers and Young Adults with Cancer Experience Their Care? A European Survey. J Adolesc Young Adult Oncol. 2017;6(1):102–10. https://doi.org/10.1089/jayao.2016.0011. Epub 2016 Jun 17. PMID:27314907.
42. Bleyer WA, et al. American Cancer Society Workshop on Adolescents and Young Adults with Cancer. Workgroup #1: long-term care and lifetime follow-up. Cancer. 1993;71(7):2413.
43. Statistics, O.f.N. Large increase in 20 to 34-year-olds living with parents since 1996. 2014. http://www.ons.gov.uk/ons/rel/family-demography/young-adults-living-with-parents/2013/sty-young-adults.html.
44. Iacovou M. Leaving home: independence, togetherness and income in Europe. New York: United Nations, Department of Economic and Social Affairs; 2011.
45. Michelagnoli MP, Pritchard J, Phillips MB. Adolescent oncology—a homeland for the "lost tribe". Eur J Cancer. 2003;39(18):2571–2.

46. Stark D, et al. Survival patterns in teenagers and young adults with cancer in the United Kingdom: comparisons with younger and older age groups. Eur J Cancer. 2015;51(17): 2643–54.
47. Smith S. Adolescent units-an evidence-based approach to quality nursing in adolescent care. Eur J Oncol Nurs. 2004;8(1):20–9.
48. Marris S, Morgan S, Stark D. 'Listening to Patients': what is the value of age-appropriate care to teenagers and young adults with cancer? Eur J Cancer Care (Engl). 2011;20(2):145–51.
49. Olsen PR, Harder I. Caring for teenagers and young adults with cancer: a grounded theory study of network-focused nursing. Eur J Oncol Nurs. 2011;15(2):152–9.
50. Perales MA, et al. Social media and the adolescent and young adult (AYA) patient with cancer. Curr Hematol Malig Rep. 2016;11(6):449–55.
51. Albritton K, Bleyer WA. The management of cancer in the older adolescent. Eur J Cancer. 2003;39(18):2584–99.
52. Ferrari A, et al. Starting an adolescent and young adult program: some success stories and some obstacles to overcome. J Clin Oncol. 2010;28(32):4850–7.
53. Bleyer A. The Quid Pro Quo of pediatric versus adult services for older adolescent cancer patients. Pediatr Blood Cancer. 2010;54(2):238–41.
54. Whiteson M. The Teenage Cancer Trust—advocating a model for teenage cancer services. Eur J Cancer. 2003;39(18):2688–93.
55. Ferrari A, Trama A, De Paoli A, Bergeron C, Merks JHM, Jenney M, Orbach D, Chisholm JC, Gallego S, Glosli H, De Salvo GL, Botta L, Gatta G, Bisogno G; RARECAREnet Working Group. Access to clinical trials for adolescents with soft tissue sarcomas: Enrollment in European pediatric Soft tissue sarcoma Study Group (EpSSG) protocols. Pediatr Blood Cancer. 2017;64(6). https://doi.org/10.1002/pbc.26348. Epub 2016 Nov 24.
56. Goyal S, et al. Symptom interval in young people with bone cancer. Eur J Cancer. 2004;40(15):2280–6.
57. Martin S, et al. Delays in cancer diagnosis in underinsured young adults and older adolescents. Oncologist. 2007;12(7):816–24.
58. Desandes E, et al. Pathways of care for adolescent patients with cancer in France from 2006 to 2007. Pediatr Blood Cancer. 2012;58(6):924–9.
59. Veneroni L, et al. Symptom interval in pediatric patients with solid tumors: adolescents are at greater risk of late diagnosis. Pediatr Blood Cancer. 2013;60(4):605–10.
60. Fern LA, et al. Why can't we improve the timeliness of cancer diagnosis in children, teenagers, and young adults? BMJ. 2013;347:f6493.
61. Lyratzopoulos G, et al. Variation in number of general practitioner consultations before hospital referral for cancer: findings from the 2010 National Cancer Patient Experience Survey in England. Lancet Oncol. 2012;13(4):353–65.
62. Ahrensberg JM, Fenger-Gron M, Vedsted P. Primary care use before cancer diagnosis in adolescents and young adults—a Nationwide Register Study. PLoS One. 2016;11(5):e0155933.
63. Forbes LJ, et al. Differences in cancer awareness and beliefs between Australia, Canada, Denmark, Norway, Sweden and the UK (the International Cancer Benchmarking Partnership): do they contribute to differences in cancer survival? Br J Cancer. 2013;108(2):292–300.
64. Magni C, et al. Adolescents' health awareness and understanding of cancer and tumor prevention: when and why an adolescent decides to consult a physician. Pediatr Blood Cancer. 2016;63(8):1357–61. https://doi.org/10.1002/pbc.25985.
65. Magni C, et al. "There's no reason why": a campaign to raise cancer awareness among adolescents. Tumori. 2016;2016(3):270–5. https://doi.org/10.5301/tj.5000493.
66. Rose PW, et al. Explaining variation in cancer survival between 11 jurisdictions in the International Cancer Benchmarking Partnership: a primary care vignette survey. BMJ Open. 2015;5(5):e007212.
67. Jensen H, et al. Diagnostic intervals before and after implementation of cancer patient pathways - a GP survey and registry based comparison of three cohorts of cancer patients. BMC Cancer. 2015;15:308.

68. Ingeman ML, et al. The Danish cancer pathway for patients with serious non-specific symptoms and signs of cancer-a cross-sectional study of patient characteristics and cancer probability. BMC Cancer. 2015;15:421.
69. Larsen MB, et al. Secondary care intervals before and after the introduction of urgent referral guidelines for suspected cancer in Denmark: a comparative before-after study. BMC Health Serv Res. 2013;13:348.
70. Committee LFR. Livestrong young adult alliance implementation plan. Austin: Livestrong; 2014.
71. Livestrong. Closing the gap: a strategic plan. Austin: Livestrong; 2007.
72. Fern LA, Stark DP, Phillips B, Morgan S, Azzim A, Gibson F. Benchmarking teenage and young adult cancer professional developments across Europe: A Delphi Survey. In European cancer congress. Amsterdam; 2013.
73. Smith S. In: Case L, editor. A blueprint of care for teenagers and young adults with cancer. London, UK: Teenage Cancer Trust; 2013.
74. GMC (UK). Curriculum for specialty training in medical oncology. 2010. http://www.gmc-uk.org/Medical_Oncology_curriculum_2010.pdf_32731045.pdf.
75. Hayes-Lattin B, Mathews-Bradshaw B, Siegel S. Adolescent and young adult oncology training for health professionals: a position statement. J Clin Oncol. 2010;28(32):4858–61.
76. Ercan O, et al. Demography of adolescent health care delivery and training in Europe. Eur J Pediatr. 2009;168(4):417–26.
77. Ramphal R, et al. Practices and resources devoted to the care of adolescents and young adults with cancer in canada: a survey of pediatric and adult cancer treatment centers. J Adolesc Young Adult Oncol. 2011;1(3):140–4.
78. Bernig T, et al. Treatment of adolescents and young adults (AYA) with cancer in a multidisciplinary setting: on the way to a highly specialized AYA unit. Klin Padiatr. 2013;225(6):335–8.
79. Ferrari A, et al. Adolescents with cancer in Italy: entry into the national cooperative paediatric oncology group AIEOP trials. Eur J Cancer. 2009;45(3):328–34.
80. Ferrari A. The challenge of access to care for adolescents with cancer In Italy: national and local pediatric oncology programs. J Adolesc Young Adult Oncol. 2013;2(3):112–7.
81. Ferrari A. SIAMO: Italian pediatric oncologists and adult medical oncologists join forces for adolescents with cancer. Pediatr Hematol Oncol. 2014;31(6):574–5.
82. Ferrari A, et al. Adolescents with cancer in Italy: improving access to national cooperative pediatric oncology group (AIEOP) centers. Pediatr Blood Cancer. 2016;63(6):1116–9.
83. Aben KK, et al. Cancer in adolescents and young adults (15-29 years): a population-based study in the Netherlands 1989-2009. Acta Oncol. 2012;51(7):922–33.
84. Lassaletta A, Andión M, Garrido-Colino C. The current situation of adolescents with cancer in pediatric hematology-oncology units in Spain. Results of a national survey. An Pediatr (Barc). 2013;78(4):268.e1–7.
85. Bleyer A. The adolescent and young adult gap in cancer care and outcome. Curr Probl Pediatr Adolesc Health Care. 2005;35(5):182–217.
86. Bleyer A, O'Leary M, Barr R, LAG R. Cancer epidemiology in older adolescents and young adults 15 to 29 years of age, including SEER incidence and survival, 1975–2000. Bethesda: National Cancer Institute; 2006.
87. Johnson RH. AYA in the USA. International perspectives on AYAO, part 5. J Adolesc Young Adult Oncol. 2013;2(4):167–74.
88. Smith AW, et al. Health-related quality of life of adolescent and young adult patients with cancer in the United States: the Adolescent and Young Adult Health Outcomes and Patient Experience study. J Clin Oncol. 2013;31(17):2136–45.
89. Mathews-Bradshaw B, et al. The history and accomplishments of the livestrong young adult alliance. J Adolesc Young Adult Oncol. 2011;1(1):43–7.
90. Zebrack B, Mathews-Bradshaw B, Siegel S. Quality cancer care for adolescents and young adults: a position statement. J Clin Oncol. 2010;28(32):4862–7.
91. Reed D, Block RG, Johnson R. Creating an adolescent and young adult cancer program: lessons learned from pediatric and adult oncology practice bases. J Natl Compr Canc Netw. 2014;12(10):1409–15.

92. Teen Cancer America. State of the nation. 2016. https://www.teencanceramerica.org/state-of-the-nation-our-hospital-partners/.
93. Keegan TH, et al. Comparison of cancer survival trends in the United States of adolescents and young adults with those in children and older adults. Cancer. 2016;122(7):1009–16.
94. Parsons HM, et al. Who treats adolescents and young adults with cancer? A report from the AYA HOPE Study. J Adolesc Young Adult Oncol. 2015;4(3):141–50.
95. Smith, A.W., et al., Next steps for adolescent and young adult oncology workshop: an update on progress and recommendations for the future. Cancer, 2016.
96. Parsons HM, et al. Young and uninsured: Insurance patterns of recently diagnosed adolescent and young adult cancer survivors in the AYA HOPE study. Cancer. 2014;120(15):2352–60.
97. Parsons HM, et al. Clinical trial participation and time to treatment among adolescents and young adults with cancer: does age at diagnosis or insurance make a difference? J Clin Oncol. 2011;29(30):4045–53.
98. Roth ME, et al. Low enrollment of adolescents and young adults onto cancer trials: insights from the community clinical oncology program. J Oncol Pract. 2016;12(4):e388–95.
99. Shaw PH, et al. Improved clinical trial enrollment in adolescent and young adult (AYA) oncology patients after the establishment of an AYA oncology program uniting pediatric and medical oncology divisions. Cancer. 2012;118(14):3614–7.
100. Weiss AR, Nichols CR, Freyer DR. Enhancing adolescent and young adult oncology research within the national clinical trials network: rationale, progress, and emerging strategies. Semin Oncol. 2015;42(5):740–7.
101. Freyer DR, Felgenhauer J, Perentesis J. Children's Oncology Group's 2013 blueprint for research: adolescent and young adult oncology. Pediatr Blood Cancer. 2013;60(6):1055–8.
102. Olson TA, et al. Pediatric and adolescent extracranial germ cell tumors: the road to collaboration. J Clin Oncol. 2015;33(27):3018–28.
103. Fernandez C, et al. Principles and recommendations for the provision of healthcare in canada to adolescent and young adult-aged cancer patients and survivors. J Adolesc Young Adult Oncol. 2011;1(1):53–9.
104. Rogers PC, et al. A process for change in the care of adolescents and young adults with cancer in canada. "Moving to action": the Second Canadian International Workshop. International perspectives on AYAO, part 1. J Adolesc Young Adult Oncol. 2013;2(2):72–6.
105. Ramphal R, et al. Active therapy and models of care for adolescents and young adults with cancer. Cancer. 2011;117(10 Suppl):2316–22.
106. Baxter NN, et al. The initiative to maximize progress in adolescent and young adult cancer therapy (IMPACT) cohort study: a population-based cohort of young Canadians with cancer. BMC Cancer. 2014;14:805.
107. White V, et al. The Australian-Canadian adolescent and young adult collaborative cohort initiative: initial meeting report. J Adolesc Young Adult Oncol. 2016,6(1):1–5.
108. Gupta AA, et al. Reimagining care for adolescent and young adult cancer programs: moving with the times. Cancer. 2016;122(7):1038–46.
109. Xu Y, et al. Quantifying treatment delays in adolescents and young adults with cancer at McGill University. Curr Oncol. 2015;22(6):e470–7.
110. Palmer S, Patterson P, Thompson K. A national approach to improving adolescent and young adult (AYA) oncology psychosocial care: the development of AYA-specific psychosocial assessment and care tools. Palliat Support Care. 2014;12(3):183–8.
111. Magrath I, Epelman S. Cancer in adolescents and young adults in countries with limited resources. Curr Oncol Rep. 2013;15(4):332–46.
112. ESMO. European Society for Medical Oncology. 2013. http://www.esmo.org/About-Us/Who-We-Are/Educational-Committee/Educational-Committee-Major-Achievements.
113. SIOP-E. SIOP-E Strategic plan 2015-2020. 2015. http://www.siope.eu/2015/10/05/3505/.

4 Psychological Support and Social Care

Lucy Holland and Kate Thompson

4.1 Introduction

A cancer diagnosis and its treatment during the AYA years is highly challenging, with the timing of this significant health crisis coinciding with critical transformations of growth and development [1–5]. For young people experiencing cancer during these formative years, disruption to the normal developmental trajectory can have significant impacts on physical growth, fertility and body image; identity, self-esteem, mental health and distress; family, peer and partner relationships; school and career plans; life perspectives and future prospects for adulthood [6–12]. These impacts overlie the threat to prospective life lived and known survival detriments experienced for young people diagnosed with particular cancer types [13–15]. They are also accompanied by significant impacts for parents, siblings, partners and peers.

Recognition of the unique impacts experienced by young people and their families has seen growing appreciation of the need for health services to deliver care that is orientated to the developmental needs of young people. This is a concept referred to as 'youth friendly,' 'youth responsive' or 'quality youth' healthcare [5, 6, 8–12, 16]. Such care is founded on the recognition that health services and healthcare professionals have a responsibility to understand and support young people's development and emerging capacity for self-management, in the face of challenges to health and wellbeing [16–18]. The premise of youth friendly cancer care is a founding principle underlying the provision of psychological support and social care for young people living with cancer.

L. Holland
The University of Newcastle, University Drive, Callaghan, Newcastle, NSW, Australia

K. Thompson (✉)
Victorian Adolescent and Young Adult Cancer Service, Peter MacCallum Cancer Centre, Melbourne, VIC, Australia
e-mail: Kate.Thompson@petermac.org

J. Chisholm et al. (eds.), *A Practical Approach to the Care of Adolescents and Young Adults with Cancer*, https://doi.org/10.1007/978-3-319-66173-5_4

This chapter will begin with an overview of the unique developmental and psychosocial impacts experienced by young people. It will define what is meant by psychological support and social care, before addressing the foundations of practice required to deliver youth friendly cancer care including those related to: practice philosophy; engagement; communication; consent, capacity and confidentiality; psychosocial assessment; the environment and culturally safe practice. It will conclude by addressing the key domains of psychological and social care including: psychological support; relationships; education and vocation; finances; practical considerations; existential and spiritual care; self-management; health promotion and transitions in care.

4.2 Impact of a Cancer Diagnosis and Treatment During the AYA Years

4.2.1 AYA Development

A thorough understanding of the rapid change that occurs across physical, neurobiological, cognitive, psychological, social and existential domains is essential to understand the unique complexities that young people with cancer experience compared to children and older adults. Youth specific care encompasses the appreciation that processes of development are not linear and understands that there is huge heterogeneity in the rate and progress of development for each individual, across each domain. This will be evident in practice, where you may encounter a 19-year-old patient who is financially autonomous, living independently and is married or has limited emotional reliance on their parents. This young person may well receive care alongside a 23-year-old patient who is immature, whether economically, in terms of cognitive maturity or independence. It is essential to understand these trajectories and the corresponding impacts of cancer to ensure that young people are assessed individually and supported appropriately, on the basis of developmental stage, not just age and according to the nature of the health crisis they are experiencing and the associated psychological and social impacts.

4.2.1.1 Physical Development

The physical transformations that occur during adolescence and young adulthood are significant and result from complex hormonal change. The onset of puberty sees a period of rapid physical growth and physiological change that typically occurs at age 10–11 for females and at age 11–12 for males. Puberty is usually complete by age 15–17 for females and by age 16–17 for males [19, 20]. This pubertal change culminates in sexual maturity which is defined as the achievement of fertility and the development of secondary sexual characteristics, including body hair and voice changes [21, 22]. This change is accompanied by an increase in sexual desire and arousal [22]. Complete physical maturation is marked by the attainment of an adult balance of hormonal functioning, completed physical growth, the attainment of fertility and the development of adult body image and physical sense of self.

4.2.1.2 Neurobiological and Cognitive Development

Over recent decades, our understanding of adolescent behaviour has significantly increased through research that explains processes of neurobiological and cognitive development that occur during the AYA years. Within the brain, the striatal regions develop first in early adolescence. These are crucial for detecting and learning about novel and rewarding cues in the environment and determining positive affect. They are therefore also responsible for a heightened propensity for sensation seeking and risk taking during the adolescent years [23]. The prefrontal cortex undergoes later development, with full maturation occurring during the mid-20s [23, 24]. This is responsible for higher order executive functions including the ability to comprehend and interpret information; analyse situations logically in terms of cause and effect; consider options and hypothetical or abstract consequences; consider present and future implications; inhibit behaviour; plan for the future and set personal goals [21, 23]. As a result, in early adolescence, the response to reward and novel stimuli is heightened, influencing risk taking and sensation seeking behaviour. In parallel, the pre-frontal cortex is still maturing which means that young people lack adult capacity to consistently enact higher order cognitive functions, especially in the context of heightened responses to social, physical or neurobiological reward. This does not mean that young people are completely unable to make informed decisions, plan or inhibit behaviour. Rather, their ability to enact these functions consistently, especially in light of a situation that may offer a significant reward, is yet to mature [23].

4.2.1.3 Psychological Development

Psychological development involves the search for personal identity and independence including determining self-concept, needs, values and beliefs and understanding one's place in the world [21]. During the rapid growth that characterises the AYA years, young people experience a range of new emotions and their coping strategies evolve in response. Emotional maturation involves recognizing and managing emotional responses, developing empathy, learning to resolve conflict constructively, the ability to cooperate and the development of self-esteem [21, 25, 26]. However, adolescence is also now recognised as a time of significant risk for the onset of mental ill-health both within Australia and globally [27, 28]. Within Australia, mental health problems account for the highest burden of disease among young people [28]. In addition, 75% of all mental health issues present before the age of 25 years; adolescents experience higher than average rates of suicide compared to adult counterparts and; mental health and substance use disorders account for at least 50–70% of the burden of disease among 15–24 year olds [28–30]. However, only 1 in 4 young people experiencing mental ill-health receives professional help [28] and young people are known to not access services for mental ill-health as often as other age groups [28]. The trajectory of psychological development for young people today can therefore be complicated and compromised by mental ill-health and a lack of appropriate support.

4.2.1.4 Social Development

Throughout development, young people traverse significant social and role changes. They navigate the transition from familial independence to autonomy and interdependence, characterised by an increased focus on peer relationships [25, 31]. Peer groups serve a number of important functions throughout adolescence, providing a reference point for developing identity and the evolution of moral judgment and values [32]. This time is also characterised by the development of romantic relationships, increased sexual activity and the development of sexual identity [33]. Social development is attained with the development of mature relationships with peers of both sexes, the adoption of social roles and achievement of socially responsible behaviour.

4.2.1.5 Education and Vocation

Education and work provide essential contexts to promote: skill development, self-confidence, developing identity, peer relationships and access to social activities. For some, it may also provide a source of safety and stability and access to reliable adults, clear boundaries and models of secure attachment [34, 35]. School participation, undergraduate study and vocational success are required to ensure economic success, solidify the young person's sense of self and contribution to the world [36, 37]. Education and vocation are typically high priorities for young people who experience evolving education, vocation and financial goals during the AYA years.

4.2.1.6 Existential Development

It is only with the combined influence of developing cognitive capabilities, psychological development, the search for identity and increased exposure to the lives of their peers, that young people become capable of existential exploration [38, 39]. It is this exploration that incorporates notions of isolation, morality, love, alienation, and taking responsibility for decision-making, which often raises questions about the meaning of life [40]. Although not universal, this process often involves the determination of religious or spiritual beliefs [38]. This search for meaning can be accompanied by feelings of confusion and vulnerability as young people look for answers to the big questions such as why things exist, why events occur and addressing the issues of mortality [41].

4.2.2 Social Influences

Young people today are the most successful generation to date. Globally, they have the greatest life expectancy, access to more resources than generations before and more economic and social opportunity [42]. The characteristics of the community in which an adolescent lives have profound impacts on development. These include factors such as demography and socioeconomic characteristics, the types of resources available, the service systems within the community and media access

[43]. Media and technology continue to play an increasing role in the lives of young people who are, on average, estimated to be exposed to some form of media for 6–8 h per day [3, 20, 44]. The increase in access to media and information has the potential for both positive and negative impacts on development, depending on the information and content involved and the young person's use of the medium [44]. Cultural and ethnic influences are particularly integral to understanding processes of development for each young person [45], with strong ethnic identity identified as contributing to high self-esteem among adolescents [43]. Specific cultural differences must be considered when assessing the developmental progress and needs of a young person particularly in relation to differences between family or community oriented cultures and those which prioritise independence and individualism [21].

4.2.3 Known Impacts of Cancer and Treatment During the AYA Years

The impacts of a cancer diagnosis and its treatment during the AYA years differ to those experienced during other life stages as they coincide with critical transformations of growth and development. It is because of this, that young people both respond differently to cancer and are impacted by it in ways that children and adults are not [3]. While often framed in the negative, it is important to understand that this experience can also have positive impacts and provide opportunities for healthy growth and the development of life skills and perspectives [46]. It is essential to remember the significant impacts experienced by parents, siblings, partners and peers [1]. Known impacts of a cancer diagnosis and its treatment during the AYA years include:

- Physical impacts including: pain; discomfort; nausea; fatigue; hair loss; hearing and visual changes; amputation and scaring; lung and cardiac dysfunction, organ dysfunction; hormonal imbalance; impacts to fertility and infertility; sexual dysfunction and increased risk of second malignancy
- Cognitive dysfunction including: altered visual and auditory function; impacts to special orientation, language and information processing; impaired concentration and increased confusion; impaired executive functions including memory dysfunction and behavioural or emotional changes
- Psychological and mental ill-health including: depression, anxiety and post-traumatic stress disorder, hopelessness, survivor guilt and anxiety associated with fear of recurrence. Positive and negative impacts to identity, body image and self-esteem may also occur
- Positive and negative changes to relationships with parents, siblings, peers, partners and children including disrupted plans for marriage and starting a family
- Disruption to education. Positive and negative changes to educational goals
- Disruption to vocation. Positive and negative changes to vocational goals

- Financial insecurity, changed financial state and challenges associated with insurance
- Impacts to economic and social contribution
- Impacts to self-efficacy and lowered sense of control over health and life in general
- Impacts to existential value systems, religion and faith
- Improved health competence, self-efficacy and self-advocacy skills
- Psychological, social, educational, vocational, financial and existential impacts for parents, siblings, partners and peers.

(Adapted from [47])

4.3 Defining Psychological Support and Social Care

Psychological support and social care are key concepts in the provision of youth friendly cancer care and must be embedded alongside medical care to promote the best health and quality of life outcomes for both young people and their families [5, 48]. Often used interchangeably with psychosocial support or psychosocial care, these terms are broadly defined to include the provision of strategies, resources and aids (including education, resources, information, emotional support and psychological support) to relieve suffering, promote mental health and wellbeing and to help a person cope with stress [49–51]. The provision of such care should be considered a team endeavour. While psychological support and social care are clearly the domains of psychologists and social workers, it is now widely recognised that psychosocial care is provided in a variety of ways, by all members of multidisciplinary teams, including those from medicine, nursing, psychology, social work, teaching and primary care. Working together in the provision of this care and to the strengths of each professional is essential to provide consistent, holistic care that best meets the needs of young people and their families. It is also essential to include the social network of the young person or client within the team of support [52]. In the end, these people remain as the young person's community of support when the cancer experience is over.

4.4 Practice Foundations

Several practice foundations underpin the provision of youth friendly psychological support and social care. Informed by literature, practice experience and the preferences of young people, these include: a developmentally specific philosophy of practice; engagement; communication; consent, confidentiality and capacity; developmentally appropriate psychosocial screening and assessment; the environment and culturally safe practice. These can be implemented regardless of the young person's unique characteristics or experience, the context of care, the stage of the cancer journey and resources available. They are essential foundations to the provision of youth friendly care that promotes partnership between the healthcare team and the young person and supports the young person's engagement in their care.

4.4.1 Practice Philosophy

Youth friendly cancer care requires a philosophy which is founded in understanding the unique value and contribution of young people, the life stage and development which characterises the AYA years and the interaction between ill-heath and development [16, 52, 53]. This philosophy should be embedded within professional practice and service and systems policy. It should:

- Recognise the unique value and contribution of young people to our present and future world
- Understand processes and trajectories of adolescent development
- Aim to maximise the health of young people
- Aim to support the development of young people and associated skills and capabilities, including self-management capabilities, using a strengths based approach
- Be both patient centred, working with where the young person is in terms of development and their health experience, and family centred, recognising that young people's social networks are the foundation of their social world and that health experiences during the AYA years impact all involved in these networks
- Involve a partnership approach to work with young people and the provision of care
- Be based on a framework of meaningful youth participation
- Provide care that is accessible, acceptable, equitable, appropriate and effective.

(Adapted from [16])

4.4.2 Engagement

Good engagement involves building rapport and trust and the establishment of a clearly defined, safe, professional relationship. This relationship is built upon mutual understanding and allows for honesty from the young person about their motivations, the barriers they perceive, changing needs and the choices they wish to make. The level of engagement determines how beneficial the relationship is between the healthcare professional and the young person throughout the care process, how well you may get to know the young person and the level of support and care that can be provided [54].

Developing good engagement with young people takes time and consistency. While adults often present to healthcare services with a willingness to engage, due to prior experience, knowledge of the healthcare system and expectations of the professional nature of the relationship, this is not always the case for young people [55, 56]. It is important to recognise that every contact with the young person, however minor, is an opportunity to begin to form and build engagement. While the following skills are useful in forming engagement with young people, good engagement fundamentally relies on an understanding of AYA development and behaviour, the ability to communicate in an open and non-judgemental way and a genuine desire to understand what is happening for the young person [56]. Skills that are recognised to assist in developing good engagement with young people are outlined in Table 4.1.

Table 4.1 Youth friendly engagement

Engagement tool	Description
The AYA client	Recognising the young person as the client empowers them in the context of the cancer experience. This is fostered through making contact with or communicating with the young person directly and encouraging their contribution and participation
Roles and expectations	Clarifying roles and expectations of the relationships at the outset alleviates anxiety associated with uncertainty and promotes a sense of trust and safety. This may involve explicit discussion about roles and experience, how the health system works, clarifying expectations and discussing confidentiality and its limits
Engender control	Engendering a sense of control is important to empower young people and fosters skills development development. This is supported through establishing clear boundaries, recognising the expertise of the young person in terms of their life, taking their perspectives and concerns seriously, promoting autonomous decision making and being willing to negotiate
Time alone	Having time alone with young people is preferable to provide opportunity for the disclosure of concerns, fears and relevant histories without the presence of family or others that young people may want to protect. This is best negotiated at the outset
Holistic perspective	Viewing and treating the young person as a whole person, within the context of their family and social life, education and vocational context, likes, dislikes and their motivations, preferences and goals, fosters engagement
Allow time	Additional time benefits engagement and allows for appropriate information provision and processing, promotes comprehension and facilitates a thorough assessment of capacity and need
Self-awareness and professional integrity	Professional awareness of assumptions, comfort levels in work with young people, strengths and limitations is essential for honest engagement and promotes confidence. Consistency and professional integrity, particularly in relation to following through on commitments made, are key to maintain trust of the young person
Advocacy	Adolescent oncology is an emerging field. Professionals may not be used to working with young people and services and systems may not best support AYA development. Young people may also present with needs that have not been disclosed or addressed before. Acting as an AYA advocate fosters trust, engagement and embodies the principles of youth friendly care

4.4.3 Communication

Healthcare professionals often cite a lack of confidence in communicating effectively with young people. They also report difficulties understanding particular characteristics of AYA communication including limited eye contact, minimal verbal responses and perceived negative body language [40, 54]. The goal of effective communication in AYA healthcare is to engage young people in a mutually beneficial process that maximises positive development, supports participation and informed decision making and allows for the identification and achievement of goals [54, 56–58]. To achieve this, communication must be age appropriate, relevant and involve a two way process which is individualised to meet the needs of the young person [59]. Truth telling is a cornerstone of effective communication in AYA care.

Effective youth specific communication skills can be considered to sit within a triad of youth friendly philosophy, the manner of the clinician and actions taken. Adopting a strengths-based approach, treating young people with respect, recognising them as the experts in the context of their lives, taking them seriously and demonstrating equity are some of the key philosophical requirements of effective communication [40, 54, 56]. It is also imperative that an engaged, professional, non-judgemental approach is used and that the communication process is cooperative, rather than competitive [40, 54, 56, 60]. Youth friendly communication tips are outlined in Table 4.2.

Table 4.2 Youth friendly communication

Youth friendly communication tips
• Take adequate time. Allow time for information processing, questions and repeat information as required. Key information may also need to be spaced out and delivered over several meetings or sessions
• Be clear, direct and honest. Use simple, clear language and avoid jargon
• Engage in active listening to both what is said and unsaid
• Use open ended questions and ask frequent questions to clarify your understanding and that of the young person
• Frequently summarise and paraphrase
• Use multiple modes of communication and information provision (written, visual, online etc.)
• Avoid misinterpreting silence or putting words in the mouth of the young person
• Maintain eye contact, open body language and demonstrate interest through non-verbal cues
• Ensure congruence between verbal and non-verbal communication and between different information methods and modes utilised
• Be prepared for, and respond appropriately to, complex emotions, content and initial disclosures. This may include responding to anger, anxiety, distress, depression and embarrassing or disturbing content. This may necessitate training in youth friendly communication and a team based approach

4.4.4 Capacity, Consent and Confidentiality

AYA capacity, consent and confidentiality are essential foundations to the provision of youth friendly cancer care. They also promote engagement through establishing clear parameters around care provision [61, 62].

4.4.4.1 Capacity

Globally, the right of legal minors to make decisions about their healthcare, when it is deemed that they have the capacity to do so, has been legally recognised in some countries. Capacity is the ability to comprehend information, consider probabilities and assess long-term advantages and disadvantages. It is the process used to come to a decision [63, 64]. There is little to indicate that young people are any less capable of making informed decisions than adult counterparts when provided with age-appropriate information and care [65–67]. Capacity requires the demonstration of comprehensive understanding of all information presented, all alternative options, all possible outcomes and the potential short term and long term consequences of each decision [2, 64, 65]. This can be assessed by presenting information in a developmentally appropriate way, at an appropriate rate, then asking questions about understanding, for a reflection of information presented and for examples [64]. Capacity should be determined on an individual basis. While these tools assist the clinician in the assessment of AYA capacity, it should be noted that this does not constitute a thorough, cognitive psychology assessment of capacity. If there is any doubt in relation to the capacity of the young person, a referral for a cognitive psychology capacity assessment should be made.

4.4.4.2 Consent

Consenting a young person to their participation is empowering and fosters engagement [68]. Ideally, young people should be consented to the following, even if in addition to parents or carers: service engagement/involvement; psychosocial assessment; treatment and care; disclosure of information and; on-referral. The ability to consent requires capacity including full understanding of the processes involved and associated requirements and outcomes.

4.4.4.3 Confidentiality

Confidentiality is an essential component of youth friendly cancer care [69]. Confidentiality means that what is discussed with the young person in the clinical context is not repeated to others, unless there is significant risk identified or it is deemed beneficial to care provision and there is express permission granted by the young person [56, 70]. In order to provide confidential, youth friendly care, it is important to understand and operate according to professional mandatory requirements, duty of care, legal responsibilities and organisational processes for reporting risk. Confidentiality and its limits should be discussed and understood at the outset to ensure clear boundaries relating to the clinical relationship with the young person and to alleviate any concerns of family members relating to confidentiality between the young person, family and healthcare professional [20, 71]. The three main limits to confidentiality are when the young person is:

- At risk of harming or killing themselves
- At risk of harming someone else or committing a serious offence, or
- Being threatened or harmed (e.g. physical, sexual or other abuse) by someone else.

4.4.5 Psychosocial Screening and Assessment

The lives of young people are complex. In order for healthcare professionals to best support AYA clients throughout their cancer experience, they must understand the whole life of the young person including their: developmental stage; strengths and stressors; goals; resources; past experiences and motivations [52, 54, 69]. For this reason regular psychosocial screening and assessment is essential component to the provision of youth friendly cancer care [1, 72]. Adopting a preventative approach enables treating teams to: identify young people at risk of a negative psychosocial outcomes; monitor their progressive coping; identify areas of need requiring additional care and support and identify factors that can promote compliance. Commonly reported risk and resilience factors, identified in many Western countries are presented in Table 4.3.

Age based screening tools and assessment measures are crucial to the provision of youth friendly cancer care [69]. Whilst international efforts are underway to develop an AYA cancer specific distress screening tool (e.g. [73–75]), the HEADSS

Table 4.3 Risk and resilience factors

Domain	Resilience factors	Risk factors
Individual	Good health and mental health	Ill health and mental ill-health
	Strong moral values	Lack clear moral values
	High self-esteem	Low self esteem
	Robust intelligence	Low intelligence
	Creative pursuits	Hyperactivity
	Sporting pursuits	Refugee experience
Family	Intact family	Family breakdown
	Effective parenting	Poor parenting
	No parental psychopathology	Parental psychopathology
	Positive relationships	Risk taking behaviour in family home
	Family rituals	Low socio economic status
Peers and school	Positive peer relationships	Bullying
	Low risk taking behaviour	High risk taking behaviour
	Achievement	Low or poor achievement
	Engagement	Isolation
	Parental interest in education	Low parental interest in education
Community	High employment	Lack of employment
	Culture of cooperation	Poor community cohesion
	Contribution to community	Racial discrimination
	Low availability of drugs and alcohol	Availability of drugs and alcohol

Assessment [76, 77] remains the foremost psychosocial assessment measure used in adolescent health and medicine and has been adapted internationally to improve its relevance for the AYA cancer population [35, 68]. The areas explored through the HEADSS assessment include: home environment, education and employment, activities, drugs and alcohol use, sexuality, suicidality, depression, anxiety and mental health. Administration of psychosocial assessments will typically fall under the domain of trained psychologists, social workers or nurses. When conducting a psychosocial assessment the following process and practice points are key:

- Establish good engagement to ensure that the young person is comfortable to be asked questions about their life
- Explain the purpose of the assessment so that the rationale for question asking is clear to all parties. This fosters the trust of the young person and professional confidence
- Ensure confidentiality and its limits have been discussed and are understood
- Employ principles of youth friendly communication to ensure that the young person understands what is being asked of them and why and is comfortable to disclose information
- Allow sufficient time. Work at the pace of the young person and be conscious that the assessment may need to be paused if information or emotional overload occurs. The assessment may require more than one session
- Have a low threshold for collaboration and on-referral. While mood variations, apathy, disturbed sleep, altered eating, drug use and anxiety are commonly taken as normal adolescent behaviour, these are often indicators of mental ill-health or significant risk. Any areas that appear to pose a significant risk to the young person or others, or to which the professional feels unable to adequately respond, should trigger discussions about referrals for psychological support or social care. This may involve on-referral to an external agency.

4.4.6 The Environment and Workplace Culture

Young people who present to adult or paediatric healthcare settings often feel alienated [56]. Youth friendly environments have been found to promote engagement, create a sense of comfort and safety for the young person and provide an opportunity for young people to meet others in a similar situation, build friendships and share mechanisms to cope with their disease [52, 78–81]. Young people prefer private consultation spaces in settings that are less clinical, have limited association with medical procedures and contain age appropriate media and magazines, art, music, activities and access to the Internet where possible [2, 35, 78, 82–85]. It is also recommended that services establish a culture that makes young people feel comfortable. This goes beyond the physical environment to include considerations about: work attire; modes of communication; information formats and availability; extended and flexible appointment times and booking systems [2, 82, 84, 85].

4.4.7 Culturally Safe Practice

Attention should be paid to the cultural context, identity and needs of any young person and their family or social network, regardless of where they live or where they present for care. While developmental stage is a clear factor in determining developmentally appropriate care, culture is equally important. Healthcare providers must recognise the cultural beliefs, values, language needs and norms relevant to each young person and their family to ensure the provision of appropriate psychological support and social care [50]. These needs should be considered in consultation with the young person and family and appropriate responses determined accordingly.

4.5 Domains of Psychological Support and Social Care

The psychological and social wellbeing of young people diagnosed with cancer should be a priority across the cancer journey, from diagnosis throughout treatment and into post treatment survivorship or end of life care [48, 52]. Now that the foundations to youth friendly psychological support and social care have been discussed, a practical approach to psychological support and social care will be provided. The Sect. 4.6 will discuss: good mental health, coping and adjustment; distress and mental ill-health and; psychological support interventions. The Sect. 4.7 will discuss: relationships; education and vocation; finances; practical considerations; existential and spiritual care; self-management; health promotion and; transitions in care.

4.6 Psychological Support

Maintaining psychological wellbeing and avoiding the onset of psychological ill-health is imperative to promote the best outcomes and quality of life for young people with cancer. While the majority of all age cancer patients experience normal psychological functioning, living through a cancer diagnosis, treatment and its myriad of significant impacts, facing mortality and fear of cancer recurrence create significant stressors that can result in new psychological distress or mental ill-health problems or, can worsen pre-existing conditions [8, 86–88]. It is also known that young people diagnosed with cancer are at higher risk of experiencing distress and poor psychological outcomes compared to older patients and their healthy peers, as they navigate the cross roads of illness and development [8, 86–90]. When coupled with the known increased risk of mental ill-health in the healthy AYA population, the importance of understanding and providing developmentally appropriate psychological support for his patient cohort is evident [87]. The ultimate aim of such support is to enable proactive identification of distress and the factors that contribute to distress, unmet need psychological mal-adjustment and mental ill-health, to enable the provision of appropriate support to promote adjustment, coping, wellbeing, quality of life and the attainment of typical developmental milestones.

4.6.1 Mental Health, Coping and Adjustment

Mental health is defined by the WHO [91] as "a state of wellbeing in which every individual realises his or her own potential, can cope with the normal stresses of life, can work productively and fruitfully and is able to make a contribution to her or his community". This definition falls within the WHO [91] definition of health that considers complete physical, mental and social wellbeing. Coping is understood to reflect the processes by which one manages stress and stressors that pose a threat to mental health or are overwhelming [49]. Adjustment is understood to be the outcome experienced by people in response to stressors and coping strategies applied. Positive coping strategies, known to promote positive adjustment and good mental health outcomes are known to include active coping strategies, seeking help and professional support, family and social support, exercise and health promotion and acceptance [46]. Negative coping strategies, known to promote mal-adjustment and worse mental health outcomes include risk taking behaviour, drug and alcohol use, avoidant coping strategies [46]. These concepts are key, to understand the goal of psychological support for young people facing a diagnosis of cancer and its treatment. They also provide a framework for discussion of a practical approach to the provision of such care that aims to promote positive adjustment, the development of positive coping strategies and mental health and wellbeing.

4.6.2 Distress and Mental Ill-Health

Distress and mental ill-health in young people can manifest as diagnosable conditions including distress, depression and anxiety or post-traumatic stress disorder. However, they can also manifest as less described episodes of: sadness or worry; anger or frustration; uncertainty about the future; adjustment difficulties; communication problems; decision making difficulties or; challenges managing daily life [8, 86–88, 92–94]. Increasing research is now illustrating the emergence of a new particular form of anxiety associated with fear of cancer recurrence for survivors of cancer [95]. Among individuals with cancer, symptoms of mental ill-health are common, although prevalence rates vary widely across studies and by patient age, diagnosis, social and demographic variables and across the cancer trajectory [88, 96]. Additionally, there is complexity inherent to the overlap between side effects of cancer and its treatment and symptoms of mental ill-health, including insomnia and sleep disturbance; anhedonia; fatigue; appetite change and difficulties with concentration [96]. This creates challenges in terms of the consistent measurement of distress and mental ill-health prevalence in the AYA oncology population. For example, rates of clinically significant distress in AYA patients have been reported as being present for between 12% to over 85% of patients [8, 46, 86–88, 90, 94, 95]. Rates of depression in cancer patients generally are reported to be between 1 in 2 and 1 in 4 [86]. These rates are likely to be higher among AYAs who are known to be at greater risk of mental ill-health due to age and life-stage [86]. Recent studies identify that between one third and one half of AYA patients have clinically significant post-traumatic stress symptomatology [8, 97] and over one third report moderate to severe symptoms of anxiety and depression [8]. Rates of fear of cancer recurrence have also been found to be higher in the AYA population compared to older patients with recent estimates place fear of cancer experienced by over 82% of AYA survivors [95]. Despite exact figures, rates of distress and mental ill-health among young people diagnosed with cancer are significant. Tailored interventions are therefore required to best support young people through the cancer journey and ensure best psychological outcomes, wellbeing and quality of life.

4.6.3 Psychological Support in Practice

The availability of evidence based psychological interventions in AYA oncology remains very limited [10]. Broadly speaking, interventions that are either known to be effective in the psychological support of young people, or those known to be effective in oncology, are applied to psychological support within the AYA oncology population. At the outset, the use of age-appropriate screening tools and assessment measures are crucial to the identification of distress, unmet need and mental ill-health. They are also crucial to understand the associated aetiology and severity and enable the formation of relevant, responsive care [72, 98]. However, it must be recognised that such tools are not diagnostic tools. Therefore, referral to a mental health professional should be made for appropriate diagnosis, using an appropriate classification and diagnostic tool such as the DSM-IV. Appropriate interventions are required if risk factors for distress or mental ill-health are identified or there are concerns about the mental health and wellbeing of a young person. In identifying and responding to distress in young people, the following practice points apply:

- Adopt a preventative approach involving psychosocial screening, assessment and care planning at diagnosis and throughout the cancer journey; particularly at points of major transition or crisis including: in the event of a new major life stressor; with changes to treatment; with changed prognosis; at the end of treatment; into post treatment survivorship and at end of life.
- Provide age appropriate information and support. These are discussed in more detail below but may include services provided within the treating team or those which necessitate on-referral to a mental health professional. The interventions applied may be provided face to face or with the use of technology. They may include:
  - Psycho-education about physical and mental health and strategies to promote good health and wellbeing
  - Individual, couple or family emotional support, counselling or psychological support which may include:

    Mindfulness
    Relaxation and stress management
    Cognitive Behavioural Therapy (CBT)
    Acceptance and Commitment Therapy (ACT)
    Supportive-Expressive Therapy

- Psychiatric support
- Pharmacological intervention through a General Practitioner or psychiatrist
- Additional interventions including:

  Practical support
  Peer or social support
  Exercise interventions
  Music therapy
  Acupuncture

4.7 Social Care

4.7.1 Relationships

Family, peers, partners and significant others all play a part in supporting a young patient throughout their cancer experience. Promoting wellbeing within these existing relationships and support networks is essential alongside building new connections with other AYAs, siblings or parents living with cancer.

4.7.1.1 Family Relationships

The AYA years see young people working to separate themselves from parents and carers and become increasingly independent and autonomous. However, a cancer diagnosis and its treatment often results in an increased reliance on family for care and support [99]. For young people who may have previously left the family home, many will be forced to return for a period of time, if not for the entirety of treatment. Throughout the cancer journey, young people and families are exposed to many illness-specific stressors. The way in which the young person copes with these stressors will have a direct impact on the coping of the family and their adjustment to the cancer experience [100]. Similarly, the way in which the family copes with these stressors will have a direct impact on the coping of the young person [100]. For this reason, the role, needs and coping of parents and carers are of prime importance to promote good psychological and social outcomes for all. It is therefore essential that healthcare professionals work within both a patient-centred and family centred model of care and have a comprehensive understanding of family functioning, coping styles, risk factors and resources available to both the young person and their family [93]. Specific areas of information need and support for parents and carers relate to: supporting the young person throughout the cancer journey; understanding the impact of the cancer, its treatment and side effects; mental health and wellbeing; distress management; relationship management, particularly relating to managing intimate relationships, marriages and the needs of other offspring; managing at home and changes to family routines, relationships and daily living; education and work; housing and accommodation; financial assistance; peer support; bereavement support and; self-care [101, 102]. Social care for families can be achieved through: regular family assessments; the provision of honest, accurate, clear information; psycho-education; linking in parents or carers with emotional or psychological support, practical and financial assistance and peer support.

4.7.1.2 Siblings

There is a growing appreciation of the impacts of an AYA cancer diagnosis on siblings [103]. These effects can be complex for the healthy sibling as the focus of parents and the healthcare team are strongly focused on the support and treatment needs of the unwell brother or sister [104]. Siblings report a number of changes to the family unit including reduction in parental time and attention; changes to roles and responsibilities; decreased sense of security; restricted communication; loss of normalcy and predictability [50, 105]. As a result they may experience a range of complex emotions including anger, guilt, resentment, fear, isolation distress and anxiety. This can place siblings at increased risk of social, emotional and behavioural problems as they themselves are often navigating the processes of adolescent development. Social care for siblings can be provided at both individual and family levels. The benefits of peer support programs; access to age appropriate and accurate medical information, communicated at regular intervals and; family orientated programs aimed at facilitating family interactions have all been identified as improving sibling's psychological adjustment [106]. Regular screening and assessment of sibling need and engaging appropriate emotional and psychological support are also of value. School psychologists and welfare coordinators are particularly good resources for providing support to school-aged siblings.

4.7.1.3 Peers

Peer relationships and social networks are central to the world of the developing young person and yet these can be significantly compromised following a cancer diagnosis. Without appropriate support, young people are at risk of peer rejection and social isolation as social groups continue to evolve while they are absent due to illness and hospitalisation [53, 98]. For some young people, a cancer diagnosis and its treatment will have a negative impact upon peer relationships and links with friends can be lost. This can occur for a range of reasons including: friends feeling overwhelmed by the cancer experience and unsure how to offer help; friends getting on with life; the young person with cancer feeling different from previously close friends; or feeling part of the sick world and loss of confidence. Supporting the young person to manage important peer relationships is critical to healthy development [39, 53]. This can be done by: encouraging peer interactions as an inpatient; making the ward environment a welcoming place to visit; providing an appropriate place for young people to gather; keeping young people connected to their peers through technology based interventions and providing information for peers that will alleviate their concerns. Providing information about how to tell friends about cancer and how to manage the response of others is also essential to support the maintenance of peer relationships during treatment and to support the young person in managing changed relationships [53].

4.7.1.4 Intimate Relationships

Cancer and its treatment have the potential to significantly interrupt romantic relationships and the psychosexual development of a young person. It is during this life stage that young people are gaining independence from their parents and forming intimate relationships with romantic partners [107]. While for some young people in relationships, they may be in newly formed, immature partnerships that are still evolving their foundations, others may be married or in secure long-term partnerships. It is imperative when providing social care to young people to work within the context of their social network, however this is defined. If a young person is in a romantic relationship, the needs of their partner must therefore be taken into account. This can provide challenges for healthcare professionals at times when the needs of the young person, their family, peers and partners all factor into the model of care. Providing regular opportunities for the young person and their partner to discuss any questions or concerns relating to the cancer diagnosis and treatment, fertility, intimacy and sexual wellbeing is imperative. Social care for partners must also involve a developmental approach to nest support this young person's development in the context of their cancer experience. This care may include: information provision; psycho-education; counselling, emotional or psychological support; practical assistance and advocacy. For young people not in relationships, the focus should be on encouraging the development of healthy relationships and maximise their potential benefits whilst equipping them with the skills and support to recognise and deal with the challenges that they might bring.

4.7.2 Practical Considerations

A cancer diagnosis can impact practically on life in many ways. The practical concerns associated with a cancer diagnosis and its treatment can cause significant worry and stress to young people and their families [47, 98, 108]. To support treatment engagement, a young person will ideally feel safe; have a safe and secure home environment, an appropriate mode of transport to travel to and from treatment and financial security including the ability to pay for the costs associated with both daily living and care [108]. These costs include the direct costs associated with cancer and its treatment (e.g. medication, high cost drugs, hospitalisations), treatment related out of pocket expenses (e.g. travel, accommodation, childcare, car parking, food) and indirect costs (e.g. the loss of income with young people or their parents either having to leave work for a period of time or negotiate a reduction in working hours) [47]. To promote the ability of the young person to engage in treatment and to enable them to cognitively, emotionally and psychologically process the cancer experience; the practical needs of young people often need to be met first [39]. The identification of practical need necessitates regular psychosocial screening and assessment. Social care for practical needs may be provided through: information provision; assisting with access to government and social security benefits; financial assistance; travel and accommodation reimbursement schemes and assistance; legal advice and referral. This care may come from within the treating team or facility or from not-for-profit organisations and community agencies.

4.7.3 Education and Vocation

Education and employment are important determinants of future health and quality of life for all young people. A diagnosis of cancer and its subsequent treatment have the potential to profoundly disrupt education and employment through interrupting physical participation, affecting cognitive maturation and functioning, inhibiting autonomy and independence and disturbing social connections with peers [34, 36, 109–111]. Education attainment is a significant predictor of future employment for cancer survivors and is key as survivors of adolescent cancer are known to be at greater risk of future unemployment [110, 112]. Healthcare professionals have been shown to play a significant role in supporting a young person's continued connection to their education following a cancer diagnosis [113]. Understanding a young person's educational goals and aspirations and working in collaboration with schools can assist in the development of individualised learning plans and support both the young person's health and engagement in the school environment [34, 53, 109]. For older AYA patients who are attending, or making the transition to college, university or other higher education institutions, assisting them to identify a key contact within the educational setting can facilitate proactive support and discussions regarding an appropriate and supportive educational pathway, the management of treatment requirements and side effects and future opportunities and goals. For those young people already engaged in the workforce, many will be employed in insecure part time or casual positions. They are likely to have limited sick and annual leave entitlements and limited flexibility in relation to work [108]. These young people may require support to liaise with employers to explore flexible working conditions and advocacy to ensure the young person, where possible, remains a valued, participating member of their workplace. Providing information regarding employment rights and responsibilities, including leave entitlements and access to social security support, is also key for young people, education institutions and workplaces alike [53].

4.7.4 Existential and Spiritual

The AYA life stage is a time of existential and spiritual growth. It is during this time in life that young people begin to question the meaning of life. This search for meaning involves grappling with notions of isolation, morality, love, alienation, morality and self-responsibility [114–116]. A cancer diagnosis can trigger existential crises and questioning that may affect how the young person makes sense of, and copes with, their cancer journey [38, 117]. Treating teams must be mindful of the existential and spiritual needs of young people and provide them with the opportunity to explore these within the context of a trusting and appropriate relationship. This may involve allowing the space and opportunity for young people to ask and explore existential questions or referral to specific religious or spiritual support through chaplaincy, spiritual or pastoral care services [38, 116].

4.7.5 Transitions in Care

Young people will experience transitions in their care across the cancer continuum, including: between care providers; from the paediatric to adult sector or; from the acute to community healthcare environment. For others, transition will be defined as the experience of moving from active therapy into follow up care and survivorship or moving from curative treatment to palliative intent treatment or to end of life care [69, 118–124]. Every point of transition presents differing psychological and social care needs for both young people and those around them. To promote positive transitions in care, it is crucial to ensure effective communication between care providers and with young people and their families. Ideally, transition between different services should occur at a time of medical stability and be discussed well ahead of the transition occurring. It is also crucial to employ ongoing psychosocial assessments, at key time points of transition or change, to identify the evolving needs of the young person and their families and enable the provision of appropriate information, support and resources to promote positive coping and ensure ongoing adjustment and wellbeing.

Conclusion

This chapter has emphasised that effective psychological and social support to young people requires an understanding of the breadth and intensity of development during this time in life and identification of the particular issues that set this population apart from children and older adults. Addressing these particular issues within a developmental approach has the potential to buffer the many negative consequences of a cancer diagnosis, build skills, capabilities and resilience that will assist young people to successfully traverse the road to adulthood and beyond.

References

1. National Institute for Health and Clinical Excellence, Guidance on Cancer Services: Improving Outcomes in Children and Young People with Cancer. The manual. London: National Institute for Health and Clinical Excellence (NICE); 2005.
2. Abrams AN, Hazen EP, Penson RT. Psychosocial issues in adolescents with cancer. Cancer Treat Rev. 2007;33(7):622–30.
3. Docherty SL, et al. The adolescent and young adult with cancer: a developmental life course perspective. Semin Oncol Nurs. 2015;31(3):186–96.
4. Harvey N, Finch A. Supportive care of adolescents and young adults during cancer treatment. In: Kelly D, Gibson F, editors. Cancer care for adolescents and young adults. Victoria: Blackwell Publishing; 2008.
5. Sawyer SM, et al. Fulfilling the vision of youth friendly cancer care: a study protocol. J Adolesc Young Adult Oncol. 2016;5(3):267–77.
6. Bolte S, Zebrack BJ. Sexual issues in special populations: adolescents and young adults. Semin Oncol Nurs. 2006;24(2):5.3.

7. Carpentier MY, et al. Prevalence of multiple health related behaviors in adolescents with cancer. J Pediatr Hematol Oncol. 2008;30(12):902–7.
8. McCarthy MC, et al. Psychological distress and posttraumatic stress symptoms in adolescents and young adults with cancer and their parents. J Adolesc Young Adult Oncol. 2016;5(4):322–9.
9. Murnane A, et al. Adolescents and young adult cancer survivors: exercise habits, quality of life and physical activity preferences. Support Care Cancer. 2015;23(2):501–10.
10. Seitz DC, Besier T, Goldbeck L. Psychosocial interventions for adolescent cancer patients: a systematic review of the literature. Psychooncology. 2009;18(7):683–90.
11. Shnorhavorian M, et al. Fertility preservation knowledge, counselling, and actions among adolescent and young adult patients with cancer: a Population-Based Study. Cancer. 2015;121(19):3499–506.
12. Zebrack BJ. Information and service needs for young adult cancer survivors. Support Care Cancer. 2009;17(4):349–57.
13. Barr RD. Common cancers in adolescents. Cancer Treat Rev. 2007;33(7):597–602.
14. Bleyer A, et al. The distinctive biology of cancer in adolescents and young adults. Nat Rev Cancer. 2008;8(4):288–98.
15. Australian Institute of Health and Welfare, Cancer in adolescents and young adults in Australia. Cancer series no. 62. 2011, Canberra: AIHW.
16. World Health Organisation. Adolescent friendly health services: an agenda for change. Geneva: World Health Organization; 2002.
17. Sawyer S, Aroni RA. Self-management in adolescents with chronic illness: what does it mean and how can it be achieved? Med J Aust. 2005;138(8):405–9.
18. Sawyer S, et al. Adolescents with a chronic condition: challenges living, challenges treating. Lancet. 2007;369(9571):1481–9.
19. Hofmann AD, Greydanus DE. Adolescent medicine. Stamford: Appleton & Lange; 1997.
20. Sawyer SM, et al. Adolescence: a foundation for future health. Lancet. 2012;6736(12):1630–40.
21. American Psychological Association. Developing adolescents: a reference for professionals. Washington, DC: American Psychological Association; 2002.
22. Patton G, Viner R. Pubertal transitions in health. Lancet. 2007;369(9567):1130–9.
23. Casey BJ, Jones RM. Neurobiology of the adolescent brain and behaviour. J Am Acad Child Adolesc Psychatry. 2010;49(12):1189–285.
24. Johnson SB, Blum RW, Giedd JN. Adolescent maturity and the brain: the promise and pitfalls of neuroscience research in adolescent health policy. J Adolesc Health. 2009;45(3):216–21.
25. Erikson EH. Identity: Youth and Crisis. New York: Norton; 1968.
26. Harter S. Self and identity development. In: Feldman SS, Elliot GR, editors. At the threshold: the developing adolescent. Cambridge: Harvard University Press; 1990.
27. Green H, et al. Mental health of children and young people in the Great Britain 2004. Norwich: Palgrave Macmillan; 2005.
28. Australian Institute of Health and Welfare. Young Australians: their Health and Wellbeing. Canberra: AIHW; 2011.
29. Department of Health and Aging. The Mental Health of Australians 2: report on the 2007 National Survey of Mental Health and Wellbeing. Canberra: Department of Health and Ageing; 2009.
30. Institute for Health Metrics and Evaluation. Global Burden of Disease Study: results by cause 1990–2010—country level. Seattle: Institute for Health Metrics and Evaluation (IHME); 2010.
31. Robinson E. Young people and their parents: supporting families through changes that occur in adolescence, In AFRC Briefing No.1. Melbourne: Australian Family Relations Clearinghouse, Australian Institute of Family Studies; 2006.
32. Gardener M, Steinberg L. Peer influence on risk-taking, risk preference and risky decision-making in adolescence and adulthood: an experimental study. Dev Psychol. 2005;41(1):625–35.

33. Micucci JA. The adolescent in family therapy: breaking the cycle of conflict and control. New York: Guilford; 1998.
34. Gravestock H, McDowell K, Mazzini M. No teenager with cancer left out, the impact on young peoples' secondary education. London: CLIC Sargent—Cancer Support for the Young; 2013.
35. Palmer S. Improving care for AYA patients treated within adult hospitals: what can be done right now? Cancer Forum. 2009;33(1):22–5.
36. Donnan BM, et al. What about school? Educational challenges for children and adolescents with cancer. Aust Educ Dev Psychol. 2015;23(32):23–40.
37. Perry CL. Preadolescent and adolescent influences on health. In: Smedley BD, Syme LS, editors. Promoting health: intervention strategies from social and behavioral research. Washington, DC: National Academy Press; 2000.
38. McNeil SB. Spirituality in adolescents and young adults with cancer: a review of the literature. J Paediatr Oncol Nurs. 2016;33(1):55–63.
39. Zebrack B, Isaacson S. Psychosocial care of adolescent and young adult patients with cancer and survivors. J Clin Oncol. 2012;30(11):1221–6.
40. Arnett JJ. Suffering, selfish, slackers? Myths and reality about emerging adults. J Youth Adolesc. 2007;36(1):23–9.
41. Piaget J. Intellectual evolution from adolescence to adulthood. In: Learner R, Jovanovic J, editors. Cognitive and moral development and academic achievement in adolescence. New York: Garland Publishing, Inc.; 1999.
42. World Health Organisation. The health of young people: a challenge and a promise. Geneva: World Health Organisation (WHO); 1993.
43. Carlson C, Uppal S, Prosser EC. Ethnic differences in processes contributing to the self-esteem of early adolescent girls. J Early Adolesc. 2000;20(1):44–68.
44. Roberts DM. Media and youth: access, exposure, and privatization. J Adolesc Health. 2000;27(Suppl):8–14.
45. Bennett DL, Chown P, Kang MS. Cultural diversity in adolescent health care. Med J Aust. 2005;183(8):436–8.
46. Turner-Sack AM, et al. Posttraumatic growth, coping strategies and psychological distress in adolescent survivors of cancer. Pediatric Oncol Nurs. 2012;29(2):70–9.
47. Bellizzi KM, et al. Positive and negative psychosocial impact of being diagnosed with cancer as an adolescent or young adult. Cancer. 2012;118(20):5155–62.
48. Osborn M, et al. Youth cancer services in Australia: development and implementation. International perspectives on AYAO, Part 3. J Adolesc Young Adult Oncol. 2012;2(3):1–8.
49. American Psychological Association. Glossary of psychological terms. 2016.
50. Cancer Australia. National service delivery framework for adolescents and young adults with cancer. Canberra: Commonwealth of Australia; 2008.
51. National Cancer Institute. NCI dictionary of cancer terms: psychosocial. 2012. https://www.cancer.gov/publications/dictionaries/cancer-terms?cdrid=648685.
52. Fernandez C, et al. Principles and recommendations for the provision of healthcare in Canada to adolescent and young adult–aged cancer patients and survivors. J Adolesc Young Adult Oncol. 2011;1(1):6.
53. Clinical Oncology Society of Australia. Psychosocial management of AYAs diagnosed with cancer: Guidance for health professionals. 2014.
54. Sacks D, Westwood M. An approach to interviewing adolescents. Paediatr Child Health. 2003;8(9):554–6.
55. Health, C.F.A. Clinical practice guideline: engaging with the adolescent patient. 2012.
56. Robinson E, Miller R. Adolescents and their families: best interests case practice model and specialist practice resource. Melbourne: The Victorian Government Department of Human Services; 2012.
57. Duncan R, Young MA. Tricky teens: are they really tricky or do genetic health professionals simply require more training in adolescent health? Pers Med. 2013;10(6):589–600.

58. Zebrack B, Chesler MA, Kaplan S. To foster healing among adolescents and young adults with cancer: what helps? What hurts? Support Care Cancer. 2010;18(1):131–5.
59. Coupey SM. Interviewing adolescents. Pediatr Clin North Am. 1997;44(6):1349–64.
60. Eccles JS, et al. Development during adolescence: the impact of stage-environment fit on young adolescents' experiences in schools and in families. Am Psychol. 1993;48(1):90–101.
61. English A, Ford C. More evidence supports the needs to protect confidentiality in adolescent healthcare. J Adolesc Health. 2007;40(1):199–200.
62. English A, et al. Health care reform for adolescents—an agenda for the lifespan: a position paper of the Society for Adolescent Medicine. J Adolesc Health. 2009;6(1):1–6.
63. Appelbaum PS, Grisso T. Assessing patients' capacity to consent to treatment. N Engl J Med. 1998;319(1):1635–8.
64. Bellhouse J, et al. Decision-making capacity in adults: its assessment in clinical practice. Adv Psychiatr Treat. 2001;7(1):294–301.
65. Royal Australian College of Physicians. Routine adolescent health psychosocial assessment - position statement. Sydney: Royal Australian College of Physicians (RACP); 2008.
66. Kuther TL. Medical decision-making and minors: issues of consent and assent. Adolescence. 2003;38(150):343–58.
67. Shaw M. Competence and consent to treatment in children and adolescents. Adv Psychiatr Treat. 2001;7(2):150–9.
68. Palmer S, Thomas DA. A practice framework for working with 15–25 year-old cancer patients treated within the adult health sector. Melbourne: ONTrac@PeterMac Victorian Adolescent & Young Adult Cancer Service; 2008.
69. Yeo MS, Sawyer SM. Psychosocial assessment for adolescents and young adults with cancer. Cancer Forum. 2009;33(1)
70. Ford C, English A, Sigman G. Confidential healthcare for adolescents: position paper for the society of adolescent medicine. J Adolesc Health. 2004;35(1):1–8.
71. Sasse RA, et al. Confidential consultations with adolescents: an exploration of Australian parents' perspectives. J Adolesc Health. 2013;52(6):786–91.
72. Palmer S, Patterson P, Thompson K. A national approach to improving adolescent and young adult (AYA) oncology psychosocial care: the development of AYA-specific psychosocial assessment and care tools. Palliat Support Care. 2014;12(3):183–8.
73. CanTeen Australia. Adolescent and young adult oncology psychosocial care manual. Sydney: sCanTeen Australia; 2011.
74. Parker A, Hetrick S, Percell R. Psychosocial assessment of young people: refining and evaluating a youth friendly assessment interview. Aust Fam Physician. 2010;39(8).585–8.
75. Recklitis CJ, Blackmon JE, Chang G. Screening young adult cancer survivors for distress with the distress thermometer: comparisons with a structured clinical diagnostic interview. Cancer. 2016;122(2):296–303.
76. Goldenring J, Cohen E. Getting into adolescents heads. Contemp Pediatr. 1988;5(1):75–90.
77. Goldenring J, Rosen D. Getting into adolescents heads: an essential update. Contemp Pediatr. 2004;21(1):64–90.
78. Hollis R, Morgan S. The adolescent with cancer—at the edge of no-man's land. Lancet Oncol. 2001;2(1):43–8.
79. Hutton A. Consumer perspectives in adolescent ward design. J Clin Nurs. 2005;15(5):537–45.
80. Morgan S, et al. Sex, drugs, and rock 'n' roll: caring for adolescents and young adults with cancer. J Clin Oncol. 2010;28(32):4825–30.
81. Sturrock T, Steinbeck K. Adolescents and youth in adult hospitals: psychosocial assessment n admission—an evaluation of the youth care plan. Aust J Adv Nurs. 2011;31(1):28–35.
82. D'Agostino NM, Penney A, Zebrack B. Providing developmentally appropriate psychosocial care to adolescent and young adult cancer survivors. Cancer. 2011;117(Supp 10):2329–34.
83. Kang M, et al. Better practice in youth health. In: SW Centre for the Advancement of Adolescent Health, The Children's Hospital at Westmead, in association with the Department of General Practice. Sydney: The University of Sydney at Westmead Hospital; 2005.

84. Kyngäs H. Patient education: perspective of adolescents with a chronic disease. J Clin Nurs. 2003;15(5):744–51.
85. Mulhall A, Kell D, Pearce A. Qualitative evaluation of an adolescent cancer unit. Eur J Cancer Care. 2004;13(1):16–22.
86. Corey AL, et al. Social support and symptom distress in adolescent/young adults with cancer. J Paediatr Nurs. 2008;25(5):275–84.
87. Kwak M, et al. Trajectories of psychological distress in adolescent and young adult patients with cancer: a 1-year longitudinal study. J Clin Oncol. 2013;31(17):2160–6.
88. Park EM, Rosenstein DL. Depression in adolescents and young adults with cancer. Dialogues Clin Neurosci. 2015;17(2):171–80.
89. Smith AW, Bellizzi KM, Keegan TH. Health-related quality of life of adolescent and young adult patients with cancer in the United States: the adolescent and young adult health outcomes and patient experience study. J Clin Oncol. 2013;31(17):2136–45.
90. Xie J, et al. A prevalence study of psychosocial distress in adolescents and young adults with cancer. Cancer Nurs. 2017;40(3):217–23.
91. World Health Organisation. Mental health: a State of Wellbeing. Geneva: World Health Organisation; 2014.
92. Dyson GJ, et al. The relationship between unmet needs and distress amongst young people with cancer. Support Care Cancer. 2012;20(1):75–85.
93. Yeo MS, Sawyer SM. ABC of adolescence. Chronic illness and disability. Br Med J. 2005;330(7493):721–3.
94. Zebrack B, et al. Psychological distress and unsatisfied need for psychosocial support in adolescent and young adult cancer patients during the first year following diagnosis. Psychooncology. 2014;23(11):1267–75.
95. Shay LA, Carpentier MY, Vernon SW. Prevalence and correlates of fear of recurrence among adolescent and young adult versus older adult post-treatment cancer survivors. Support Care Cancer. 2016;24(11):4689–96.
96. Lauer AL. Treatment of anxiety and depression in adolescents and young adults with cancer. J Pediatr Oncol Nurs. 2015;32(5):278–83.
97. Kwak M, et al. Prevalence and predictors of post-traumatic stress symptoms in AYA cancer survivors: a 1 year follow up study. Psychooncology. 2013;2(8):1798–806.
98. Ramphal R, et al. Adolescent and young adult cancer: principles of care. Curr Oncol. 2016;23(3):204–9.
99. Lynam J. Supporting one another: the nature of family work when a young adult has cancer. J Adv Nurs. 1995;22(1):116–25.
100. Zebrack B, Chesler MA, Penn A. Psychosocial support. In: Bleyer MA, Barr RD, editors. Cancer in adolescents and young adults. Heidelberg: Springer Verlag; 2007.
101. Price J. Information needs of the child with cancer and their family. Cancer Nurs Pract. 2003;2(7):35–8.
102. Trask P, et al. Parent and adolescent adjustment to paediatric cancer: associations with coping, social support and family function. J Paediatr Oncol Nurs. 2003;20(1):36–47.
103. Alderfer MA, et al. Psychosocial adjustment of siblings of children with cancer: a systematic review. Psychooncology. 2010;19(8):789–805.
104. Spinetta J, et al. Guidelines for assiatcne to siblings of children with cancer: report for the SIOP working committee on psychosocial issues in paediatric oncology. Med Paediat Oncol. 1999;33(4):395–8.
105. CanTeen Australia. Supporting adolescent and young adult siblings of cancer patients: the family context. Sydney: CanTeen Australia; 2011.
106. Patterson P, Medlow S, McDonald F. Recent developments in supporting adolescent & young adult siblings of cancer patients. Supportive Care. 2015;27(4):311–15.
107. Robertson E, Sansom-Daly UM, Wakefield CE, et al. Sexual and Romantic Relationships: Experience of Adolescnet & Young Adult Cancer Survivors. J Adolesc Young Adult Oncol. 2016;5(3):286–91.

108. Longo CJ. Financial and family burden associated with cancer treatment in Ontario, Canada. Support Care Cancer. 2006;14(11):1077–85.
109. Choquette A, Rennick J, Lee V. Back to school after cancer treatment. Cancer Nurs. 2016;39(5):393–401.
110. Pini S, Hugh-Jones S, Gardner PH. What effect does a cancer diagnosis have on the educational engagement and school life of teenagers? A systematic review. Psychooncology. 2011;21(7):685–94.
111. Zebrack BJ. Psychological, social, and behavioral issues for young adults with cancer. Cancer. 2011;117(10):2289–94.
112. Gurney JG. Social outcomes of the childhood cancer survivor study cohort. J Clin Oncol. 2009;27(14):2390–5.
113. Searle NS. Homebound schooling is the least favourable option for continued education of adolescent cancer patients: a preliminary report. Med Paediatr Oncol. 2003;40(6):380–4.
114. Jaffe ML. Adolescence. New York: Wiley; 1998.
115. Manaster GJ. Adolescent development and the life tasks. Boston: Allyn & Bacon, Inc.; 1977.
116. Taylor E, et al. Spirituality and spiritual care in adolescents and young adults with cancer. Sem Oncol Nurs. 2015;3(3):227–41.
117. Wein S, Pery S, Zer A. Role of palliative care in adolescent and young adult oncology. J Clin Oncol. 2010;28(32):4819–24.
118. Casillas J, et al. Transitioning childhood cancer survivors to adult-centred health care: insights from parents, adolescent young adult survivors. Psychooncology. 2010;19(2):982–90.
119. Doug M, et al. Transition to adult services for children and young people with palliative care needs: a systematic review. Arch Dis Child. 2011;96(1):78–84.
120. Mulder RL, et al. Transition guidelines: an important step in the future care for childhood cancer survivors. A comprehensive definition as groundwork. Eur J Cancer. 2016;54(1):64–8.
121. Nathan PC, et al. Critical issues in transition and survivorship for adolescents and young adults with cancers. Cancer. 2011;117(10 Suppl):2335–41.
122. Patterson P, et al. Emerging issues among adolescent and young adult cancer survivors. Semin Oncol Nurs. 2015;31(1):53–9.
123. Freyer DR. Transition of care for young adult survivors of childhool and adolescent cancer: Rationale and approaches. J Clin Oncol. 2010;28(32):4810–8.
124. Kinahan KE, et al. Models of cancer survivorship care for adolescents and young adults. Semin Oncol Nurs. 2015;31(3):251–9.

Health Behaviour and Adolescent and Young Adult Cancer Survivors

5

Gemma Pugh and Abigail Fisher

5.1 Introduction

The majority of adolescents and young adults (AYAs) will now survive a cancer diagnosis [1, 2]. However, as a result of their cancer diagnosis and treatment, AYA cancer survivors are at increased risk of chronic health conditions [3]. Cumulative prevalence estimates indicate that by the age of 45 years nearly 95% of childhood and AYA cancer survivors will have a chronic health problem of some kind, and 80% will have a health problem classed as disabling or life threatening [4]. Common health problems, such as cardiovascular disease, endocrine dysfunction, and metabolic syndrome (increased blood pressure, high blood sugar, excess body fat around the waist, and abnormal cholesterol or triglyceride levels) can have both transient and lifelong negative impacts on health and well-being [5]. Emerging evidence among adult cancer survivors, indicates that the adoption of healthy lifestyle habits, such as being sufficiently physically active and eating a healthy diet, may prevent or ameliorate some of the health problems faced by those who have had a cancer diagnosis [6]. As a result, there is a growing awareness of need for health behaviour promotion among young people with cancer [7]. Healthy lifestyle choices may substantially improve the long-term survivorship and quality of life of AYA cancer survivors, whereas health risk behaviours (e.g., smoking, drinking and tanning) may exacerbate survivors' underlying risk of chronic disease and of secondary malignancy [8]. Evidence from the St Jude Lifetime Cohort Study in the United States of America has shown that long-term survivors of childhood and adolescent malignancies who do not follow physical activity and diet guidance set out by the World Cancer Research Fund and American Institute of Cancer were more likely to have metabolic syndrome with a relative risk of 2.2 (95% CI 1.6–3.0) among males and 2.4 (95% CI 1.7–3.3) among females [9]. Data from Acute Lymphoblastic

G. Pugh (✉) • A. Fisher
Department of Behavioural Science and Health, University College London, London, UK
e-mail: gemma.pugh.14@ucl.ac.uk; abigail.fisher@ucl.ac.uk

J. Chisholm et al. (eds.), *A Practical Approach to the Care of Adolescents and Young Adults with Cancer*, https://doi.org/10.1007/978-3-319-66173-5_5

Leukaemia (ALL) survivors in the same cohort indicate males who smoked, and females who consumed between one and three drinks per day had increased odds (OR 1.71; 95% CI 1.02–2.85. 0R 2.09; 95% CI 1.14–3.83 respectively) of low bone mass density [10]. Given that metabolic syndrome and low bone mass density are associated with reduced longevity and poor quality of life, such data emphasizes the need to provide young people with cancer with support to make and sustain positive health behaviour choices overtime. This chapter provides an overview of the importance of health behaviour promotion among AYA cancer survivors and outlines key strategies for engaging young people with lifestyle information and health behaviour change interventions.

5.2 The Importance of Promoting Health and Lifestyle Among Teenagers and Young Adults

Adolescence and early adulthood are key stages of development where many health related habits and behaviours are established [11]. While health behaviour during childhood is strongly influenced by parental instruction, during early adolescence young people gain increasing autonomy and begin to make their own dietary and exercise choices and often experiment with 'adult' behaviours such as alcohol consumption, smoking or drug misuse [12–14]. Although such experimentation behaviour is a normal part of a young persons' development, behaviours established during the period of growth from adolescence to young adulthood 'track' throughout the life-course and can result in cumulative risk profiles for later adult onset health problems [15, 16]. For example longitudinal cohort studies consistently report that high levels of alcohol consumption in adolescence continue into adulthood and such drinking patterns associate with alcohol related health problems including alcohol dependence in later life [17]. Moreover, obesity (a condition magnified by low levels of physical activity and poor diet) during adolescence has also been shown to track into adulthood [18, 19] and has been found to be independently predictive of later adulthood cardiovascular health status [20]. Efforts to promote healthy lifestyle choices (i.e., sufficient physical activity, a healthy diet, abstinence from smoking and low levels of drinking) among adolescents and young adults have the potential to yield short term improvements in health and well-being and prevent the manifestation of non-communicable diseases later in life [21].

5.3 Lifestyle Recommendations for AYA Cancer Survivors

Lifestyle recommendations for young people with cancer are contained in the long-term follow-up guidance set out by the Children's Oncology Group and Scottish Intercollegiate Guidance Network. The focus of the recommendations, as contained within Table 5.1, is to improve the quality of life and decrease the likelihood of health problems among child, adolescent and young adult cancer survivors. Specifically, health professionals are advised to provide health behaviour counselling to

Table 5.1 Lifestyle guidance for teenage and young adult cancer survivors

Health behaviour	Guidance	
	Children's Oncology Group (October 2013)	*SIGN 132 (March 2013)*
Physical activity	Check with healthcare team before starting an exercise plan or taking part in a new sport or recreational activities	
	For adults—Engage in moderate physical activity (brisk walking, bicycling, vacuuming, gardening) ≥30 min/day for ≥5 days per week. 45–60 min is preferable	
	For children and adolescents—Engage in ≥60 min of moderate to vigorous physical activity (running, aerobics, heavy yard work) for ≥5 days per week	
Diet	Choose a variety of foods from all the food groups (fruits, grains, vegetables, and protein)	
	Use the interactive customized guide at www.choosemyplate.gov to develop a well-balanced diet and activity plan	
Fruit/Veg	Eat ≥5 servings of fruit and veg per day. Including citrus fruits and dark green and deep yellow vegetables	Eat plenty, at least five portions of a variety of fruit and vegetables a day
	When drinking juice choose 100% fruit or vegetable juice and limit to 4 oz. per day	
Milk/Dairy	Choose low fat milk and dairy products	Eat some, choose lower fat alternatives whenever possible or eat higher fat versions infrequently or in smaller amounts
Meat	Limit intake of red meat and substitute with fish, poultry and beans	Eat some, choose lower fat alternatives whenever possible or eat higher fat versions infrequently or in smaller amounts. The Food Standards Agency advises that if you eat more than 90 g of red and processed meat a day, you should cut down to 70 g
	When eating meat, select leaner, or smaller portions	Aim for at least two portions of fish a week, including a portion of oily fish

(continued)

Table 5.1 (continued)

Health behaviour	Guidance	
Fibre	Eat plenty of high-fibre foods, such as whole grain breads, rice, pasta and cereals	Eat plenty, choose wholegrain varieties when you can
	Limit refined carbohydrates, including pastries, sweetened cereals, soft drinks and sugars	
Fat	Decrease the amount fat in meals by baking, broiling or boiling foods	Foods and drinks high in fat and/or sugar consume just a small amount
	Limit fried or high fat foods	
Sugar	Limit food and beverages with added sugar	As above
	Children's Oncology Group	*SIGN*
Alcohol consumption	Adults should limit alcoholic drinks to less than two a day for men and one for women	Keep alcohol intake within government recommended limits[a]
Smoking	Do not smoke	Avoid smoking

[a]Current government recommendations advise both men and women to not regularly drink more than 14 units a week

young people in the context of late-effects management, especially when regarding the treatment of cardiac problems and metabolic syndrome [22]. The lifestyle recommendations for AYA cancer survivors are based upon recommendations made by the World Cancer Research Fund and American Cancer Society for adult cancer survivors [23] and do not differ substantially from national government recommendations on health behaviour intended for the young people within the general population. Nonetheless, clinicians and health professionals working with cancer patients and survivors are encouraged to be mindful that the nutritional needs and physical activity capabilities of cancer survivors may change over time, and will most likely be dictated by individual factors such as diagnosis type, treatment status, and age. As such lifestyle guidance for cancer survivors' of all ages stipulate that health professionals should individually tailor the advice they provide to patients and account for any individual differences in health and well-being.

Several UK child and AYA specific organisations (Children's Cancer and Leukaemia Group, TYAC, Teenage Cancer Trust) have produced information resources and position statements relating to lifestyle for the interest of clinicians and health professionals working with AYA cancer patients and survivors. While no formal or structured guidance exists for young people on cancer treatment, clinicians and health professionals caring for AYA aged cancer patients are encouraged to advocate the importance of lifestyle behaviour and discourage young people from inactivity, unhealthy eating habits, and poor lifestyle choices such as smoking, excessive drinking and excessive sun exposure.

5.4 Health Behaviour and Young People with Cancer

5.4.1 Physical Activity

Physical activity, defined as 'any bodily movement produced by skeletal muscles which results in energy expenditure' [24], is essential for adolescent and young adult health. The benefits of physical activity for cancer survivors are multifactorial, with previous studies among adult cancer survivors reporting improvements in body mass index, body weight, peak oxygen consumption, peak power output, endurance, strength and quality of life [25–27]. It has been suggested that physical activity could have the same (if not more) benefits for young people affected by cancer [28, 29]. Data from 1187 adult survivors of childhood Hodgkin lymphoma in the childhood cancer survivors study (CCSS) cohort (mean age: 31 years at the time of analysis; median years since diagnosis: 16.7 years) has shown that those meeting national vigorous intensity exercise guidelines[1] had 51% reduced risk of cardiovascular events in comparison to those not meeting the guidelines (RR 0.49, 95% CI 0.31–0.76) [30]. Moreover, associations have been found between physical activity and both the health related quality of life and the sleep quantity of AYA-aged childhood cancer survivors [31, 32]. In particular, physical activity has been outlined as the most promising management strategy for cancer-related fatigue among AYA cancer survivors [33]. Conversely, sedentary behaviour is associated with increased lethargy and decreased fitness among young people with cancer [34]. Such cross-sectional findings are important in supporting the idea that physical activity could be effective in reducing the negative consequences of cancer treatment such as pain and fatigue, whereas inactivity contributes to a self-perpetuating decline in fitness, physical function, and mental well-being [35]. However, in order to test for a causal association, randomised controlled trials (RCTs) of physical activity interventions are required.

Unfortunately, to date, very few trials have specifically examined the impact of physical activity on health outcomes among young people with cancer. A narrative review of physical activity interventions specifically targeting young people with cancer, reported only nine empirical studies of exercise or physical activity interventions designed for AYA cancer survivors [36].

In general studies report small, but significant, post-intervention improvements in strength and endurance [29, 37, 38], body composition and weight status, [37, 39, 40] health related quality of life [38], mood and self-efficacy [41, 42]. None report any negative outcomes or adverse events, suggesting that physical activity is safe and feasible for cancer survivors of this age. A systematic review investigating the feasibility of physical activity interventions conducted during the intense phase of

[1] Meeting vigorous intensity exercise guidelines equates to ≥3 sessions of vigorous intensity exercise/ week of ≥20 min in duration, the equivalent to ≥9 metabolic equivalents (MET) hours/week.

cancer treatment among children and adolescents also concluded it is both safe and feasible for young people to be active during treatment [43]. Of the included studies, the majority of physical activity interventions were tailored to the specific needs of the patient, supervised and delivered in an inpatient setting However, often young people who are medically complex are excluded from participating within intervention studies limiting the applicability of the results on the safety of physical activity interventions to the whole AYA cancer population. Moreover, existing studies investigating the benefits of physical activity among young people with cancer have several methodological limitations, such as inadequate power and difficulties in participant recruitment and retention. As a result, there is currently insufficient evidence to quantify the optimal mode, frequency, and duration of physical activity prescription for AYA cancer patients or survivors.

Nevertheless, observational data certainly highlight a need for physical activity intervention in this group. Existing data (although limited to a small number of studies with the majority of these using self-reported physical activity) suggest that a large proportion of AYA cancer survivors do not meet physical activity recommendations [44–46]. Data from the Childhood Cancer Survivor Cohort indicate 44.2% of 18–24 years olds do not meet Centre for Disease Control recommendations of being active for more than 30 min per day on more than 5 days of the week [47]. Whilst one cross-sectional survey of 74 young adult cancer survivors (mean age = 22.9 years) found that only 48.7% of the sample met physical activity guidelines and that more than half retrospectively rated their fitness as 'much worse' or 'not quite as good' compared to pre-diagnosis [48]. Studies have indicated that the physical activity levels of AYAs drop significantly following a cancer diagnosis, and typically do not return to pre-diagnosis levels of activity following treatment completion [48, 49]. In one study of 40 childhood cancer haematopoietic stem cell transplant survivors (mean age: 12.5 ± 3.2 years) more than two thirds of participants reported spending three or more hours per day on sedentary activities during leisure time [50]. A recent Dutch study 'Quality of Life in Motion,' found AYA cancer survivors (n = 60, mean age: 13.8 years) were sedentary for more than 80% of all waking hours (median 869/1080 min per day) [51].

The impact of a cancer diagnosis, its subsequent treatment, and low self-esteem may partially explain the low levels of physical activity seen among AYA cancer survivors. However, decreased physical activity often leads to a cycle of increasing fatigue and muscular deconditioning. Efforts to support young people with cancer to be sufficiently active both during and after cancer are needed. Moreover, further work is required to explore how physical activity intervention may be integrated and adopted into standard clinical practice as there is some confusion among health professionals on the safety of prescribing physical activity and exercise to young people with cancer [43, 52].

5.4.2 Diet

There is a general consensus that, among adult cancer survivors, a diet rich in fruit, vegetables, complex whole grains and lean proteins should be recommended, as this may reduce chronic health problems and prevent cancer recurrence (although the literature has mainly focussed on survivors of breast, prostate and colorectal cancer survivors) [53]. For instance, one prospective study of 1009 adult colorectal cancer survivors found those with western diets (high intake of red meat, saturated fat and refined sugar) had three times the risk of cancer recurrence or death compared with those who had the lowest intake of red meat, saturated fat and refined sugar (Hazard Ratio, HR: 3.25, 95% CI 2.05–5.19) [54]. Findings from the European Prospective Investigation into Cancer and Nutrition Study (a study of nearly 400,000 adults) report that death from chronic disease and cancer mortality is 34% lower among adult cancer survivors who have healthy diet (high fruit and veg intake, complex whole grains and lean proteins) than cancer survivors with a poor diet [55]. Such evidence underscores the importance of providing nutritional counselling to cancer survivors in order to reduce the manifestations of chronic disease and cancer recurrence.

Although evidence linking diet to health outcomes among AYA cancer survivors is very limited, there is potential that common treatment related late-effects experienced by young people with cancer such as diabetes and high blood pressure could be managed through effective dietary interventions [28, 56, 57]. Adherence to a Mediterranean diet has been found to be associated with lower body mass index (BMI) ($p = 0.04$), lower visceral adiposity ($p = 0.07$), lower subcutaneous adiposity ($p < 0.001$) and a 31% (OR 0.69, 95% CI 0.50, 0.94) risk reduction in developing metabolic syndrome among AYA-aged childhood cancer survivors ($n = 117$, mean age: 24 years; mean time since diagnosis: 17.6 years) [58]. Moreover, adherence to dietary guidance has also been found to be significantly associated with improved quality of life and reduced fatigue among AYA aged childhood cancer survivors ($n = 179$ mean age = 17.7 years) [59].

However, despite growing recognition of the importance of diet in AYA cancer survivorship, as observed for physical activity levels, existing evidence, although also limited to a few studies, suggests that dietary patterns and nutritional intake among young people with cancer is typically poor. Cross-sectional data have indicated that more than half of AYA cancer survivors do not meet national dietary recommendations [59–61]. For instance, one study of AYA aged childhood cancer survivors ($n = 209$; mean age = 20.3 years) in the United States found 79% of young people did not meet recommended daily fruit intake, 68% fell below guidelines for calcium intake, and 84% did not comply with guidelines for dietary fat intake [62]. Worryingly, previous studies of young people with cancer have found that energy intake often exceeds energy expenditure by more than 10% [63] and energy intake from sweets can be up to 70% higher than recommended, [64]. Such data emphasizes the need to provide AYA cancer survivors with nutrition and diet intervention. Given that poor dietary intake is one of the main factors contributing to weight gain, tailored interventions which use diet as a weight management strategy developed specifically for AYA cancer survivors are warranted [65]. However, akin to studies investigating physical activity, data on dietary patterns gathered from self-report food frequency questionnaires is subject to a high level of biased reporting and systematic error [66]. As a result of these dietary data collection limitations, and the lack of randomised controlled trials within this area, there is currently insufficient evidence to draw conclusions about the role of nutrition and dietary intake on health and cancer outcomes among AYAs. Nevertheless the emerging evidence among AYA cancer survivors does suggest diet is a core part of health and well-being among young people who have had cancer.

5.4.3 Weight Management

Although dramatic weight loss and cachexia is a concern among AYA cancer patients, obesity, defined as an excessive accumulation of body weight resulting in body mass index (BMI) >30 kg of body weight per square meter of height (kg/m^2), and overweight body status (BMI 25–29 kg/m^2), is common among young people who have had a cancer diagnosis [67]. One meta-analysis of the obesity prevalence among acute lymphoblastic leukaemia survivors found the prevalence of obesity among survivors 5–9 years post treatment (n = 14 studies, mean/median age = 13.2–19.4 years) ranged between 29–69%; and the prevalence of obesity among survivors more than 10 years post treatment (n = 5 studies, mean/median age = 20.5 = 24.1 years) to be within the range of 34–46% [68]. Weight gain often occurs during, and is maintained post, treatment such that the prevalence of overweight and obesity in AYA aged cancer survivors is greater than among the young people within the general population [67].

Box 5.1 outlines mechanisms for obesity among AYA cancer patients and survivors. Earlier age at diagnosis, diagnosis of acute lymphoblastic leukaemia, cranial radiation, glucocorticoid exposure, growth hormone deficiency and female gender have been identified as high risk groups for weight gain and obesity [69]. The prevalence of obesity and AYA cancer survivors' elevated risk of weight gain is a cause for concern as many of the long-term physical, metabolic, and endocrine effects of AYA cancer such as cardiovascular dysfunction, hypertension, and glucose intolerance are heavily influenced by weight status [70]. Additionally, among young people with cancer, specifically those who have had a diagnosis of leukaemia, obesity has been associated with poorer overall and event-free survival [71, 72]. Within one study of high-risk acute lymphoblastic leukaemia patients (n = 2008, age range: 0–21 years) being obese at diagnosis was associated with greater treatment related toxicity. However, encouragingly, in individuals whose weight status returned to healthy BMI ranges during treatment, this risk of poor event free survival and treatment related toxicity was mitigated [73]. This study provided evidence that, unlike previous reports, survival and treatment related toxicity is not solely influenced by weight status at diagnosis but is moderated by weight status during treatment. Such findings indicate that efforts should be made to address young peoples' weight status from the point of diagnosis onwards. Whilst treatment-related energy imbalance may be unavoidable, health behaviour especially high levels of energy consumption (high calorie intake) and low levels of energy expenditure (low levels of physical activity) are likely to amplify energy imbalance and lead to further weight gain. Findings from the Childhood Cancer Survivor Cohort Study (n = 9283) indicate adult survivors of childhood cancer who are physically active had a reduced risk of obesity than those who were inactive (RR 0.90; 95% CI 0.82–0.97) [74]. Likewise, high intake of fruit, vegetables, fish and legumes has been found to be associated with significantly lower adiposity and BMI among young adult aged survivors of childhood ALL, (mean age: 23 years; mean years since treatment: 17.5) [58].

However, weight status is a notoriously difficult issue for health professionals to address. Health professionals report lower levels of enquiry about or providing advice on weight status than any other lifestyle behaviour [75]. This is despite 86% of young people reporting interest in receiving such advice [76]. Lifestyle interventions for AYA cancer patients and survivors should target energy balance and weight management through diet and physical activity in order to prevent and manage weight gain or obesity. Addressing the weight status of AYA cancer patients and AYA aged survivors of cancer throughout the cancer care pathway has the potential to prevent morbidity and mortality within this population group [65, 77].

Box 5.1: Mechanisms for Obesity Among AYA Cancer Survivors

Weight gain is a result of energy imbalance caused by greater energy intake than energy expenditure [78]. Although AYA cancer survivors' weight status may be fuelled by high calorie dietary intake and low levels of physical activity, common AYA cancer treatments can often contribute to excessive weight gain among young people with cancer. For example, steroids, often prescribed to treat haematological malignancies such as leukaemia, result in dose-response increase in appetite and hence energy intake [79, 80]. Although it is assumed that appetite will return to normal following the end of steroid treatment young people often report difficulties breaking dietary patterns and habits formed during treatment. A second common obesity risk treatment for young people with cancer is cranial radiation. Cranial radiation can inadvertently damage the hypothalamic region of the brain and impair the production and regulation of appetite related hormones such as ghrelin and leptin leading to increased energy intake and subsequent weight gain [81]. Moreover, cranial radiation can cause postural imbalance and some chemotherapeutic drugs and steroids are linked to neuropathy and degenerative bone conditions such avascular necrosis. Such treatment related side-effects can cause difficulties in physical function and mobility which in turn have been associated with weight gain and obesity among both young people with cancer and those in the general population [74].

5.4.4 Smoking

Smoking is the most preventable cause of lung cancer and is linked to 20% of all cancers among adults in the UK each year [82]. It is well established that smoking causes a plethora of chronic diseases including stroke, gum disease, high blood pressure, heart disease, pneumonia, hardening of the arteries, chronic lung disease, asthma and bone thinning. Among adult cancer survivors, smoking and tobacco use has been strongly associated with an increased risk of cancer recurrence and second primary lung cancer (Hazard Ratio: 6.69, 95% CI 2.00–22.42) [83]. Among young people who have been treated for cancer, smoking may exacerbate cardiopulmonary toxicities and respiratory infection risks associated with thoracic radiation exposure and some antineoplastic therapies [84]. Data from the United States indicate adult aged survivors of AYA cancer (n = 1019) who smoke are more likely to report health problems (OR = 1.62; 95% CI = 1.06–2.47; P 5.03) than general population controls [85]. Specifically, smoking has been identified as a risk factor for low bone mass density among adult aged Acute Lymphoblastic Leukaemia survivors [10]. As outlined within Table 5.1 young people with cancer are advised to either abstain or quit smoking following their diagnosis.

Data on smoking patterns among AYA cancer survivors is extremely limited. The data from comparative studies concerning smoking prevalence among AYA cancer survivors compared to age-matched population controls vary. Some studies indicate that the prevalence of smoking among childhood and AYA cancer survivors is lower than general population controls (Observed/Expected: 0.72, 95% CI 0.69–0.75) [86] whereas other studies have shown no significant difference between survivors and population control groups [61, 87]. Such discrepancies in findings can be attributed to variation in smoking status measures used, recall bias and use of convenience sampling. A recent meta-analysis of smoking among childhood cancer survivors, siblings and age-matched peers found survivors of childhood cancer (defined as young people diagnosed <21 years of age) were less likely than siblings (OR 0.68, 95% CI 0.49–0.96) or peers (OR 0.54, 95% CI 0.42–0.77) to smoke [88]. These findings are consistent with previous narrative reviews within this field [8, 89].

Nevertheless, although AYA cancer survivors appear to be less likely to smoke than peers it is estimated that 16–22% of young people who have had a cancer diagnosis are current smokers [88, 90] and almost a third of AYA cancer survivors have tried or experimented with smoking [87]. Cognitive factors, such as emotional distress and perceived risk, and environmental factors, such as friends or family who smoke, heavily influence whether a young person experiments with cigarettes. Worryingly, within one study of AYA cancer survivors who smoke (n = 374, age range: 18–55 years) 21% of young people did not perceive themselves at risk of a serious health problems in the future despite acknowledging that smoking increases the likelihood of serious health difficulties [91]. Given that poor decision making is a risk factor for smoking, tailored efforts to support young people with cancer to understand the risks of smoking, and make the decision to subsequently quit, are required [92].

5.4.5 Alcohol Consumption

Alcohol consumption rises during adolescence and peaks during young adulthood [93]. Although there are currently very limited available data linking alcohol consumption and health outcomes among AYA cancer survivors it is important to monitor and counsel young people on alcohol consumption because of their elevated risk of chronic disease and cancer recurrence. Alcohol consumption, specifically binge drinking, may exacerbate treatment related late effects experienced by AYA cancer survivors such as cardiovascular dysfunction, osteoporosis, and liver damage. Among adults it has been well established that lifelong excessive alcohol consumption is associated with increased risk of myocardial dysfunction, liver damage, osteoporosis, and cancers of the oral cavity, larynx, oesophagus, breast, and colon [53].

The evidence of patterns of alcohol consumption among AYA cancer survivors is heterogeneous and confounded by country-specific laws concerning alcohol purchase, recall bias, and variability in the classification of alcohol consumption. The reported prevalence of binge drinking among young people with cancer varies widely from 8 to 54% [94, 95]. A recent meta-analysis of comparative studies indicates that childhood and AYA cancer survivors are less likely to report binge drinking (OR 0.77, 95% CI 0.68–0.88) when compared to siblings but equally likely to binge drink when compared to peers (0R 0.97, 95% CI 0.38–2.49) [88]. However, one cross-sectional survey of AYA cancer survivors (n = 178; mean age: 25.2 years) in the UK found that when looking at alcohol consumption over a week, although AYA cancer survivors within this sample were less likely to binge drink, both male and female AYA cancer survivors (43% and 68%, respectively) reported higher levels of light drinking (i.e., up to 8 units over a week) than controls or siblings [61]. Such data, which suggest AYA cancer survivors drink at comparable rates to young people within the general population, is concerning given their heightened risk of hepatic dysfunction.

It has been hypothesized that AYA cancer survivors may engage in health risk behaviours (e.g., smoking and drinking) to cope with life stressors or as a method of normalisation [96]. Moreover, although there is no quantitative evidence to support the notion, it has previously been suggested that the observed differences in smoking and alcohol consumption behaviours between AYA cancer survivors and general population AYAs may be reflective of a less active social life among survivors [61]. Factors associated with binge drinking among AYA cancer survivors include male gender, educational status, substance use-related coping style, and worse parent-reported family functioning [97, 98].

5.4.6 Sun Safety

Exposure to sunlight or ultraviolet light is the primary risk factor for both melanoma and non-melanoma skin cancers [99]. Efforts to reduce sunlight exposure during AYA years are unlikely to reduce the incidence of cancer among young people, but may reduce the incidence rate of cancer among adults [100]. This is specifically true for childhood and AYA cancer survivors: data from the Childhood Cancer Survivor Study in the United States indicate young people who have undergone cancer treatment with radiotherapy are at a 6.3-fold increased risk of melanoma and non-melanoma skin cancers [101]. Safe sun practices such as minimizing sun exposure, applying sunscreen and wearing protective clothing, hats, and sunglasses may mitigate some of this risk.

Data on sun exposure or sun safety practices among AYA cancer survivors are extremely limited but, like studies of smoking and alcohol consumption, results do suggest that young people with cancer engage in poor sun-related health behaviour. One study (n = 175, mean age: 14.2 years; time since diagnosis; 9 years) found that non-adherence to skin protection was the most common harmful lifestyle behaviour among AYA cancer survivors [102] and data from the United States indicate 29% of AYA cancer survivors (n = 44/153; mean age: 26 years; time since diagnosis: 14 years) reported >5 h per week of tanning or reported using a sun bed twice within the last year [103]. However, when compared to siblings, adult-aged childhood cancer survivors are significantly less likely to report sunbathing (RR = 0.92 95% CI = 0.89–0.95) [104]. These findings suggest AYA-aged and adult-aged AYA cancer survivors may be more aware of the importance of sun-safe behaviours in preventing cancer recurrence. However, there is no concrete evidence to suggest that perceived risk of cancer recurrence is associated with improved health behaviour choice among AYA cancer survivors. Nevertheless, despite the lack of evidence, it is generally considered that health promotion efforts which incorporate counselling regarding the risks of sun exposure among AYAs may prompt an affective behavioural response, and trigger positive behaviours change, which in turn may mitigate AYA cancer survivors risk of malignant and non-malignant melanoma occurring as second primary cancers [15].

5.5 AYA Cancer Survivors Interest in Receiving Lifestyle Information

Although the health behaviours of young people with cancer appear to be sub-optimal, encouragingly their interest in receiving information and support on health behaviour is high. In a survey of 216 AYA cancer survivors in the UK (mean age: 20 years), over 80% of young people were interested in advice on physical activity, diet, and weight management [76]. In the United States, surveys of AYA aged childhood cancer survivors indicate similar levels of interest in receiving lifestyle information and support [48, 59, 105]. One study exploring the psychosocial program preferences of young people with cancer (n = 111, mean age = 17 years) found a greater proportion of AYAs were interested in information and support on reintegration into sport and improving body image than information about school or employment (48.1 vs. 29.9%, respectively) [105]. Young peoples' high level of interest in information and support on physical activity, diet and weight management is thought to be a reflection of their desires to regain normalcy and cultivate a personal identity [106]. Often young people with cancer advocate that being active and eating a healthy diet are important in managing treatment related side-effects of cancer and that these behaviours and allow them to regain control over their health [107]. AYA cancer survivors (mean age: 22.9 years) have reported specific interest in information on physical activity, diet, and weight management which relate to the impact and effect cancer has had upon their health and well-being; for example the impact of steroid treatment upon weight or the effects of chemotherapy drugs on taste and food preferences [108]. Although young people with cancer report less interest in advice on alcohol consumption, smoking and sun safety it is still imperative to provide AYA cancer patients and survivors with information on these topics given the well-established links these behaviours have to current and future health status. Adult aged AYA cancer survivors have indicated that during adolescence they were ambivalent to the importance of their health behaviour or their need for information on certain topics such as alcohol consumption and only now as adults do they fully appreciate the need to lead a healthy lifestyle or be provided with lifestyle information [109].

5.6 Health Promotion Among Young People with Cancer

Health professionals working with AYA cancer patients and survivors are well positioned to provide young people with the right support and guidance to make healthy lifestyle choices [7, 110]. The long-term and trusting relationships young people often have with health professionals provide a strong foundation on which discussions about health behaviour may be introduced. However, health professionals must be mindful of the ways in which they communicate lifestyle information and deliver health behaviour interventions. Young people typically do not respond well to paternalistic approaches to counselling and mistimed or inappropriate advice may damage patient relationships, specifically when regarding health risk behaviours [111]. Equally, if education or information on health behaviour is not followed by practical advice on strategies to make or sustain changes in health behaviour it is unlikely young people will make any attempts to change their health behaviour.

To date, very few health behaviour change interventions have been developed for or specifically piloted among AYA cancer survivors [112]. The majority of interventions which have been piloted have been conducted as small feasibility studies among AYA aged childhood cancer survivors in the United States. So far, no interventions targeting health behaviour change among AYAs' either on treatment or off treatment for cancer have been conducted or evaluated in the United Kingdom. Existing health behaviour interventions vary substantially in terms of the target health behaviour, content, format, and delivery mode. For example, while some intervention studies have been resource intensive and heavily incentivised [113–116] others have been delivered remotely using online resources such as specially designed websites or social networking websites [40, 113, 116, 117]. Similarly, while some interventions simply involve written information materials in the form of leaflets or guidebooks [37, 118–120] other interventions involved social support from peers, family and health professionals [38, 41, 115]. As a result of the heterogeneity of existing interventions, combined with the lack of research within this area of AYA cancer care, it is not possible to draw definitive conclusions about the most effective means of promoting behaviour change among young people with cancer. Nevertheless, drawing from health behaviour change interventions conducted among young people within the general population and the small but growing body of literature within the AYA cancer field it is clear that there are several key aspects of health behaviour promotion among AYA cancer survivors.

Firstly, as per the COM-B model of behaviour change, lifestyle interventions designed for young people with cancer must enhance young peoples' *capability* to regulate their own behaviour; maximise young peoples' *opportunities* to support self-regulation of behaviour; and increase young peoples' *motivation* to engage in the desired behaviour [121, 122]. This model recognises that health behaviour is multidimensional and centres upon the premise that an individuals' *capability* to change their health behaviour (e.g., become more active, stop smoking, have a healthier diet) is determined by both their physical and psychological capacity; that an individual will only carry out a behaviour or change their behaviour if the *opportunity* is presented within either their 'physical' environment and/or 'social' environment; and that an individuals' *motivation* to carry out a change in behaviour is influenced by self-conscious planning and evaluation (reflective motivation) and emotional desires, reactions and impulses (automatic motivation). These components of health behaviour are interactive, for example an increase in knowledge (psychological capability) of the benefits of physical activity for cancer survivors is likely to increase motivation to seek opportunities to be active. Addressing these six tenets (physical capability, psychological capability, physical opportunity, social opportunity, reflective motivation and automatic motivation) of behaviour is likely to lead to an increase in receptivity to health and lifestyle information and health behaviour change intervention efficacy among young people with cancer.

Secondly, lifestyle information provision is passive, and unlikely to prompt behaviour change alone. Lifestyle information materials and health behaviour change interventions developed for AYA cancer survivors must include functional components, i.e., 'active ingredients' to facilitate the desired change in health behaviour. These 'active ingredients' to behaviour change are commonly referred to as behaviour change techniques (BCTs) [123]. Typically behaviour change interventions are based upon formal theories of behaviour and contain BCTs relevant to the behavioural theory being used. Common behaviour change theories such as the Transtheoretical Model, Theory of Reasoned Action, Social Cognitive Theory, and Health Belief Model have underpinned the development and design of health behaviour interventions for AYA cancer survivors in the past [112]. However, despite the promising efficacy of existing health behaviour interventions, there is currently insufficient evidence to draw conclusions on what the most promising BCT or strategy would be to promote behaviour change among young people with cancer. This is primarily because there have been very few studies investigating behaviour change among AYA aged cancer survivors and there is very little consistency between studies so common elements of success cannot be clearly identified. Nevertheless, again, drawing from health behaviour change interventions conducted among young people within the general population and the small but growing body of literature within the AYA cancer field it is clear that there are several promising behaviour change techniques which may be somewhat important in changing the health behaviour of young people with cancer (Table 5.2).

Table 5.2 COM-B model of behaviour change and promising BCTs which have shown efficacy among young people with cancer

COM-B	COM-B model Subcomponents	Common behaviour change techniques	AYA cancer specific examples
Capability	**Physical capability**	Demonstration of the behaviour	**Belanger et al.** [124]. **(n = 212, Ages: 18–39 years**
	Physical skills, strength and stamina	Instruction on how to perform a behaviour	Study Design: Randomized Control Trial
		Behavioural practice/Rehearsal/ Repetition	Target Behaviour: Physical Activity
			Behaviour Change Techniques: Instruction on how to perform the behaviour, repetition
			Intervention: Targeted physical activity guidance, including advice on how to engage in physical activity, tips on how to make physical activity enjoyable, how much physical activity is recommended, how to determine physical activity intensity, guidance to recognize physical activity opportunities, and information about goal setting
	Psychological capability	Information about social consequences	**Cox et al.** [45] **and Hudson et al** [27]. **(n = 266, Ages: 12–28 years)**
	Knowledge or psychological skills, strength or stamina to engage in the necessary mental processes	Information about health consequences	Study Design: Randomized Control Trial
		Feedback on behaviour	Target Behaviour: Physical Activity, Diet, Smoking and Alcohol Consumption
		Goal Setting (Behaviour)	Behaviour Change Techniques: Goal setting, information about health consequences, action planning
		Goal Setting (Outcome)	Intervention: Health behavior training in health goal chosen by the survivor and encouragement to make a commitment to a health goal for ensuing year. Health behavior training session included a review of the advantages and disadvantages of the health behavior, an explanation of how to engage in the health behavior, problem solving of potential barriers, and an encouraged commitment to engage in the health behavior. Participants were also given reinforcement at 3 and 6 months via telephone
		Problem Solving	Results: Junk food consumption decreased in the intervention group and smoking abstinence remained unchanged. No effect on physical activity or alcohol use
		Action Planning	
		Self-monitoring	

(continued)

Table 5.2 (continued)

COM-B	COM-B model Subcomponents	Common behaviour change techniques	AYA cancer specific examples
Opportunity	**Physical opportunity**	Adding objects to the environment	**Huang et al.** [91] **(n = 38, Mean Age: 13 years)**
	Opportunity afforded by the environment, involving time, resources, locations, cues, physical 'affordance'	Prompts/Cues	Study Design: Randomized Control Trial
			Target Behaviour: Physical Activity and Diet
			Behaviour Change Techniques: Prompt
			Intervention: Weight maintenance intervention tailored for cancer survivors providing weekly nutritional tips and physical activity goals and skills. Participants were given weekly messages containing relevant lifestyle tips and set short text messages twice daily to their mobile phone
	Social opportunity	Restructuring social environment	**Mays et al.** [80] **(N = 75, Mean Age: 14.2 years)**
	Opportunity afforded by interpersonal influences, social cues and cultural norms that influence the way that we think about things, e.g., the words and concepts that make up our language	Modelling	Study Design: Randomized Control Trial
		Social Support	Target Behaviour: Diet
			Behaviour Change Technique: Social Support, Information about health consequences, Instruction on how to perform the behaviour
			Intervention: A group-based bone health behavioural intervention involving a half day interactive workshop that included messages and skill building exercises addressing relevant risk reducing and health promoting behaviours

Motivation	**Reflective motivation**	Reviewing behaviour goals	**Tyc et al.** 125
	Reflective processes involving plans (self-conscious intentions) and evaluations (beliefs about what is good and bad)	Self-Reward	Study Design: Randomized Control Trial
		Self-monitoring	Target Behaviour: Smoking
		Information about health consequences	Behaviour Change Technique: Information about health consequences, Goal setting, feedback on behaviour
		Feedback on behaviour	Intervention: Risk counselling intervention providing late-effects counselling, educational videos, goal setting, physician feedback, tobacco literature, and follow up telephone counselling
		Credible Source of information	Results: Significant increase in knowledge-perceived vulnerability, and lower intention to smoke scores at 12 months
		Biofeedback	
	Automatic motivation	Prompts/Cues	
	Automatic processes involving emotional reactions, desires (wants and needs), impulses, inhibitions, drive states and reflex responses	Goal setting	
		Self-monitoring	
		Feedback on behaviour	

5.6.1 Key Behaviour Change Techniques

Among children and adolescents health interventions which include behaviour change techniques such as goal setting, feedback and self-monitoring are more effective in initiating behaviour change than interventions solely based on education [126]. Health professionals working with AYAs affected by cancer must be mindful of this and must provide practical support to young people with cancer to help them make and sustain positive health behaviour changes.

5.6.1.1 Goals and Planning

Within the context of behaviour change, goals refer to a specific aim or desired result. The process of goal setting often involves planning specific actions which result in the goal being achieved. It is proposed that goal setting directs an individuals' effort towards a positive outcome and boosts self-efficacy through mastery. Goal setting has been effectively incorporated into health behaviour change interventions piloted among AYA cancer survivors [112]. For example, within the Fit4Life intervention piloted by Haung and colleagues among 38 overweight and obese adolescent survivors of childhood cancer (median age at study: 13 years; median age at diagnosis 5 years) young people and their families were encouraged to set specific goals and identify strategies for weight reduction such as achieving 15,000 steps daily. Results, although not statistically significant, indicated young people who received the intervention and had set specific goals became more active, reduced calorie intake, and lost weight when compared to controls [40]. AYAs' with cancer should be encouraged to set specific health behaviour goals and prompted to plan exactly how and when they will carry out the behaviour.

5.6.1.2 Feedback and Monitoring

Self-monitoring and feedback (awareness of standards and efforts) allow individuals to track their progress and compare their current behaviour to the specific goal they have set. In line with social cognitive theory [127] self-monitoring and feedback on behaviour develops self-efficacy through validating the individuals' belief that they are capable of carrying out the behaviour (enactive attainment). Self-monitoring typically involves measuring and then recording the behaviour in the form of a diary or chart.

5.6.1.3 Information About Health Consequences

According to long-term follow up guidance set by the Children's Oncology Group, young people, specifically those with metabolic syndrome or cardiovascular disease, should be provided with comprehensive and detailed information on the importance of health behaviours and be fully informed of the benefits of physical activity and healthy dietary behaviours and the risks of smoking, heavy alcohol consumption and sun exposure. Incorporating risk-based counselling into health behaviour interventions for young people with cancer may motivate young people to make positive behaviour changes, as young people who are unaware of their heightened risk of chronic health problems are likely to be passive towards health information and unable commit to specific health goals [91, 128]. For example a young person with Hodgkins lymphoma treated with chest irradiation who is unaware of their increased risk of cardiopulmonary sequelae is unlikely to identify smoking abstinence as a health priority. However, information about smoking exacerbating cardiopulmonary health problems may trigger an affective behavioural response and greater consciousness regarding their health behaviour. Risk-based education and counselling has been successfully integrated into existing health behaviour interventions piloted among AYA cancer survivors [112]. Specifically, intensive late-effects counselling, which includes specific information about the risks of tobacco use for AYA cancer survivors, has been found to be effective at improving health knowledge and lowering intentions to smoke among AYA aged childhood cancer survivors (n = 103, age range: 10–18 years) [125]. Given that intention has been found to predict physical activity behaviour among young people with cancer [129] risk-based counselling which increases the intentions of young people to make health behaviour changes could be effective across the spectrum of health behaviours. The more informed young people are of the benefits of healthy lifestyle choices, the more engaged they will be in making and sustaining positive behaviour changes. On the other hand, vague information, misinformation, or information overload is likely to lead to confusion, indifference and frustration towards behaviour change [130, 131].

5.6.1.4 Tailored Information and Intervention Delivery

Despite the need for information to be comprehensive and detailed, lifestyle information and behaviour change interventions should be delivered sensitively in the context of a young persons' cancer diagnosis, treatment history, and current health status [132]. Young people require information and support on health behaviour across the cancer care continuum from the point of diagnosis onwards and often (both during and after treatment) young people will experience one or more distinct physical and psychological problems at any given time [124]. As such a 'one-size-fits-all' approach to behaviour change is unlikely to be effective. Tailoring information provision and health behaviour interventions specifically to young people with cancer are likely to be more effective as they are likely to perceive information as more personally relevant if it is reflective of their individual needs [133]. For example, information on healthy dietary intake for haematological cancer survivors, which includes guidance and reference to neutropenia, will likely be more effective at prompting engagement and behaviour change than generic information materials about eating a healthy balanced diet. Several narrative reviews and one meta-analysis have demonstrated the efficacy of tailored health messages on health behaviour change [134]. Although empirical data in the AYA cancer sphere is limited, a small study of 23 AYA cancer survivors (mean age = 23.38 years) found tailored graphical depictions of daily health behaviour to significantly reduce binge drinking behaviour [113]. In this study participants logged into a custom made website where they were asked to fill in a log of their health behaviour (number of minutes of physical activity, number of alcoholic drinks and number of cigarettes smoked) in the last 3–4 days. Following this, participants were routed to graphical depictions of their behaviour alongside health related information and video messaging. This seems a promising area for future research.

5.6.1.5 Social Support

Multiple individual, interpersonal and environmental factors influence the development and maintenance of health behaviour [135]. Specifically among AYAs' family and peer-group behaviour can influence the lifestyle choices and health behaviour decisions a young person makes. Consistent with studies conducted among AYAs within the general population, social influences (friends and family) have been found to independently predict AYA cancer survivors physical activity levels [136]. Moreover, young people with cancer (n = 118, Mean age: 21.6 years) have cited having friends with poor diets as one of the many barriers to eating healthily [137]. Evidence from the Partnership for Health Study in the United States indicates adult aged-AYA cancer survivors (mean age: 31 years; SD = 6.66) who report receiving social support to stop smoking make more quit attempts and have greater self-efficacy [138]. This is consistent with a meta-analysis of behaviour change techniques applied in mobile apps targeting diet and physical activity behaviour change among children and adolescents which found mobile apps which included modelling (e.g., demonstration of the behaviour) and/or social support had greater effect than those which did not [139]. Efforts to deliver lifestyle information and behaviour change interventions to AYAs with cancer should take social influences on behaviour into account and provide means by which young people with cancer can access both emotional and practical social support.

5.6.2 Other Factors to Consider in Behaviour Change Among Young People with Cancer

5.6.2.1 Design and Visual Features

If health behaviour information and intervention resources are not stimulating or attractive to young people it is likely AYA cancer patients and survivors will not engage with the materials and quickly lose interest in the idea of making or sustaining healthy lifestyle choices. Good visual design has been suggested to be as important, if not more important, than the message content itself in health promotion [140]. Content and visual design features such as topic sections, lists, imaginative page layout, colour and infographics are likely to make information resource easier to navigate which in turn is likely to enhance young peoples' receptivity to the information being provided. Providing written information in smaller blocks in multiple formats means young people have the option to seek the specific information they are looking for. Multiple modes of health behaviour information delivery (e.g., leaflets, websites, posters, phone helplines, mobile phone texts) increases the likelihood that young people will be able to access the information in a format which appeals to them. Lifestyle information and behaviour change interventions which are designed and developed in partnership with AYA cancer patients and survivors are an important step in ensuring young people with cancer receive the patient centred care and support they require.

5.6.2.2 Age and Developmentally Appropriate

Addressing health behaviour with young people is a challenge because of the unique and distinct characteristics of this age group. Young people mature socially, emotionally and cognitively at different rates and often display individual differences in their ability to handle sensitive information. Individual differences in neurological development mean some young people may not yet have the ability to comprehend abstract information or control their emotional impulses and affective responses to cues [141, 142]. As a result, they may lack the ability to comprehend the long-term consequences of their health choices and may be most responsive to health behaviours which provide immediate gratification, such as sweet un-healthy food or binge drinking [143, 144]. Moreover, during the transition from adolescence into young adulthood young people become more autonomous and parental influence on health behaviour choice often subsides. Friends and peer group influences become increasingly important as young people strive to fit in with young people of a similar age. Engagement with health care can often dwindle during this period as the demands of school, university, work and new friendships take over. Health professionals providing lifestyle advice and health behaviour counselling to young people with cancer must consider these age-related challenges in patient education and engagement. Children and younger adolescents respond best to health behaviour information and interventions which are structured and provide modelling opportunities whereas behaviour change support which targets intention formation and self-efficacy to carry out a particular behaviour has been found most effective among adolescents [139]. Health professionals must also be mindful of age –related differences in information need. It is unlikely that a young person with cancer at the age of 13 will need comprehensive advice or information about smoking, alcohol consumption or illicit drug use, but by age 16–18 years the need for this information will become imperative.

5.6.2.3 Timing

'Teachable moments' refer to particular events or circumstances which motivate individuals to learn about, adopt, and maintain positive health behaviours [145]. In the context of health behaviour promotion among young people with cancer; cancer diagnosis, treatment and survivorship may provide opportunities, or a 'teachable moment' to convey health behaviour information to young people with maximal impact. However, very little is currently known as to whether 'teachable moments' exist among young people with cancer and whether receptivity to health behaviour intervention is related to individual personal factors, stage of treatment or age. Understanding the precise point at which young people would like to receive health behaviour information is likely to increase young peoples' receptivity to the prospect of health behaviour change. Young people with cancer, when surveyed, have expressed an interest in receiving lifestyle information and health behaviour change interventions throughout the cancer pathway [76]. Nonetheless, while intervention delivery appears to be acceptable at any point within the cancer pathway from diagnosis to survivorship, there is potential that the most effective interventions in terms of health would be those that are implemented and delivered prior to the onset of health problems or noted declines in health behaviour which often occur during treatment. Specifically, among young people with cancer there is argument that lifestyle interventions, particularly those targeting physical activity, delivered during treatment or at an early stage of survivorship may be effective at mitigating the onset and development common late effects and chronic health problems [146]. Early introductions to health behaviour change interventions may trigger behaviour change among some young people and prime those who are not ready for lifestyle change [6, 147].

5.6.3 The Potential of New Technologies

The rise of the internet and e-health technologies has widened the reach of health promotion efforts among AYAs with cancer. Among young people with cancer, technology based interventions (often referred to as e-health or m-health) have emerged as promising and innovative strategies for delivering health behaviour change information and support [148]. Information delivery strategies such as email alerts, text message reminders, push messaging services, and videoconferencing provide health professionals with a means to communicate information to young people with cancer in a more likeable and engaging manner. Such additional messaging features have been found enhance the effectiveness of internet-based health behaviour change interventions among the general population [149]. In addition, automated output functions provide an opportunity for young people with cancer to receive tailored feedback about their health and well-being. For example, as within the 6 week feasibility trial of a web-based health behaviour change intervention conducted by Berg et al. [113] interactive websites which allow young people to enter logs of their health behaviour can easily be designed to generate personalized tailored messages which relate to the input health behaviour data. Moreover, online based forums and group chat features offer young people the potential to access peer-to-peer support in a safe and supportive environment. One study examining the feasibility and preliminary efficacy of a 12-week, Facebook based physical activity intervention (FITNET) among AYA cancer survivors (Mean age: 30 years: Mean time since diagnosis: 58.2 months) found young people commonly shared messages of encouragement [116]. Furthermore, content analyses of discussion threads relating to diet and physical activity within an online AYA cancer support forum indicate young people often communicate concerns between each other about the impact cancer has had upon their ability to achieve diet or physical activity goals [107]. The finding that a high proportion of young people with cancer seek empathetic support about their lifestyle from their peers online supports the rationale behind the design and development of digital health promotion resources for young people with cancer. Moreover, technology based intervention programs may overcome the commonly reported geographical distance barrier to intervention participation. However, despite young peoples' high level of interest in health and lifestyle information available online [44, 150] young people with cancer do acknowledge that such mediums of information delivery lack the valuable personal support health professionals provide during one-to-one consultations [108]. Moreover, web-based health interventions often have a number of user related governance issues to contend with, particularly among vulnerable population groups such as AYA cancer patients and survivors [151]. Although technology-based interventions are considered an effective means of increasing intervention reach and decreasing cost further research is required to establish the utility and effectiveness of novel technologies in health promotion among AYA cancer survivors [152].

5.7 Future Priorities for Research and Care on Health Behaviour for Adolescent and Young Adult Cancer Survivors

To date, existing literature provides promising evidence that health behaviour promotion is needed and feasible among young people with cancer. However there is a paucity of literature within this area of AYA cancer research: in particular, evidence of the direct and indirect effects of health behaviour upon cancer and health outcomes among AYAs is a severely lacking. Such data are essential to mandate the importance of providing young people with cancer with health behaviour information and counselling. In addition, further research efforts to identify 'best practices' in adolescent and young adult health promotion are warranted. Continued research within this area will lead to evidence-based approaches to health promotion among teenage and young adult cancer patients and survivors which move beyond existing programs based upon general principles gathered from intuition or studies conducted among adult cancer survivors or general population adolescents and young adults.

References

1. O'Hara C, Moran A, Whelan JS, Hough RE, Stiller CA, Stevens MCG, Stark DP, Feltbower RG, McCabe MG. Trends in survival for teenagers and young adults with cancer in the UK 1992–2006. Eur J Cancer. 2015;51:2039–48.
2. Ward E, DeSantis C, Robbins A, Kohler B, Jemal A. Childhood and adolescent cancer statistics, 2014. CA Cancer J Clin. 2014;64:83–103.
3. Oeffinger KC, Mertens AC, Sklar CA, Kawashima T, Hudson MM, Meadows AT, Friedman DL, Marina N, Hobbie W, Kadan-Lottick NS, Schwartz CL, Leisenring W, Robison LL. Chronic health conditions in adult survivors of childhood cancer. N Engl J Med. 2006;355:1572–82.
4. Hudson MM, Ness KK, Gurney JG, Mulrooney DA, Chemaitilly W, Krull KR, Green DM, Armstrong GT, Nottage KA, Jones KE, Sklar CA, Srivastava DK, Robison LL. Clinical ascertainment of health outcomes among adults treated for childhood cancer. JAMA. 2013;309:2371–81.
5. Robison LL, Hudson MM. Survivors of childhood and adolescent cancer: life-long risks and responsibilities. Nat Rev Cancer. 2014;14:61–70.
6. Demark-Wahnefried W, Pinto BM, Gritz ER. Promoting health and physical function among cancer survivors: potential for prevention and questions that remain. J Clin Oncol. 2006;24:5125–31.

7. Daniel CL, Emmons KM, Fasciano K, Fuemmeler BF, Demark-Wahnefried W. Needs and lifestyle challenges of adolescents and young adults with cancer: summary of an Institute of Medicine and Livestrong Foundation Workshop. Clin J Oncol Nurs. 2015;19:675–81.
8. Clarke S-A, Eiser C. Health behaviours in childhood cancer survivors: a systematic review. Eur J Cancer. 2007;43:1373–84.
9. Smith WA, Li C, Nottage KA, Mulrooney DA, Armstrong GT, Lanctot JQ, Chemaitilly W, Laver JH, Srivastava DK, Robison LL, Hudson MM, Ness KK. Lifestyle and metabolic syndrome in adult survivors of childhood cancer: a report from the St.Jude Lifetime Cohort Study. Cancer. 2014;120:2742–50.
10. Wilson CL, Chemaitilly W, Jones KE, Kaste SC, Srivastava DK, Ojha RP, Yasui Y, Pui C-H, Robison LL, Hudson MM, Ness KK. Modifiable factors associated with aging phenotypes among adult survivors of childhood acute lymphoblastic leukemia. J Clin Oncol. 2016;34:2509–15.
11. Viner R, Macfarlane A. Health promotion. BMJ. 2005;330:527–9.
12. Birch LL, Fisher JO. Development of eating behaviors among children and adolescents. Pediatrics. 1998;101:539–49.
13. Kohl HW, Hobbs KE. Development of physical activity behaviors among children and adolescents. Pediatrics. 1998;101:549–54.
14. Steinberg L, Morris A. Adolescent development. Annu Rev Psychol. 2001;52:83–110.
15. Murphy MH. Health promotion in adolescent and young adult cancer survivors: mobilizing compliance in a multifaceted risk profile. J Pediatr Oncol Nurs. 2013;30:139–52.
16. Ness KK, Gurney JG. Adverse late effects of childhood cancer and its treatment on health and performance. Annu Rev Public Health. 2007;28:279–302.
17. McCambridge J, McAlaney J, Rowe R, Lanphear B. Adult consequences of late adolescent alcohol consumption: a systematic review of cohort studies. PLoS Med. 2011;8:e1000413.
18. Deshmukh-Taskar P, Nicklas TA, Morales M, Yang SJ, Zakeri I, Berenson GS. Tracking of overweight status from childhood to young adulthood: the Bogalusa Heart Study. Eur J Clin Nutr. 2006;60:48–57.
19. Herman KM, Craig CL, Gauvin L, Katzmarzyk PT. Tracking of obesity and physical activity from childhood to adulthood: the Physical Activity Longitudinal Study. Int J Pediatr Obes. 2009;4:281–8.
20. Freedman DS, Khan LK, Dietz WH, Srinivasan SR, Berenson GS. Relationship of childhood obesity to coronary heart disease risk factors in adulthood: the Bogalusa Heart Study. Pediatrics. 2001;108:712–8.
21. Sothern SM, Loftin M, Suskind MR, Udall NJ, Blecker U. The health benefits of physical activity in children and adolescents: implications for chronic disease prevention. Eur J Pediatr. 1999;158:271–4.
22. Scottish Intercollegiate Guidelines Network, SIGN (2013). Long term follow up of childhood cancer (SIGN publicaiton no. 132).
23. Rock CL, Doyle C, Demark-Wahnefried W, Meyerhardt J, Courneya KS, Schwartz AL, Bandera EV, Hamilton KK, Grant B, McCullough M, Byers T, Gansler T. Nutrition and physical activity guidelines for cancer survivors. CA Cancer J Clin. 2012;62:242–74.
24. Caspersen CJ, Powell KE, Christenson GM. Physical activity, exercise, and physical fitness: definitions and distinctions for health-related research. Public Health Rep. 1985;100:126–31.
25. Fong DYT, Ho JWC, Hui BPH, Lee AM, Macfarlane DJ, Leung SSK, Cerin E, Chan WYY, Leung IPF, Lam SHS, Taylor AJ, Cheng K-K. Physical activity for cancer survivors: meta-analysis of randomised controlled trials. BMJ. 2012;344:e70.
26. Lahart IM, Metsios GS, Nevill AM, Carmichael AR. Physical activity, risk of death and recurrence in breast cancer survivors: a systematic review and meta-analysis of epidemiological studies. Acta Oncol. 2015;54:635–54.
27. Schmid D, Leitzmann MF. Association between physical activity and mortality among breast cancer and colorectal cancer survivors: a systematic review and meta-analysis. Ann Oncol. 2014;25:1293–311.

28. Barnes MJ, Demark-Wahnefried W. Importance of balanced diet and physical activity during and after cancer treatment in adolescent patients. Clin Oncol Adolesc Young Adults. 2014;2014:13–20.
29. Gilliam MB, Schwebel DC. Physical activity in child and adolescent cancer survivors: a review. Health Psychol Rev. 2013;7:92–110.
30. Jones LW, Liu Q, Armstrong GT, Ness KK, Yasui Y, Devine K, Tonorezos E, Soares-Miranda L, Sklar CA, Douglas PS, Robison LL, Oeffinger KC. Exercise and risk of major cardiovascular events in adult survivors of childhood hodgkin lymphoma: a report from the Childhood Cancer Survivor Study. J Clin Oncol. 2014;32:3643–50.
31. Orsey AD, Wakefield DB, Cloutier MM. Physical activity (PA) and sleep among children and adolescents with cancer. Pediatr Blood Cancer. 2013;60:1908–13.
32. Paxton RJ, Jones LW, Rosoff PM, Bonner M, Ater JL, Demark-Wahnefried W. Associations between leisure-time physical activity and health-related quality of life among adolescent and adult survivors of childhood cancers. Psychooncology. 2010;19:997–1003.
33. Spathis A, Booth S, Grove S, Hatcher H, Kuhn I, Barclay S. Teenage and young adult cancer-related fatigue is prevalent, distressing, and neglected: it is time to intervene. A systematic literature review and narrative synthesis. J Adolesc Young Adult Oncol. 2015;4:3–17.
34. Braam KI, van Dijk-Lokkart EM, Kaspers GJL, Takken T, Huisman J, Bierings MB, Merks JHM, van de Heuvel-Eibrink MM, van Dulmen–den Broeder E, Veening MA. Cardiorespiratory fitness and physical activity in children with cancer. Support Care Cancer. 2016;24:2259–68.
35. Walter L, et al. Sleep and fatigue in pediatric oncology: a review of the literature. Sleep Med Rev. 2015;24:71–82.
36. Barnes M, Casazza K, Austin H. Strategies to promote regular exercise in adolescent and young adult cancer survivors. Clin Oncol Adoles Young Adults. 2015;2015:103–13.
37. Jarvela LS, Kemppainen J, Niinikoski H, Hannukainen JC, Lahteenmaki PM, Kapanen J, Arola M, Heinonen OJ. Effects of a home-based exercise program on metabolic risk factors and fitness in long-term survivors of childhood acute lymphoblastic leukemia. Pediatr Blood Cancer. 2012;59:155–60.
38. Keats MR, Culos-Reed SN. A community-based physical activity program for adolescents with cancer (project TREK): program feasibility and preliminary findings. J Pediatr Hematol Oncol. 2008;30:272–80.
39. Hartman A, te Winkel ML, van Beek RD, de Muinck Keizer-Schrama SM, Kemper HC, Hop WC, van den Heuvel-Eibrink MM, Pieters R. A randomized trial investigating an exercise program to prevent reduction of bone mineral density and impairment of motor performance during treatment for childhood acute lymphoblastic leukemia. Pediatr Blood Cancer. 2009;53:64–71.
40. Huang JS, Dillon L, Terrones L, Schubert L, Roberts W, Finklestein J, Swartz MC, Norman GJ, Patrick K. Fit4Life: a weight loss intervention for children who have survived childhood leukemia. Pediatr Blood Cancer. 2014;61:894–900.
41. Li HCW, Chung OKJ, Ho KY, Chiu SY, Lopez V. Effectiveness of an integrated adventure-based training and health education program in promoting regular physical activity among childhood cancer survivors. Psychooncology. 2013;22:2601–10.
42. Rabin C, Dunsiger S, Ness KK, Marcus BH. Internet-based physical activity intervention targeting young adult cancer survivors. J Adolesc Young Adult Oncol. 2011;1:188–94.
43. Grimshaw SL, Taylor NF, Shields N. The feasibility of physical activity interventions during the intense treatment phase for children and adolescents with cancer: a systematic review. Pediatr Blood Cancer. 2016;63:1586–93.
44. Belanger LJ, Plotnikoff RC, Clark A, Courneya KS. A survey of physical activity programming and counseling preferences in young-adult cancer survivors. Cancer Nurs. 2012;35:48–54.
45. San Juan AF, Wolin K, Lucia A. Physical activity and pediatric cancer survivorship. Recent Results Cancer Res. 2011;186:319–47.

46. Stolley MR, Restrepo J, Sharp LK. Diet and physical activity in childhood cancer survivors: a review of the literature. Ann Behav Med. 2010;39:232–49.
47. Florin TA, Fryer GE, Miyoshi T, Weitzman M, Mertens AC, Hudson MM, Sklar CA, Emmons K, Hinkle A, Whitton J, Stovall M, Robison LL, Oeffinger KC. Physical inactivity in adult survivors of childhood acute lymphoblastic leukemia: a report from the childhood cancer survivor study. Cancer Epidemiol Biomarkers Prev. 2007;16:1356–63.
48. Murnane A, Gough K, Thompson K, Holland L, Conyers R. Adolescents and young adult cancer survivors: exercise habits, quality of life and physical activity preferences. Support Care Cancer. 2015;23:501–10.
49. Keats MR, Culos-Reed SN, Courneya KS, McBride M. An examination of physical activity behaviors in a sample of adolescent cancer survivors. J Pediatr Oncol Nurs. 2006;23:135–42.
50. Bogg TF, Shaw P, Cohn R, Wakefield C, Hardy L, Broderick C, Naumann F. Physical activity and screen-time of childhood haematopoietic stem cell transplant survivors. Acta Paediatr. 2015;104:e455–9.
51. Braam KI, van Dijk-Lokkart EM, Kaspers GJL, Takken T, Huisman J, Bierings MB, Merks JHM, van de Heuvel-Eibrink MM, van Dulmen–den Broeder E, Veening MA. Cardiorespiratory fitness and physical activity in children with cancer. Support Care Cancer. 2015;24:2259–68.
52. Spreafico F, Murelli M, Ferrari A, Terenziani M, Giacon B, Veneroni L, Massimino M. Should we encourage exercise and sports in children and adolescents with cancer? Pediatr Blood Cancer. 2014;61:2125.
53. WCRF & AICR, W. C. R. F. A. I. C. R. Food, nutrition, physical activity and the prevention of cancer: a global perspective [Online]. Washington, DC: AICR; 2007.
54. Meyerhardt JA, Niedzwiecki D, Hollis D, Saltz LB, Hu FB, Mayer RJ, Nelson H, Whittom R, Hantel A, Thomas J, Fuchs CS. Association of dietary patterns with cancer recurrence and survival in patients with stage III colon cancer. JAMA. 2007;298:754–64.
55. Vergnaud AC, Romaguera D, Peeters PH, van Gils CH, Chan DS, Romieu I, Freisling H, Ferrari P, Clavel-Chapelon F, Fagherazzi G, Dartois L, Li K, Tikk K, Bergmann MM, Boeing H, Tjonneland A, Olsen A, Overvad K, Dahm CC, Redondo ML, Agudo A, Sanchez MJ, Amiano P, Chirlaque MD, Ardanaz E, Khaw KT, Wareham NJ, Crowe F, Trichopoulou A, Orfanos P, Trichopoulos D, Masala G, Sieri S, Tumino R, Vineis P, Panico S, Bueno-de-Mesquita HB, Ros MM, May A, Wirfalt E, Sonestedt E, Johansson I, Hallmans G, Lund E, Weiderpass E, Parr CL, Riboli E, Norat T. Adherence to the World Cancer Research Fund/American Institute for Cancer Research guidelines and risk of death in Europe: results from the European Prospective Investigation into Nutrition and Cancer cohort study1,4. Am J Clin Nutr. 2013;97:1107–20.
56. Ladas E. Nutritional counseling in survivors of childhood cancer: an essential component of survivorship care. Children. 2014;1:107.
57. Phillips-Salimi CR, Lommel K, Andrykowski MA. Physical and mental health status and health behaviors of childhood cancer survivors: findings from the 2009 BRFSS survey. Pediatr Blood Cancer. 2012;58:964–70.
58. Tonorezos ES, Robien K, Eshelman-Kent D, Moskowitz CS, Church TS, Ross R, Oeffinger KC. Contribution of diet and physical activity to metabolic parameters among survivors of childhood leukemia. Cancer Causes Control. 2013;24:313–21.
59. Badr H, Chandra J, Paxton RJ, Ater JL, Urbauer D, Cruz CS, Demark-Wahnefried W. Health-related quality of life, lifestyle behaviors, and intervention preferences of survivors of childhood cancer. J Cancer Surviv. 2013;7:523–34.
60. Hansen J, Stancel H, Klesges L, Tyc V, Hinds P, Wu S, Hudson M, Kahalley L. eating behaviour and bmi in adolescent survivors of brain tumor and acute lymphoblastic leukemia. J Pediatr Oncol Nurs. 2014;31:9.
61. Larcombe I, Mott M, Hunt L. Lifestyle behaviours of young adult survivors of childhood cancer. Br J Cancer. 2002;87:1204–9.
62. Demark-Wahnefried W, Werner C, Clipp EC, Guill AB, Bonner M, Jones LW, Rosoff PM. Survivors of childhood cancer and their guardians. Cancer. 2005b;103:2171–80.

63. Cohen J, Wakefield CE, Fleming CA, Gawthorne R, Tapsell LC, Cohn RJ. Dietary intake after treatment in child cancer survivors. Pediatr Blood Cancer. 2012;58:752–7.
64. Tylavsky FA, Smith K, Surprise H, Garland S, Yan X, McCammon E, Hudson MM, Pui CH, Kaste SC. Nutritional intake of long-term survivors of childhood acute lymphoblastic leukemia: evidence for bone health interventional opportunities. Pediatr Blood Cancer. 2010;55:1362–9.
65. Zhang F, Parsons S. Obesity in childhood cancer survivors: call for early weight management. Adv Nutr. 2015;6:611–9.
66. Natarajan L, Pu M, Fan J, Levine RA, Patterson RE, Thomson CA, Rock CL, Pierce JP. Measurement error of dietary self-report in intervention trials. Am J Epidemiol. 2010;172:819–27.
67. Garmey EG, Liu Q, Sklar CA, Meacham LR, Mertens AC, Stovall MA, Yasui Y, Robison LL, Oeffinger KC. Longitudinal changes in obesity and body mass index among adult survivors of childhood acute lymphoblastic leukemia: a report from the Childhood Cancer Survivor Study. J Clin Oncol. 2008;26:4639–45.
68. Zhang FF, Liu S, Chung M, Kelly MJ. Growth patterns during and after treatment in patients with pediatric ALL: a meta-analysis. Pediatr Blood Cancer. 2015;62:1452–60.
69. Gibson TM, Ehrhardt MJ, Ness KK. Obesity and metabolic syndrome among adult survivors of childhood leukemia. Curr Treat Options Oncol. 2016;17:1–13.
70. Guh D, Zhang W, Bansback N, Amarsi Z, Birmingham CL, Anis A. The incidence of co-morbidities related to obesity and overweight: a systematic review and meta-analysis. BMC Public Health. 2009;9:88.
71. Amankwah EK, Saenz AM, Hale GA, Brown PA. Association between body mass index at diagnosis and pediatric leukemia mortality and relapse: a systematic review and meta-analysis. Leuk Lymphoma. 2016;57:1140–8.
72. Butturini A, Dorey F, Gaynon P, Fu C, Franklin J. Obesity and body weight independently predict relapse and survival in preadolescents and teenagers with acute lymphoblastic leukemia (ALL). A retrospective analysis of five children cancer group (CCG) studies. Blood. 2004;104:284A.
73. Orgel E, Sposto R, Malvar J, Seibel NL, Ladas E, Gaynon PS, Freyer DR. Impact on survival and toxicity by duration of weight extremes during treatment for pediatric acute lymphoblastic leukemia: a report from the Children's Oncology Group. J Clin Oncol. 2014;32:1331–7.
74. Green DM, Cox CL, Zhu L, Krull KR, Srivastava DK, Stovall M, Nolan VG, Ness KK, Donaldson SS, Oeffinger KC, Meacham LR, Sklar CA, Armstrong GT, Robison LL. Risk factors for obesity in adult survivors of childhood cancer: a report from the Childhood Cancer Survivor Study. J Clin Oncol. 2012;30:246–55.
75. Pugh G, Hough R, Williams K, Gravestock HL, Fisher A. Lifestyle advice provision to teenage ad young adult cancer patients: the Perspective of Health Professionals in the UK Support Care. Cancer. 2017.; (in press).
76. Pugh G, Hough RE, Gravestock HL, Jackson SE, Fisher A. The health behavior information needs and preferences of teenage and young adult cancer survivors. J Adolesc Young Adult Oncol. 2017;6:318–26.
77. Armstrong GT, Oeffinger KC, Chen Y, Kawashima T, Yasui Y, Leisenring W, Stovall M, Chow EJ, Sklar CA, Mulrooney DA, Mertens AC, Border W, Durand J-B, Robison LL, Meacham LR. Modifiable risk factors and major cardiac events among adult survivors of childhood cancer. J Clin Oncol. 2013;31(29):3673–80.
78. Hall KD, Heymsfield SB, Kemnitz JW, Klein S, Schoeller DA, Speakman JR. Energy balance and its components: implications for body weight regulation. Am J Clin Nutr. 2012;95:989–94.
79. Jansen H, Postma A, Stolk RP, Kamps WA. Acute lymphoblastic leukemia and obesity: increased energy intake or decreased physical activity? Support Care Cancer. 2009;17:103–6.
80. Reilly JJ, Brougham M, Montgomery C, Richardson F, Kelly A, Gibson BE. Effect of glucocorticoid therapy on energy intake in children treated for acute lymphoblastic leukemia. J Clin Endocrinol Metab. 2001;86:3742–5.

81. von Deneen KM, Liu Y. Obesity as an addiction: why do the obese eat more? Maturitas. 2011;68:342–5.
82. Parkin DM, Boyd L, Walker LC. 16. The fraction of cancer attributable to lifestyle and environmental factors in the UK in 2010. Br J Cancer. 2011;105:S77–81.
83. Bishop JD, Killelea BK, Chagpar AB, Horowitz NR, Lannin DR. Smoking and breast cancer recurrence after breast conservation therapy. Int J Breast Cancer. 2014;2014:5.
84. Klosky J, Tyc V, Garces Webb D, Buscemi J, Klesges R, Hudson M. Emerging issues in smoking among adolescent and adult cancer survivors. Cancer. 2007;110:2408–19.
85. Kaul S, Veeranki SP, Rodriguez AM, Kuo YF. Cigarette smoking, comorbidity, and general health among survivors of adolescent and young adult cancer. Cancer. 2016;122:2895–905.
86. Emmons K, et al. Predictors of smoking initiation and cessation among childhood cancer survivors: a report from the childhood cancer survivor study. J Clin Oncol. 2002;20(6):1608–16.
87. Kahalley LS, Robinson LA, Tyc VL, Hudson MM, Leisenring W, Stratton K, Mertens AC, Zeltzer L, Robison LL, Hinds PS. Risk factors for smoking among adolescent survivors of childhood cancer: a report from the childhood cancer survivor study. Pediatr Blood Cancer. 2012;58:428–34.
88. Marjerrison S, Hendershot E, Empringham B, Nathan PC. Smoking, binge drinking, and drug use among childhood cancer survivors: a meta-analysis. Pediatr Blood Cancer. 2016;63(7):1254–63.
89. Rabin C. Review of health behaviors and their correlates among young adult cancer survivors. J Behav Med. 2011;34:41–52.
90. Gibson TM, Liu W, Armstrong GT, Srivastava DK, Hudson MM, Leisenring WM, Mertens AC, Klesges RC, Oeffinger KC, Nathan PC, Robison LL. Longitudinal smoking patterns in survivors of childhood cancer: an update from the Childhood Cancer Survivor Study. Cancer. 2015;121:4035–43.
91. Ford JS, Puleo E, Sprunck-Harrild K, deMoor J, Emmons KM. Perceptions of risk among childhood and young adult cancer survivors who smoke. Support Care Cancer. 2014;22:2207–17.
92. Hollen PJ, Hobbie WL, Donnangelo SF, Shannon S, Erickson J. Substance use risk behaviors and decision-making skills among cancer-surviving adolescents. J Pediatr Oncol Nurs. 2007;24:264–73.
93. Britton A, Ben-Shlomo Y, Benzeval M, Kuh D, Bell S. Life course trajectories of alcohol consumption in the United Kingdom using longitudinal data from nine cohort studies. BMC Med. 2015;13:47. https://doi.org/10.1186/s12916-015-0273-z.
94. Bauld C, Toumbourou JW, Anderson V, Coffey C, Olsson CA. Health-risk behaviours among adolescent survivors of childhood cancer. Pediatr Blood Cancer. 2005;45:706–15.
95. Lown EA, Goldsby R, Mertens AC, Greenfield T, Bond J, Whitton J, Korcha R, Robison LL, Zeltzer LK. Alcohol consumption patterns and risk factors among childhood cancer survivors compared to siblings and general population peers. Addiction (Abingdon, England). 2008;103:1139–48.
96. Martin A, Kadan-Lottick N. Hazardous drinking: childhood cancer survivors at heightened risk as young adults. Pediatr Blood Cancer. 2012;58:161–2.
97. Rebholz CE, Kuehni CE, Strippoli M-PF, Rueegg CS, Michel G, Hengartner H, Bergstraesser E, von der Weid NX, for the Swiss Pediatric Oncology, Group. Alcohol consumption and binge drinking in young adult childhood cancer survivors. Pediatr Blood Cancer. 2012;58:256–64.
98. Szalda DE, Brumley LD, Danielson CK, Schwartz LA. Exploratory analyses of substance use in adolescents with and without cancer. J Adolesc Young Adult Oncol. 2013;2:77–82.
99. Kricker A, Armstrong BK. Epidemiology of sun exposure and skin cancer. Cancer Surv. 1996;26:133–53.
100. Balk SJ. Ultraviolet radiation: a hazard to children and adolescents. Pediatrics. 2011;127:e791–817.
101. Perkins JL, Liu Y, Mitby PA, Neglia JP, Hammond S, Stovall M, Meadows AT, Hutchinson R, Dreyer ZE, Robison LL, Mertens AC. Nonmelanoma skin cancer in survivors of childhood and adolescent cancer: a report from the Childhood Cancer Survivor Study. J Clin Oncol. 2005;23:3733–41.

102. Tercyak KP, Donze JR, Prahlad S, Mosher RB, Shad AT. Multiple behavioral risk factors among adolescent survivors of childhood cancer in the Survivor Health and Resilience Education (SHARE) program. Pediatr Blood Cancer. 2006;47:825–30.
103. Zwemer E, Werchniak A, Recklitis C, Mahler HIM. Sun exposure in young adult cancer survivors on and off the beach: results from Project REACH. J Cancer Surviv. 2012;6:63–71.
104. Buchanan N, Leisenring W, Mitby PA, Meadows AT, Robison LL, Hudson MM, Mertens AC. Behaviors associated with ultraviolet radiation exposure in a cohort of adult survivors of childhood and adolescent cancer. Cancer. 2009;115:4374–84.
105. Barakat L, Galtieri L, Szalda D, Schwartz L. Assessing the psychosocial needs and program preferences of adolescents and young adults with cancer. Support Care Cancer. 2016;24:823–32.
106. D'Agostino NM, Penney A, Zebrack B. Providing developmentally appropriate psychosocial care to adolescent and young adult cancer survivors. Cancer. 2011;117:2329–34.
107. Love B, Moskowitz MC, Crook B, Thompson CM, Donovan-Kicken E, Stegenga K, Macpherson CF, Johnson RH. Defining adolescent and young adult (AYA) exercise and nutrition needs: concerns communicated in an online cancer support community. Patient Educ Couns. 2013;92:130–3.
108. Pugh G, Hough R, Gravestock HL, Haddrell J, Beeken RJ, Fisher A. The lifestyle information and intervention preferences of teenage and young adult cancer survivors: a Qualitative Study. Cancer Nurs. 2017.; [Epub ahead of print].
109. Lie HC, Loge JH, Fosså SD, Hamre HM, Hess SL, Mellblom AV, Ruud E, Finset A. Providing information about late effects after childhood cancer: lymphoma survivors' preferences for what, how and when. Patient Educ Couns. 2015;98:604–11.
110. Wurz A, Brunet J. Promoting physical activity in adolescent cancer survivors. Univ Ottawa J Med. 2015;5:29.
111. Morgan S, Davies S, Palmer S, Plaster M. Sex, drugs, and rock 'n' roll: caring for adolescents and young adults with cancer. J Clin Oncol. 2010;28:4825–30.
112. Pugh G, Gravestock HL, Hough RE, King WM, Wardle J, Fisher A. Health behavior change interventions for teenage and young adult cancer survivors: a systematic review. J Adolesc Young Adult Oncol. 2016;5:91–105.
113. Berg CJ, Stratton E, Giblin J, Esiashvili N, Mertens A. Pilot results of an online intervention targeting health promoting behaviors among young adult cancer survivors. Psychooncology. 2014;23:1196–9.
114. Hollen PJ, Hobbie WL, Finley SM. Testing the effects of a decision-making and risk-reduction program for cancer-surviving adolescents. Oncol Nurs Forum. 1999;26:1475–86.
115. Mays D, Black JD, Mosher RB, Heinly A, Shad AT, Tercyak KP. Efficacy of the survivor health and resilience education (SHARE) program to improve bone health behaviors among adolescent survivors of childhood cancer. Ann Behav Med. 2011;42:91–8.
116. Valle CG, Tate DF, Mayer DK, Allicock M, Cai J. A randomized trial of a Facebook-based physical activity intervention for young adult cancer survivors. J Cancer Surviv. 2013;7:355–68.
117. Hollen PJ, Tyc VL, Donnangelo SF, Shannon SV, O'Laughlen MC, Hinton I, Smolkin ME, Petroni GR. A substance use decision aid for medically at-risk adolescents: results of a randomized controlled trial for cancer-surviving adolescents. Cancer Nurs. 2013;36:355–67.
118. Belanger LJ, Mummery WK, Clark AM, Courneya KS. Effects of targeted print materials on physical activity and quality of life in young adult cancer survivors during and after treatment: an exploratory randomized controlled trial. J Adolesc Young Adult Oncol. 2014;3:83–91.
119. Cox CL, McLaughlin RA, Rai SN, Steen BD, Hudson MM. Adolescent survivors: a secondary analysis of a clinical trial targeting behavior change. Pediatr Blood Cancer. 2005;45:144–54.
120. Hudson MM, Tyc VL, Srivastava DK, Gattuso J, Quargnenti A, Crom DB, Hinds P. Multi-component behavioral intervention to promote health protective behaviors in childhood cancer survivors: the Protect Study. Med Pediatr Oncol. 2002;39:2–11.
121. Abraham C, Kelly MP, West R, Michie S. The UK national institute for health and clinical excellence public health guidance on behaviour change: a brief introduction. Psychol Health Med. 2009;14:1–8.

122. Michie S, van Stralen MM, West R. The behaviour change wheel: a new method for characterising and designing behaviour change interventions. Implement Sci. 2011;6:42.
123. Michie S, Richardson M, Johnston M, Abraham C, Francis J, Hardeman W, Eccles MP, Cane J, Wood CE. The behavior change technique taxonomy (v1) of 93 hierarchically clustered techniques: building an international consensus for the reporting of behavior change interventions. Ann Behav Med. 2013;46:81–95.
124. Ruland CM, Hamilton GA, Schjodt-Osmo B. The complexity of symptoms and problems experienced in children with cancer: a review of the literature. J Pain Symptom Manage. 2009;37:403–18.
125. Tyc, VL, et al. Intervention to reduce intentions to use tobacco among pediatric cancer survivors. J Clin Oncol. 2003;21(7):1366–72.
126. Cushing CC, Steele RG. A meta-analytic review of eHealth interventions for pediatric health promoting and maintaining behaviors. J Pediatr Psychol. 2010;35(9):937–49.
127. Bandura A. Social foundations of thought and action: a social cognitive theory. Englewood Cliffs, NJ: Prentice-Hall; 1986.
128. Tyc VL, Hudson MM, Hinds P. Health promotion interventions for adolescent cancer survivors. Cogn Behav Pract. 1999;6:128–36.
129. Keats MR, Culos-Reed SN, Courneya KS, McBride M. Understanding physical activity in adolescent cancer survivors: an application of the theory of planned behavior. Psychooncology. 2007;16:448–57.
130. Nagler RH. Adverse outcomes associated with media exposure to contradictory nutrition messages. J Health Commun. 2014;19:24–40.
131. Tan ASL, Lee C-J, Chae J. Exposure to health (Mis)information: lagged effects on young adults' health behaviors and potential pathways. J Commun. 2015;65:674–98.
132. Hudson MM, Findlay S. Health-risk behaviors and health promotion in adolescent and young adult cancer survivors. Cancer. 2006;107:1695–701.
133. Hawkins RP, Kreuter M, Resnicow K, Fishbein M, Dijkstra A. Understanding tailoring in communicating about health. Health Educ Res. 2008;23:454–66.
134. Noar S, et al. Does tailoring matter? Meta-analytic review of tailored print health behavior change interventions. Psychol Bull. 2007;133(4):673–93.
135. Cohen DA, Scribner RA, Farley TA. A structural model of health behavior: a pragmatic approach to explain and influence health behaviors at the population level. Prev Med. 2000;30:146–54.
136. Gilliam MB, Madan-Swain A, Whelan K, Tucker DC, Demark-Wahnefried W, Schwebel DC. Social, demographic, and medical influences on physical activity in child and adolescent cancer survivors. J Pediatr Psychol. 2012;37:198–208.
137. Arroyave WD, Clipp EC, Miller PE, Jones LW, Ward DS, Bonner MJ, Rosoff PM, Snyder DC, Demark-Wahnefried W. Childhood cancer survivors' perceived barriers to improving exercise and dietary behaviors. Oncol Nurs Forum. 2008;35:121–30.
138. Emmons KM, Butterfield RM, Puleo E, Park ER, Mertens A, Gritz ER, Lahti M, Li FP. Smoking among participants in the childhood cancer survivors cohort: the Partnership for Health Study. J Clin Oncol. 2003;21:189–96.
139. Brannon E, Cushing C. A systematic review: is there an app for that? translational science of pediatric behavior change for physical activity and dietary interventions. J Pediatr Psychol. 2015;40:373–84.
140. Whittingham JRD, Ruiter RAC, Castermans D, Huiberts A, Kok G. Designing effective health education materials: experimental pre-testing of a theory-based brochure to increase knowledge. Health Educ Res. 2008;23:414–26.
141. Bava S, Tapert SF. Adolescent brain development and the risk for alcohol and other drug problems. Neuropsychol Rev. 2010;20:398–413.
142. Wetherill R, Tapert SF. Adolescent brain development, substance use, and psychotherapeutic change. Psychol Addict Behav. 2013;27:393–402.
143. Moore S, Gullone E. Predicting adolescent risk behavior using a personalized cost-benefit analysis. J Youth Adolesc. 1996;25:343–59.

144. Parsons JT, Siegel AW, Cousins JH. Late adolescent risk-taking: effects of perceived benefits and perceived risks on behavioral intentions and behavioral change. J Adolesc. 1997;20:381–92.
145. Lawson PJ, Flocke SA. Teachable moments for health behavior change: a concept analysis. Patient Educ Couns. 2009;76:25–30.
146. Barnes M, Plaisance E, Hanks L, Casazza K. Pre-habilitation-promoting exercise in adolescent and young adult cancer survivors for improving lifelong health – a narrative review. Cancer Res Front. 2016;2:22–32.
147. Demark-Wahnefried W, Aziz NM, Rowland JH, Pinto BM. Riding the crest of the teachable moment: promoting long-term health after the diagnosis of cancer. J Clin Oncol. 2005a;23:5814–30.
148. Kopp LM, Gastelum Z, Guerrero CH, Howe CL, Hingorani P, Hingle M. Lifestyle behavior interventions delivered using technology in childhood, adolescent, and young adult cancer survivors: a systematic review. Pediatr Blood Cancer. 2017;64(1):13–7.
149. Webb LT, et al. Using the internet to promote health behavior change: a systematic review and meta-analysis of the impact of theoretical basis, use of behavior change techniques, and mode of delivery on efficacy. J Med Internet Res. 2010;12(1):e4.
150. Rabin C, et al. Recruiting young adult cancer survivors for behavioral research. J Clin Psychol Med Settings. 2013;20(1):33–6.
151. Moody L, et al. Web-based self-management for young cancer survivors: consideration of user requirements and barriers to implementation. J Cancer Surviv. 2015;9(2):188–200.
152. Pugh G, McCann L. Assessing the quality, feasibility, and efficacy of electronic patient platforms designed to support adolescents and young adults with cancer: a systematic review protocol. JMIR Res Protoc. 2017;6:e4.

6 AYA Survivorship

Victoria Grandage, Susan Mehta, and Rachael Windsor

6.1 Introduction

Since the 1970s, the incidence of cancer in 15–24 year olds in the UK has increased by 55% with 2,405 new cases each year from 2012 to 2014. Recent data indicates that more than 80% of teenagers and young adults diagnosed with cancer will now survive for longer than 5 years [1]. Overall survival has almost doubled in the last four decades, although this ranges from almost 100% for thyroid carcinomas to 55% for acute myeloid leukaemia or bone sarcoma [2]. Consequently, the majority of adolescent and young adult cancer patients will become long-term survivors. Most will have been treated with combinations of multi-agent chemotherapy, radiotherapy and surgery and may develop health complications that become apparent at the end of treatment or many years later, so-called 'Late Effects'.

An in-depth review of every systemic treatment-related adverse effect is beyond the scope of this chapter and the authors direct you to a number of excellent reviews on the subject [3–6]. Notwithstanding the paucity of robust, research-based evidence on late effects in adolescent and young adult (AYA) cancer survivors, this chapter aims to explore the impact of age on treatment-related toxicity, report on national and international strategies for improving the long term care of AYA cancer survivors and provides practical advice on delivering AYA-specific survivorship care. The chapter will also reflect collective decades of medical and nursing experience accrued in providing complex medical and psychosocial care to childhood, AYA and adult survivors within the largest survivorship service in the UK.

The burden of late effects after childhood cancer is dependent on tumour, treatment and host-related factors, such as age at diagnosis, gender and genetic predisposition. Detailed knowledge of these has been gained from two important cohort

V. Grandage (✉) • S. Mehta • R. Windsor
University College London Hospitals NHS Foundation Trust, London, UK
e-mail: victoria.grandage@uclh.nhs.uk; susan.mehta@uclh.nhs.uk; rachael.windsor@uclh.nhs.uk

J. Chisholm et al. (eds.), *A Practical Approach to the Care of Adolescents and Young Adults with Cancer*, https://doi.org/10.1007/978-3-319-66173-5_6

studies in the USA and UK. These cohorts have focused predominantly on adult survivors of childhood and adolescent cancers and data specific to survivors of AYA cancer is lacking. At 30 years after a cancer diagnosis, the US Childhood Cancer Survivor Study (CCSS) reported 73% patients had at least one chronic health condition; classified as severe, disabling or life-threatening in over 40% [7]. Data derived from the CCSS is being further scrutinized to identify survivor sub-populations at high risk for specific organ toxicity that can be used to inform clinical screening practices. For example, the data has revealed that females aged >12 years at diagnosis are at increased risk of acute ovarian failure and those aged >15 years are at increased risk of hypothyroidism [8]. The UK Department of Health, National Institute for Health and Clinical Excellence and the National Institute for Health Research are currently collaborating on a large population-based investigation addressing the spectrum of fatal and non-fatal adverse health outcomes among survivors of cancer diagnosed in teenage and young adulthood. This should provide an evidence base for all aspects of clinical follow-up, screening protocols and professional education [9].

Survivors may require lifelong holistic care focusing on medical issues, psychosocial, educational and vocational implications of living beyond cancer. Adolescent and young adult cancer patients frequently experience diagnostic delays [10, 11], manifest more aggressive tumour biology [12], experience inferior access to clinical trials [13] and excessive treatment-related toxicity [14]. These factors, coupled with the unknown long-term impact of novel therapies, mean that AYA survivorship is a rapidly evolving field.

6.2 Do AYA Cancer Survivors Experience Late Treatment-Related Toxicities That Are Distinct from Childhood Cancer Survivors?

Woodward et al. undertook an extensive literature review to determine whether the risk of a particular treatment late-effect was related to the age and type of cancer diagnosis [15]. Medline data was extracted from a 10 year period and strikingly, within this time frame, no study primarily aimed to correlate the AYA age group to late treatment effects. Despite the paucity of data, the authors reported a differential risk of late effects in AYA survivors that, in some instances, was dependent on the primary cancer diagnosis.

Within the CCSS cohort, second malignancy was one of the highest treatment related risks [7]. Hudson et al. reviewed data derived from all CCSS investigations and reported an increased risk of any subsequent malignant histology with young age at diagnosis [16]. However, the challenge lies in discerning a potential contribution of age at diagnosis against a background of increasing cancer risk with age. Woodward et al. found no literature reports of increased risk of subsequent primary cancer in AYA survivors of haematological malignancies or central nervous system tumours [15]. On the contrary, the risk of second malignant neoplasm was higher in leukaemia and lymphoma patients diagnosed <10 years compared to older patients and the risk of glioma was increased with young age at initial therapy [16]. However, AYA survivors of germ cell tumours had a slightly greater excess risk of second cancer compared to those diagnosed in childhood [17]. Overall, survivors of germ cell tumours diagnosed at <30 years are at significantly increased risk of second cancers, particularly gastric, pancreatic and connective tissue tumours and the risk at age 20 years is even higher [18].

According to Woodward et al., a diagnosis of haematological cancer before adolescence confers a greater risk for cardiovascular disorders than in older adulthood [15]. Several studies found the risk of congestive heart failure, angina and death from myocardial infarction decreased with increasing age at first treatment [19–21] although in Hodgkin's disease, a higher risk of radiation-induced ischaemic heart disease was associated with increasing age at diagnosis [22]. The authors postulated that higher relative rates of cardiovascular disease observed in those treated at a younger age may be due to low background incidence and increased vulnerability of immature cardiovascular tissue to chemo- and radiotherapy exposure. In germ cell tumour survivors, the risk of premature myocardial infarction was a particular risk for AYA compared to older adults [23].

Other common late effects including changes in bone mineral density and obesity showed conflicting results, perhaps reflecting the paucity of studies in this age group. However, some late effects were strikingly increased in AYA cancer survivors. Hypothyroidism was one such example, with a relative risk of 1.5 in patients aged >15 years at diagnosis compared to a younger age group [24]. Osteonecrosis was strongly related to age of diagnosis in survivors of acute lymphoblastic leukaemia with an incidence of 2.8% in those aged over 16 years at diagnosis compared to 0.2% of patients aged less than 10 at diagnosis [25].

On behalf of the AYACSS, Bright et al. recently investigated the risk of hospitalisation for a cerebrovascular event in 5 year survivors aged from 15 to 39 years at cancer diagnosis. The risk of hospitalisation was 40% higher than expected; the highest risk seen in survivors of CNS tumours, head and neck tumours and leukaemia. Among CNS tumour survivors, the risk of cerebral infarction increased with age but remained high across all ages for survivors of head and neck tumours [26].

Psychological morbidity and poor social functioning in AYA survivors is a familiar challenge faced by clinicians involved in their care. Tai et al. found 20% of AYA survivors had experienced >14 days of poor mental health in the previous 30 days compared to 10% of respondents with no history of cancer [27]. Furthermore, 24% of survivors were out of work or unable to work compared to 14% of controls. They also reported a significantly higher prevalence of smoking, obesity, chronic ill health and lack of medical care due to cost in the AYA survivors. Barnett et al. undertook a systematic review of psychosocial outcomes and interventions in cancer survivors diagnosed as an AYA and reported high levels of unmet emotional and psychological need, antidepressant use, symptoms of post-traumatic stress, depression and anxiety and fear of recurrence [28]. Moreover, survivors feel underprepared for survivorship and find it difficult to come to terms with being "neither sick nor healthy" [29]. Warner et al. reviewed social wellbeing in AYA with cancer, revealing difficulties related to employment, educational attainment and financial stability. Furthermore, developing and maintaining peer, family, intimate and marital relationships was problematic [30].

6.3 Aims of Survivorship Care

The aims of long term follow up/survivorship care are to identify and manage treatment-related toxicities, enabling the patient to reach their optimal physical, psychological and social potential. Survivorship care should aim to minimise further deterioration in established organ dysfunction but also provide surveillance for new predictable systemic late effects including second malignancies. The management of symptoms such as pain, fear, fatigue and psychological distress is a very common challenge. Such care should also address concerns relating to education and employment and facilitate coordination between all healthcare providers to ensure that all the survivor's needs are met.

AYA cancer survivors present unique issues relating to their age. Not all patients will have been treated within specialist AYA treatment centres with an established long-term follow up service. Historically, those treated within paediatric services or currently within an AYA service are more likely to have access to dedicated late-effects follow-up. Surveillance may be less rigorous outside such services and medical teams may be unfamiliar with national and international guidelines about recommended surveillance related to specific treatments. Patients in this age group are more likely to be geographically mobile, suffer isolation from their peers and are more likely to express concerns about fertility. As a group they also have a tendency to see themselves as invincible and may not engage in follow up until they are experiencing health problems. It is therefore important for them to have a point of contact with an expert team when needed.

Predictors of attendance at specialised survivor clinics include female gender, higher treatment intensity, radiation therapy and higher socio-economic status [31]. In this study, only 43.3% of the cohort attended an adult follow-up clinic and living more than 50 km from the clinic meant follow up was less likely. Potential barriers included cost of travel, lack of clear follow up schema, wishing to move on with life, fear of recurrent cancer diagnosis and competing life responsibilities. Alternative models of follow are required that allow flexible appointment times or virtual follow up and clear follow up guidelines need to be developed and communicated with young people, primary and secondary care providers.

6.4 Transition

The need for good transitional care for adolescents with chronic conditions originating in childhood is becoming well recognised and successful transfer from paediatric to adult health services is a complex journey involving many key elements. A position statement from the Society for Adolescent Medicine in 1993 defined transition as "the purposeful, planned movement of adolescents and young adults with chronic physical and medical conditions from child-centred to adult-orientated healthcare systems" [32], but it has taken many years for transitional care to be implemented in practice. Using a systematic and rigorous evidence-based approach, PanCare, a multidisciplinary pan-European collaborative late-effects network, recently re-defined transitional care of childhood cancer survivors as; "Transition of childhood cancer survivors is an active, planned, co-ordinated, comprehensive, multi-disciplinary process to enable childhood and adolescent cancer survivors to effectively and harmoniously transfer form child-centred to adult-oriented healthcare systems. The transition of care process should be flexible, developmentally appropriate and consider the developmental, medical, psychosocial, educational and vocational needs of survivors, their families and care-givers, and promote a healthy lifestyle and self-management" [33].

It is widely accepted that planned transitional care should be fully integrated into a well-managed cancer survivorship program to ensure teenagers and young adults transfer safely and effectively from AYA to adult services where they will need to negotiate adult healthcare independently. Transitional care should be implemented as the risk of cancer recurrence diminishes and young people move to long-term surveillance.

Transitional care was therefore included on the model pathway developed during the National Cancer Survivorship Initiative (NCSI) [34]. Time and extent of the expert input required for a successful transition are dependent on many factors including diagnosis, the age of the young person, and nature of the original diagnosis, degree of parental involvement, the patient's knowledge of their diagnosis and burden of treatment-related sequelae. Transfer to age appropriate services is only part of the process as there are multiple transition points in the aftercare pathway, all of which require appropriate planning, preparation and patient preparation.

Expert nurse-led transitional care can provide young people with information about their previous cancer diagnosis and risk for developing long term effects of treatment, empowering them to manage potential long-term sequelae as they transfer to adult healthcare services. Transitional care is one of the core competencies for nursing in long-term follow-up. Nurses can lead transitional care and this is recognized in many professional and department of health publications including the RCN nursing competency document for late effects care [35]. Extensive planning and adequate administrative support is essential for successful transition clinics and this was identified during the NCSI testing of models of care [34, 36].

Transitional care is a complex process and successful completion involves many key elements. Transfer between age appropriate services such as from paediatric to AYA or onward to adult services is only part of the process, as there are multiple transition points in the aftercare pathway, all of which require appropriate planning and preparation: These include:

- End of treatment
- Surveillance for disease recurrence
- Surveillance for late effects of treatment
- Discharge to supported self-management

The NCSI was supported by NHS Improvement in a partnership between The Department of Health, and Macmillan Cancer Support. The Children and Young People (CYP) workstream aimed to ensure that children and young people living with and beyond the acute phase of cancer treatment would be offered the care and support they needed to lead as healthy and active a life as possible, for as long as possible. The workstream tested and implemented models of care that aimed to ensure consistency for all patients. Both national clinical leads and patient representatives endorsed a dynamic teenage and adult aftercare pathway. The design of the pathway was intended to be adapted for use by individual services to ensure key elements of care were provided [34].

Within the NCSI, a model of transitional care was piloted at Great Ormond Street Hospital, London, UK [37]. Young people were referred to a nurse-led transition clinic and encouraged to attend these hospital appointments independently of their parents. At the appointment they received information about their cancer treatment, risks for developing late effects, advice about leading a healthy life style and how to negotiate adult health care. The aim was to empower young people to seek timely interventions if late effects of treatment occurred, make healthy lifestyle choices and manage their own healthcare as young adults. As an outcome measure, young people were asked to complete a questionnaire about the transition appointment. This new initiative and the service was positively evaluated by the young people attending. Young people valued an opportunity to learn more about their cancer diagnosis and reported improved knowledge after the appointment. They also preferred a face to face consultation in addition to receiving written information. General practitioners (GP) reported the value of receiving in-depth written information [36, 37].

Establishing that good transitional care improves long-term outcomes for childhood and AYA cancer is challenging compared to other long term conditions. For example, if a patient with a renal transplant stops attending appointments, the outcome may be catastrophic and fairly immediate. Transplant survival data after childhood chronic kidney disease therefore offers a powerful argument for providing transitional care [38]. If appropriate information about past treatment, risk for developing late effects and advice on self-management is not provided to AYA cancer survivors, the outcome may still be catastrophic but delayed for many years. However from experience, we know that those young people and adults treated for cancer who have received planned transitional care, seek expert advice when faced with new health concerns that may be associated with past treatment. General practitioners who have received treatment summaries and care plans are alerted to emerging health concerns and are able to contact a late effects service for advice. Treatment summaries and care plans are an essential component of good transitional care [35].

6.5 Consequences of Treatment and Transition

The effects of treatment for childhood, teenage and young adult cancer are varied and include educational and psychological difficulties, organ dysfunction and endocrinopathies that develop over time, often occurring decades after treatment has been completed. It is difficult to gauge the impact of transitional care on long term outcomes but young people have a right to be well informed. Older adults treated for teenage cancer decades previously, frequently deal with complex late effects of treatment but may have never received expert preparation for the consequences of that treatment. Complex multiple health problems that have emerged over time may be entirely unexpected. Good transitional care and education enables prompt diagnosis of emerging late effects, ameliorating extreme levels of distress. A GP will recognize how to support an adult patient with a disease such as asthma or diabetes that originates in childhood and then continues into adult life as both conditions occur in childhood and adulthood. However a young adult with a multitude of symptoms after childhood cancer may not have a diagnosis made promptly. Indeed, sometimes their symptoms may not be recognised and diagnosed until they are referred to an expert service.

6.6 Paediatric, AYA and Adult Services Working Together at Transition

It is essential for services across both paediatric, teenage and adult healthcare to understand the purpose of follow-up depending on where the young person is on the pathway. An agreed operational policy written together by paediatric, AYA and adult services should identify the needs of young adults in relation to their follow-up for late effects surveillance in an age appropriate service.

"Think transition" is a freely available document that emphasises the importance of transitional care across many childhood conditions that continue into adult life. There is an extensive section about transition and childhood cancer [39].

6.7 Treatment Summaries and Care Plans

All patients (0–24 years) should receive a treatment summary and care plan at the end of treatment [40]. This should detail patient demographics, diagnosis, date and age at diagnosis, diagnostic staging, family history or congenital conditions and relapse history. It should also detail treatment protocols used, including chemotherapy agents received and cumulative doses. Radiotherapy fields, dose and fractionation, surgical and transfusion history are also essential. If the patient has had a stem cell transplant, the donor source, conditioning and graft versus host disease (GVHD) prophylaxis should be recorded. Significant complications, grade and extent of GVHD and end of treatment organ toxicity assessment should also be documented. The care plan should detail the frequency and intensity of surveillance required for established and predicted late effects. Best practice requires the treatment summary and care plan to be available at the end of treatment, revised at key points on the pathway including transition into long term follow up and discharge to self-management [36].

Casillas et al. studied cancer survivors aged 18–39, with self-reports indicating that 71 percent attended an oncology survivorship clinic at the time of the survey, 48 percent did not have a treatment summary, and 55 percent had not received a survivorship care plan. 70% felt an oncologist was the “most important” provider for test and treatment decisions and 10 percent reported receiving care in a “shared-care model” that involved both primary care physicians and oncologists [41].

It is important that the patient understands this summary and has a copy to present at any medical review outside the long-term follow up service. The patient will need to act as their own advocate when being reviewed by teams not familiar with their treatment and late effects. These discussions can be used as teachable moments to educate survivors about treatment and its’ potential impact on their future health thereby empowering patients by educating them on their particular surveillance requirements (e.g. breast surveillance for women who have received chest radiotherapy or echocardiographic monitoring after treatment with anthracyclines).

6.8 Health Promotion

Cancer treatment confers an increased risk of premature mortality secondary to coronary artery disease, diabetes mellitus, cerebrovascular disease, hypertension and hyperlipidaemia. With this knowledge, it becomes clear that behaviour modification is an essential part of long-term follow up. Smoking prevention programmes are important because of the synergistic risk of lung cancer and the risk of lung disease with drugs such as bleomycin [42].

Clinicians advocate a healthy balanced diet and regular exercise for weight management, maintenance of bone density and a feeling of well-being. Patients should be advised against drinking excess alcohol to due to its’ negative effects on mood, causing depression and anxiety as well as leading to an increased risk of head and neck, breast, oesophageal and liver cancers.

Patients may not surprisingly question, “What’s in it for me?” and in particular, “Are cancer survivors at extra risk from certain health behaviours?” A lack of evidence makes a robust response challenging. Indeed, a recent systematic review aimed to appraise the effects of health promotion and psychological interventions for AYA after cancer treatment [43]. The authors found no conclusive evidence favouring specific interventions due to the lack of high-quality studies although they did identify promising interventions to be implemented in future. To address this in part, evidence-based guidance on health promotion is currently being compiled by PanCare (personal communication). PanCare aims to reduce the frequency, severity and impact of late side-effects of the treatment of children and adolescents with cancer (www. Pancare.eu). It was founded in 2008 and grew from informal collaborations of professionals and national groups involved in long-term follow-up. With an estimated 300,000–500,000 childhood cancer survivors in Europe [44], the Network aim was simple—to perform collaborative research and establish a research resource to try and answer many of the questions relating to late effects of treatment. The long-term strategic aim was to achieve equity of access to holistic care, ensuring that every European survivor of childhood and adolescent cancer receives optimal long-term care. Applying a robust, standardised evidence-based approach, the consortium has so far published guidance on transition, gonadotoxicity and surveillance for breast cancer and cardiomyopathy [33, 45–48].

Some thought needs to be given to how information in a treatment summary and care plan is delivered. It is important to be proactive in the delivery of information and honest about the risks to enable young people to make healthy life style choices. Modification of risky health behaviours is important but health care professionals need to be mindful that survivors' hope of a normal life is not diminished and that they are not isolated from their peers [49].

6.9 Models of Survivorship Care

The challenge of survivorship care is to design a flexible service with capacity to meet the health needs of an increasing number of survivors. Each region will have different local health needs and resources and so 'one size' does not fit all. There is not the capacity to provide face to face lifelong follow up for all survivors of AYA cancer. The best model for follow up is uncertain and models need to be developed and formally evaluated. Models of care may be classified depending on the setting of care, who is carrying out the care and may also be disease specific.

Much can be learnt from paediatric cancer survivors although many may be lost in transition to adult late effects services. As time elapses, survivors are more likely to use primary care and not infrequently find their own route back into a secondary or tertiary service. As patients age, there is an increase in co-morbidities meaning an increase in healthcare providers. This will impact further on time off work or away from education lending value to models of multidisciplinary follow up.

Wallace et al. described three levels of care based on the intensity of treatment received by the survivor [50]. Level 1 patients were treated with surgery alone or low risk chemotherapy and were at low risk of long term sequelae. These patients could safely be discharged from the long-term follow up service into the care of their GP. Although there are an increasing number of survivors, it is likely that each GP or local health provider will only see a handful of survivors of AYA cancer. Therefore, for the primary care team to be involved in the management of these patients, there would need to be clear guidance and follow up pathways as well as a single contact point at the Principal Treatment Centre for clinical advice. Treatment summaries and care plans are essential for safe transfer to primary care. Level 3 patients are those who have received intensive chemo-radiotherapy such as survivors of bone marrow transplant, brain and bone tumours and who will require expert medically-led follow up every 1–2 years. A group of patients remain that may benefit from clinical follow up, nurse or doctor led every 1–2 years (level 2). It should be emphasised that the risk of psychosocial late effects does not always relate to the intensity of treatment. Even patients who have had lower intensity treatments are at risk and this may relate to having a cancer diagnosis, disruption of schooling and family dynamics.

There is a significant variation across the UK in the provision of long term follow up, with some adults continuing to be followed up by paediatric oncologists/haematologists, others being followed up in a specific adult long-term follow up service and a proportion having no follow up at all. These differences need to be addressed at a national level.

All patients should have access to high quality survivorship care. Miedema et al. studied survivors diagnosed with cancer as young adults and reported a lack of age-specific survivorship care, such as fertility treatment; family, couples, and sexuality counselling; and assistance with re-entry into the workplace [51]. This can be achieved by promotion of successful models of survivorship care, promoting ways to ensure that treatment summaries and care plans are completed and shared with the survivors and healthcare providers. There are currently no service specifications for survivors of AYA cancer and these should be developed along with quality metrics. The best model of late effects care for survivors of AYA cancer is uncertain although a variety of models have been described. Kain et al. evaluated a joint adult/paediatric clinic for cancer survivors and suggested this approach provided continuity of care and reduced the incidence of lost to follow up (4% vs. 43–45% reported in the literature) [52]. Opportunities should be made to expand survivorship related education and training resources for all clinical staff including allied health professionals (Table 6.1).

Evidence based guidelines should be developed, disseminated and adhered to. Guidelines may be therapy based, disease based or organ based [53–56] and are clinically valuable in providing guidance for individualized patient care plans based on treatment burden. The International Late Effects of Childhood Cancer Guideline Harmonization Group, IGHG, is a worldwide endeavor to collaborate in guideline development to optimize care in childhood and adolescent cancer survivors. They are developing pan-European evidence-based guidelines for monitoring and surveillance of late effects [45–48]. The guidance needs to be freely available to all healthcare providers who provide care to cancer survivors and can form a foundation to develop quality metrics.

Providing survivorship care requires a variety of approaches to meet the needs of the growing population of survivors. Determining the model of survivorship care needs to take into consideration the practice setting, the complexity of the patients, their needs and risks. As discussed above, routine follow up may not be necessary for all patients. Recurrence of the underlying disease or emergence of late effects frequently occurs between appointments and may be identified by the patient themselves. Follow up pathways should be risk stratified based on the treatment summary and care plan. The care plan should be dynamic, taking into consideration the treatment as well as the personal circumstances which may change.

Supported self -management (SSM) empowers patients to play a key role in managing their own health in partnership with their medical team. This requires information and support from the team, including discussion of treatment summary and care plan, advice on necessary surveillance and coordination of care across different settings. Some patients, particularly those that have been followed since childhood, find this transition daunting and require additional emotional support and reassurance. They should have the ability to re-access the service promptly if a problem arises. There is evidence that this approach can have a beneficial effect on patient's health, social outcomes, personal experience and use of services [57].

A multidisciplinary 'one stop shop' approach to follow up has been shown to improve outcomes [58, 59]. In this setting, care is usually provided by multiple specialist teams in a separate area. The team will often comprise of an oncologist/haematologist and endocrinologist, but may also include cardiology, psychology, nephrology and fertility experts. This method of follow-up is suited to the intensively treated survivors of childhood and adolescent cancers, e.g. bone marrow transplant survivors. It has the advantage for the patients that multiple appointments can be provided on the same day in the same location. It provides ready access to specialists committed to survivorship care. It improves communication and coordination between the specialists; however it is resource and time intensive and not all centres will have access to a wider multidisciplinary team.

Despite increasing recognition of its importance, some young adults will not have access to a late effects service. For them, third sector support is vital, through initiatives such as the Macmillan Recovery Package (https://be.macmillan.org.uk/be/s-689-recovery-package.aspx). This is a series of key interventions designed to improve the lives of people living with and beyond cancer and includes a holistic needs assessment, treatment summary, health and wellbeing events and a GP-led cancer care review within 6 months of diagnosis.

Multidisciplinary team meetings are an integral part of cancer care: however they are often difficult to set up, challenging to maintain attendance and they are costly both in time and money. Not all centres offering late effects follow up will have access to all the necessary specialists. A virtual MDT may be a possible solution. With a virtual MDT all the team members do not need to be in the same room at the same time. They may interact using shared clinical data on a bespoke IT platform and this interaction maybe non simultaneous. This solution gives the team members an opportunity to interact with specialists beyond their geographic area and for the patient allows opinions on their care without the necessity to travel to different appointments. The platform facilitates the capture of data for audit and education [60]. A virtual MDT for consequences of cancer treatment was piloted by Macmillan Cancer Support in 2014. This has since been rolled out nationally as a 2 year project in conjunction with the Christie NHS Foundation Trust. There is also a European project ExpoRnet that is due to go live later this year.

6.10 Personal Insights from a UK Late Effects Service

The authors work within one of the largest Late Effects Services in the UK. It is based in a main central London cancer centre and the 300 or more new-patient referrals per year originate from a variety of sources. The majority are transitioned from London paediatric principal treatment centres or from the hospital's own Children and Young People's Cancer Service. A small number of patients are referred directly from primary care and some self-refer, often having been lost to follow up at other centres. Referrals are accepted by a care coordinator and are triaged by the multidisciplinary team. All patients transitioning in from paediatric services are seen in a nurse-led transition clinic. A proportion of this consultation time is with the young

Table 6.1 Key elements of a late effects service

Case coordinator to act as a central point of contact and to allow rapid re-entry into the service
Well-designed pathways into and out of the service
Flexible transition from acute to long term follow up care and from Paediatric to AYA and Adult services
Agility between levels of care based on clinical need
A robust system for completing treatment summary and care plans to facilitate planning and assignment of level of care
MDT to facilitate treatment decisions
Access to clinicians experienced in managing late effects
Access to psychology, occupational therapy and physiotherapy
Access to a Key Worker
IT systems-database
Managerial support/funding

person alone, something parents may find extremely challenging. Young people who have been treated for teenage and young adult cancer at the base hospital are offered an opportunity to meet with clinical nurse specialists who have expertise in late effects after cancer treatment.

At these appointments the focus is on information about previous treatment for cancer and the surveillance needed in the future. Most importantly, young people are given an opportunity to tell their story and explore some of the difficult emotions that intensive treatment for cancer causes. Young people tell us that they value an opportunity to reflect on the experience and the affect it has had on their life. They often describe how difficult it has been especially if treated at key stages in education pre-university or during university courses. Some will express regret that they are no longer the person they might have been if they had not had cancer. The depth of resilience is extremely variable and some young people are motivated to achieve highly despite such a difficult experience.

Young people value being able to speak openly and honestly, often discussing issues that they have not been comfortable talking about with their parents present. This is commonly the first opportunity the patient has had to discuss their treatment summary and care plan and there is also an opportunity for education not only on the possible late effects of treatment but also on positive lifestyle behaviours. This appointment frequently generates referrals to other teams, most commonly to psychology.

Following the transition appointment, a level of care is assigned to the patient and future follow up is dependent on this. Level 3 complex patients are reviewed within a multidisciplinary clinic that takes place monthly and includes specialist fertility and reproductive medicine, endocrinology and nephrology teams. Psychosocial difficulties are managed by specialist AYA or adult psych-oncology teams. Level 1 or 2 patients are seen within consultant-led age-appropriate clinics. If continued follow up is not required, the patient is seen in a further nurse-led discharge clinic to ensure they are aware of their treatment information, health and wellbeing, surveillance needs and contact details for the service.

Patients who require ongoing echocardiographic surveillance alone are referred into an echocardiogram telephone follow-up clinic. This is a novel service and every

3–5 years, provides the patient with a flexible echo appointment 7 days a week, followed by a nurse-led telephone consultation. This clinic excludes patients with known cardiac compromise who are followed up by cardiologists.

With increasing numbers of survivors, the most predictable and pressing service issue is lack of capacity. The focus is therefore on discharging appropriate patients to self-management and increasing collaboration with primary care. By definition, patients remaining within the service are the most complex and demanding on resources, nursing and medical time.

As a team, we observe a high degree of need in young adult and adult cancer survivors, even in those with low intensity treatments. There is a significant burden of psychological distress observed especially in AYA treated for cancer as a young child. These patients may transition from paediatric to AYA or adult cancer care with no knowledge or recollection of their diagnosis and treatment. This is frequently due to protective parents who have had complete ownership of their child's cancer journey. Encouraging a young patient to take responsibility for their own health requires the health professional to impart sufficient knowledge of the diagnosis and treatment burden, something that parents and carers may strongly resist. Young people who have been treated as teenagers have often undergone intensive cancer treatment at a crucial time in their education. Young people commonly express sadness that they are not the adult person they might have been, feeling that cancer treatment has changed them as a person and affected opportunities for further study, work and relationships. A focussed transition appointment with an experienced nurse specialist is critical in promoting knowledge and self-care but must allow one-to-one discussion without the presence of a parent or carer.

The spectre of recurrence recedes but may never leave some patients, leading to heavy reliance on a late-effects service for advice, reassurance or investigation of new symptoms. Whilst we encourage patients to access their primary carer initially, maintaining open-access and a single point of contact is hugely beneficial for both the patient and primary care-giver.

Peer support is of immense importance to this group of patients. Young people frequently identify a need to meet with others who have experienced cancer as children, teenagers or as young adults. They convey how lonely it can feel, simply because their peer group tends not to have experienced serious illness and are unable to understand how it feels to deal with complex and long-term health conditions in young adult life. Our first service-run late effects education day for young people provided an opportunity to learn about late effects and be advised about healthy life style choices from both clinicians and allied health professionals. Young people reported the benefit of meeting others who understand what they have been through. In response to this, there are now regular events and the patients groups and education events that are always evaluated very highly, mainly due to the opportunity to meet other patients and share experiences.

Conclusions

"There are known knowns" was the response given by the then US Secretary for Defence, Donald Rumsfeld at a news briefing in 2002 [61]. He went on to say, "We also know there are known unknowns; that is to say we know there are some things we do not know. But there are also unknown unknowns—the ones we don't know we don't know. And if one looks throughout history, it is the latter category that tend to be the difficult ones".

When considering AYA survivorship, we may have confidence in well-researched "known knowns" such as drug-related gonado-, cardio- and pulmonary toxicity. However, it may not be unreasonable to question even these, particularly as evidence is based mainly on paediatric populations and there is increasing recognition that drug metabolism may be altered in AYA patients.

The challenge of delivering AYA survivorship care lies with the known and unknown unknowns. Whereas patients would previously have died, they are now being treated with second, third and fourth lines of chemotherapy thereby exposing them not only to multiple known drug toxicities but also the unknown of whether these may be synergistic and amplify late effects in the future. The advent of targeted therapies and novel agents has also heralded an unknown as currently, follow up is too short to identify late effects with any significant lag-time. Now that cancer survival is improving, further research into the late effects of AYA cancer should be a priority.

Adaptability and flexibility is key to delivering a successful survivorship service to AYA patients. A single point of contact through a late-effects co-ordinator is possibly the single most important requirement of such a service, particularly as patients are more mobile and have higher expectations than ever before. We should aim to harness social media and online platforms to track, educate and connect patients with their peers. Clinicians must maintain vigilance for emerging late-effects that may manifest in an unexpected manner and the service itself must utilise patient experience to educate clinical staff and improve care that is offered. It cannot be denied that for some patients, the price of cure is extremely high. However, there are few things more rewarding than with the help of expert survivorship care, enabling a patient to reach their full potential following an AYA cancer diagnosis.

References

1. O'Hara C, et al. Trends in survival for teenagers and young adults with cancer in the UK. Eur J Cancer. 2015;51(14):2039–48.
2. https://www.cancerresearchuk.org.
3. Chemaitilly W, Cohen LE. Diagnosis of endocrine disease: endocrine late-effects of childhood cancer and its treatment. Eur J Endocrinol. 2017;176(4):R183–203.
4. PDQ Cancer Information Summaries. Late effects of treatment for childhood cancer health professionals version. 2017.
5. O'Sullivan D. Late effects of chemotherapeutic agents on renal function in childhood cancer survivors: a review. Ir J Med Sci. 2017;186(1):49–55.
6. Akam-Venkata J, Franco VI, Lipshultz SE. Late cardiotoxicity: issues for childhood cancer survivors. Curr Treat Options Cardiovasc Med. 2016;18(7):47.
7. Oeffinger KC, et al. Chronic health conditions in adult survivors of childhood cancer. N Engl J Med. 2006;355:1572–82.

8. Hudson MM, et al. High-risk populations identified in Childhood Cancer Survivor Study Investigations: implications for risk based surveillance. JCO. 2009;27(14):2405–14.
9. http://www.birmingham.ac.uk/research/activity/mds/projects/HaPS/PHEB/CCCSS/TYACSS/index.aspx.
10. Lethaby CD, et al. A systematic review of time to diagnosis in children and young adults with cancer. Arch Dis Child. 2013;98:349–55.
11. Fern L, et al. Why can't we improve timeliness of cancer diagnosis in children, teenagers and young adults? BMJ. 2013;347:f6493.
12. van der Graaf WT, et al. Soft tissue sarcomas in adolescents and young adults: a comparison with their paediatric and adult counterparts. Lancet Oncol. 2017;18(3):e166–75.
13. Gaspar N, Fern L. Increasing access to clinical trials and innovative therapy for teenagers and young adults with cancer – a multiple stakeholders and multiple steps process. Prog Tumor Res. 2016;43:38–49.
14. Hough R, Rowntree C, Goulden N, Mitchell C, Moorman A, Wade R, Vora A. Efficacy and toxicity of a paediatric protocol on teenagers and young adults with Philadelphia chromosome negative acute lymphoblastic leukaemia: results from UKALL 2003. Br J Haematol. 2016;172(3):439–51.
15. Woodward E, Jessop M, Glaser A, Stark D. Late effects in survivors of teenage and young adult cancer: does age matter? Ann Oncol. 2011;22(12):2561–8.
16. Hudson MM, et al. High-risk populations identified in Childhood Cancer Survivor Study Investigations: implications for risk based surveillance. J Clin Oncol. 2009;27(14):2405–14.
17. MacArthur AC, Spinelli JJ, Rogers PC, et al. Risk of a second malignant neoplasm among 5-year survivors of cancer in childhood and adolescence in British Columbia. Pediatr Blood Cancer. 2007;48(4):453–9.
18. Travis LB, Fossa SD, Schonfeld SJ, et al. Second cancers among 40576 testicular cancer patients: focus on long term survivors. J Natl Cancer Inst. 2005;97(18):1354–65.
19. Mulrooney DA, et al. Cardiac outcomes in a cohort of adult survivors of childhood and adolescent cancer: retrospective analysis of the Childhood Cancer Survivor Study cohort. BMJ. 2009;339:b4606.
20. Swerdlow AJ, et al. Myocardial infarction mortality risk after treatment for Hodgkin disease: a collaborative British cohort study. J Natl Cancer Inst. 2007;99(3):206–14.
21. Aleman BM, et al. Late cardiotoxicity after treatment for Hodgkin lymphoma. Blood. 2007;109(5):1878–86.
22. Reinders JG, et al. Ischemic heart disease after mantlefield irradiation for Hodgkin's disease in long-term follow-up. Radiother Oncol. 1999;51(1):35–42.
23. van den Belt-Dusebout A, Nuver J, de Wit R, et al. Long-term risk of cardiovascular disease in 5-year survivors of testicular cancer. J Clin Oncol. 2006;24(3):467–75.
24. Sklar C, Whitton J, Mertens A, et al. Abnormalities of the thyroid in survivors of Hodgkin's disease: data from the Childhood Cancer Survivor Study. J Clin Endocrinol Metab. 2000;85(9):3227–32.
25. Kadan-Lottick NS, et al. Osteonecrosis in adult survivors of childhood cancer: a report from the childhood cancer survivor study. J Clin Oncol. 2008;26(18):3038–45.
26. Bright C, Hawkins M, Guha J, Henson K, Winter D, Kelly J, Feltbower R, Hall M, Cutter D, Edgar A, Frobisher C, Reulen R. Risk of cerebrovascular events in 178 962 five-year survivors of cancer diagnosed at 15 to 39 years of age: the TYACSS (Teenage and Young Adult Cancer Survivor Study). Circulation. 2017;135(13):1194–210.
27. Tai E, et al. Health status of adolescent and young adult cancer survivors. Cancer. 2012;118:4884–91.
28. Barnett M, McDonnell G, DeRosa ST, Philip E, Peterson L, Touza K, Jhanwar S, Atkinson T, Ford J. Psychosocial outcomes and interventions among cancer survivors diagnosed during adolescence and young adulthood (AYA): a systematic review. J Cancer Surviv. 2016;10(5):814–31.
29. Hauken M, Larsen TMB, Holsen I. Meeting reality: young adult cancer survivors' experiences of reentering everyday life after cancer treatment. Cancer Nurs. 2013;36:E17–26.

30. Warner E, Kent E, Trevino K, Parsons H, Zebrack B, Kirchoff A. Social well-being among adolescents and young adults with cancer: a systematic review. Cancer. 2016;122:1029–37.
31. Smits-Seemann RR, Kaul S, Zamora ER, Wu YP, Kirchhoff AC. Barriers to follow up care among survivors of AYA cancer. J Cancer Surviv. 2017 Feb;11(1):126–32.
32. Blum R, Garell D, Hodgman C, Jorissen T, Okinow N, Orr D, Slap G. Transition from child-centred to adult health-care systems for adolescents with chronic conditions. A position paper for the society of adolescent medicine. J Adolesc Health. 1993;14:570–6.
33. Mulder R, Van der Paul H, Levitt G, Skinner R, Kremer L, Brown M, Bardi E, Windsor R, Michel G, Frey E. Transition guidelines: an important step in the future care for childhood cancer survivors. A comprehensive definition as groundwork. Eur J Cancer. 2016;54:64–8.
34. National Cancer Survivorship Initiative. Teenage and young adult aftercare pathway. http://webarchive.nationalarchives.gov.uk/20130221101407/http://www.improvement.nhs.uk/cancer/SurvivorshipLivingWithandBeyondCancer/TeenageandAdultAftercarePathway.aspx. Archived May 13, 2013.
35. Competences. An integrated career and competence framework for nurses working in the field of long-term follow-up and late effects care of children and young people after cancer. Published by RCN and NHS improvement. Publication code 004172. 2011.
36. Models of care to achieve better outcomes for children and young people living with and beyond cancer. http://webarchive.nationalarchives.gov.uk/20130221101407/http://www.improvement.nhs.uk/LinkClick.aspx?fileticket=Y1CGhGEoXsg%3d&tabid=56. March 2011.
37. National Cancer survivorship Initiative – Children and Young People Workstream. 4th Children and Young people National Survivorship Workshop. 2010.
38. McQuillan RF, Toulany A, Kaufman M, Schiff JR. Benefits of a transfer clinic in adolescent and young adult kidney transplant patients. Can J Kidney Health Dis. 2015;2:45.
39. Royal College of Physicians of Edinburgh. Think transition: developing the essential link between paediatric and adult care. Edinburgh. 2008. www.cen.scot.nhs.uk.
40. Cancer Services for Children and Young People. Quality standard [QS55]. 2014. https://www.nice.org.uk/guidance/qs55.
41. Casillas J, Syrjala KL, Ganz PA, et al. How confident are young adult cancer survivors in managing their survivorship care? A report from the LIVESTRONG Survivorship Center of Excellence Network. J Cancer Surviv. 2011;5(4):371–81.
42. Haugnes HS, Oldenburg J, Bremnes RM. Pulmonary and cardiovascular toxicity in long-term testicular cancer survivors. Urol Oncol. 2015;33(9):399–406.
43. Bradford NK, Chan RJ. Health promotion and psychological interventions for adolescent and young adult cancer survivors: A systematic literature review. Cancer Treat Rev. 2017;55:57–70.
44. Mariotto AB, et al. Long term survivors of childhood cancers in the United States. Cancer Epidemiol Biomarkers Prev. 2009;18:1033–40.
45. Mulder R, Kremer L, Hudson M, Bhatia S, Landier W, Levitt G, Constine L, Wallace H, Leeuwen F, Ronckers C, Henderson T, Dwyer M, Skinner R, Oeffinger K. Recommendations for breast cancer surveillance for female survivors of childhood, adolescent and young adult cancer given chest radiation: a report from the International Late Effects of Childhood Cancer Guideline Harmonization Group. Lancet Oncol. 2013;14(13):e621–9.
46. Skinner R, Mulder R, Kremer L, Hudson M, Constine L, Bardi E, Boekhout A, et al. Recommendations for gonadotoxicity surveillance in male childhood, adolescent and young adult cancer survivors: a report from the International Late Effects of Childhood Cancer Guideline Harmonization Group in collaboration with the PanCareSurFup Consortium. Lancet Oncol. 2017;18(2):e75–90.
47. van Dorp W, Mulder R, Kremer L, Hudson M, van den Heuvel-Eibrink M, van den Berg M, Levine J, et al. Recommendations for premature ovarian insufficiency surveillance for female survivors of childhood, adolescent and young adult cancer survivors: a report from the International Late Effects of Childhood Cancer Guideline Harmonization Group in collaboration with the PanCareSurFup Consortium. J Clin Oncol. 2016;34(28):3440–50.
48. Armenian S, Hudson M, Mulder R, Chen M, Constine L, Dwyer M, Nathan P, Tissing W, et al. Recommendations for cardiomyopathy surveillance for survivors of childhood cancer: a report

from the International Late Effects of Childhood Cancer Guideline Harmonization Group. Lancet Oncol. 2015;16(3):e123–36.
49. Cox A, Faithfull S. 'They're survivors physically but we want them to survive mentally as well': health care professionals' views on providing potential late effect information. Support Care Cancer. 2013;21(9):2491–7.
50. Wallace H, Blacklay A, Eiser C, Davies H, Hawkins M, Levitt G, Jenney ME. Late effects committee of the United Kingdom Children's Cancer Study Group (UKCCSG). Developing strategies for long term follow up of survivors of childhood cancer. BMJ. 2001;323(7307):271–4.
51. Miedema B, Easley J, Robinson LM. Do current cancer follow-up care practices meet the needs of young adult cancer survivors in Canada? A qualitative inquiry. Curr Oncol. 2013;20(1):14–22.
52. Kam V, Hendershot E, Anderson L, Marjerrison S. Evaluation of a joint adult and pediatric clinic for cancer survivorship care. Pediatr Blood Cancer. 2017; https://doi.org/10.1002/pbc.26476. [Epub ahead of print].
53. Skinner R, Wallace H, Levitt G. Therapy based long term follow up. Practice statement. United Kingdom's Children's Cancer Study Group. 2nd edition. 2005. www.cclg.org.uk/write/MediaUploads/Member%20area/.../LTFU-full.pdf.
54. Scottish Intercollegiate Guidelines Network 76. Long term follow up of survivors of childhood cancer Quick Reference Guide. www.rcpch.ac.uk/sites/.../files/.../Endorsed%20guidelines/.../quick%20ref%20guide76.p Jan 2004.
55. Late Effects of Treatment for Childhood Cancer – Health Professional Version. https://www.cancer.gov/types/childhood-cancers/late-effects-hp-pdq.
56. Children's Oncology Group Long Term Follow Up Guidelines version 4.0 2014. www.survivorshipguidelines.org/.
57. Self-management approaches for people with chronic conditions patient education and counselling. NHS England - NHS Five Year Forward View. 48:177–187. October 2014.
58. Komenda P, Levin A. Analysis of cardiovascular disease and kidney outcomes in multidisciplinary chronic kidney disease clinics: complex disease requires complex care models. Curr Opin Nephrol Hypertens. 2006;15(1):61–6.
59. Wright F, De Vito C, Langer B, Hunter A. Expert panel on multidisciplinary cancer conference standards. multidisciplinary cancer conferences: a systematic review and development of practice standards. Eur J Cancer. 2007;43(6):1002–10.
60. Munro A, Swartzman S. What is a virtual multidisciplinary tea (vMDT)? Br J Cancer. 2013;108(12):2433–41.
61. Defense.gov News Transcript. DoD News Briefing – Secretary Rumsfeld and Gen. Myers, United States Department of Defense (defense.gov). 2012.

7 Transitional Care: Best Practices for Adolescent Cancer Care

Faith Gibson

7.1 Introduction

The *'transition to adulthood'* is a critical stage of human development during which young people leave childhood behind and take on new roles and responsibilities. It is a period of social, psychological, economic, and biological transition. For many young people, it also involves demanding emotional challenges and important life choices, and for some, health choices. To a large degree, the nature and quality of young people's future lives depend on how successfully they negotiate this critical period. To consider this period as 'transition' suggests a brief period, and focuses our attention on what young people are *becoming*, at the expense of neglecting what they *are* [1]. Re-thinking this critical time and re-framing it in the context of a 'transitional period,' establishes the notion of this phase as a separate life-stage, and one more closely aligned to the work of Arnett and 'emerging adulthood' [1]. For young people with a long-term health condition and ongoing health needs we know that this transitional period can be less than straightforward [2–4]. A chronic illness may complicate this process: the young person must assume increasingly independent responsibility for the management of their condition, at the same time they may be required *'to transition from child to adult services'* [3]. Both these transitional processes require changes in the relationship between the patient and the healthcare provider [5].

Long-term health conditions vary widely in their impact: those living with and beyond a cancer diagnosis may face challenges that are both common to other

F. Gibson
Great Ormond Street Hospital for Children NHS Foundation Trust (GOSH) and University of Surrey, London, UK
e-mail: Faith.Gibson@gosh.nhs.uk; f.gibson@surrey.ac.uk

J. Chisholm et al. (eds.), *A Practical Approach to the Care of Adolescents and Young Adults with Cancer*, https://doi.org/10.1007/978-3-319-66173-5_7

health conditions and specific to cancer. The diagnosis itself may allow anticipation of the possible impact on physical health and associated disabilities, but what about the impact on mental health, perceived prognosis, and what impact is there also on personal identity, sexuality, education and vocational choices? Health care consequences of a cancer diagnosis can in the main be anticipated by health care professionals and therefore planned for. For young people the consequences are never planned for, and some have spoken about the unexpected medical, psychological and social challenges that arose over time, and that often remained unresolved [6]: indeed, 'stumbling from one problem to the next,' was a dominant theme in this particular study.

There is no doubt that cancer disrupts lives: young people seek to regain a sense of control over their lives as a means to attain long-term adjustment and well-being [7]. There is a growing body of evidence that describes the 'unmet needs' of young people, with many psychosocial themes relevant to emerging adults living with cancer being described [8–10]. When contrasted to adult survivors, young people have reported different needs. These include: needing help with self-esteem; to be positive and feel good at an emotional level; social and family support; healthy lifestyle; and support for a full return to life [11]. More than 5 years off therapy unmet needs remain, with emotional and psychological issues such as life direction and psychosocial support continuing to feature highly [9]: stressing the need for long-term monitoring, risk-adapted assessment, tailored interventions, ongoing care and support for young people in age-appropriate care settings [11, 12]. Survivorship focussed care is essential across the age continuum, but despite an acknowledgement of its importance cancer survivors often become lost to follow-up and report non-adherence to care recommendations [13, 14]. It has been suggested that life changes and the responsibilities that are part of being 'an adult', may undermine or interact with a young person's needs for follow-up medical care [15]. But there is also a suggestion that young people make a conscious decision to reject services, because they do not meet their needs [6]. The enablers and barriers for continuing care into adulthood are emerging as we begin to examine and report on a range of models of survivorship care [16]. The core elements of these models may indeed vary and there will be natural variation that is influenced by geography, health insurance, and healthcare provider roles. What can however be anticipated, and indeed should be planned for, is the transition to a different model of care, i.e., for the young person to receive cancer-specific follow-up care beyond the children's cancer setting [17].

The focus in this chapter is on transitional care. Some transitions are determined by age or development, others by 'systems,' i.e. healthcare both are considered here. Young people with cancer will be involved in many more 'systems' (e.g. primary, secondary, tertiary medical care, social care, housing, benefits, education, etc.) than their healthy peers, and these systems have age requirements for discharge and transfer which will vary from country to country, and even vary within one country. These transitions add an additional layer of stress on the young person with cancer and emphasise the need for 'adolescent-friendly' health care as an approach to better orientate health services to the needs of young people [18, 19].

To help explore these transitions and structure this chapter the 'Benchmarks for Transition' [20] have been used. These benchmarks were developed with and for young people receiving ongoing care from a number of different specialists, not just those with cancer, highlighting the factors necessary for adolescents to become effective partners in their own healthcare communication. They are used here to illustrate their universal potential as indicators for transitional care, irrespective of the health need of the population [21]. Woven through this chapter are some reflections on the benchmarks, and comments regarding transitional care from the perspective of those who receive and deliver this care in countries other than the UK: *their words are in italics* and their individual contributions acknowledged at the end of this chapter.

7.2 Definition of Transition

The concept of transition includes a gradual purposeful process of empowerment that equips young people with the skills necessary to manage their own healthcare in children's and adult services [22]. Ladores ([23] p126), as a result of a concept analysis, offers the following definition:

> 'a potentially stressful and emotional process in which flexibility and negotiation between the patient, parents, paediatric healthcare providers, and adult health care providers are necessary in order to facilitate achievement of autonomous health-related decision-making and self-care within the adult health care setting'.

A second helpful definition is also proposed, based on a systematic review undertaken by Mulder and colleagues [24] from the guideline development workpackage of PanCareSurFup, an EU-funded research programme under the 7th FP of the EU (www.pancaresurfup.eu), under the auspices of the network Pan-European Network for Care of Survivors after Childhood and Adolescent Cancer (PanCare, www.pancare.eu):

> '….an active planned, coordinated, comprehensive, multidisciplinary process to enable childhood and adolescent cancer survivors to effectively and harmoniously transfer from a child-centred to adult-orientated healthcare system. The transition of care process should be flexible, developmentally appropriate and consider the medical, psychosocial, educational, and vocational needs of survivors, their families and care-givers, and promote a healthy lifestyle and self-management' (p66).

Both are offered here in order to emphasize key elements of the process and the possible consequences that reflect the need for an holistic approach to transitional care [25]. However, despite the growing evidence base and apparent universal acceptance of the concept of transition, the implementation of transitional care remains a challenge [26]. In fact, some healthcare providers are unclear about the difference between transfer and transition [27]: clearly a significant barrier to transitional care.

7.3 Transition Not Transfer

Despite some promising and innovative practice, evidence continues to highlight that young people often struggle to transition to new services [28]. Current problems with transition are often described within three categories [29]:

1. An abrupt transfer to adult services.
2. Staying in the paediatric area longer than is appropriate.
3. Leaving medical supervision altogether, voluntarily or by default.

All three are associated with significant adverse impact, short and long term, on young people with a chronic illness. Simple transfer may result in increasing anxiety for young people. This immediate change in a relationship with professionals, often one that is long-standing, can leave them feeling isolated from their normal support mechanisms, and they may worry that the adult healthcare team will not be able to meet their needs. So, for some, remaining with a healthcare team they know maybe their preferred choice. There is however the potential for delayed development into adulthood, and although they may feel safe in an environment and with people they know, some of their needs may not be met if they stay with a child health team too long. Disrupted care, or care that no longer meets their needs, can lead to disengagement from services and may result in deterioration in health. In the Netherlands for example:

> "survivor clinics have been setup according to the evidence based Dutch nationwide guideline for follow-up after childhood cancer (https://www.skion.nl/voor-patienten-en-ouders/late-effecten/533/richtlijn-follow-up-na-kinderkanker/) developed by the national Dutch Childhood Oncology Group (DCOG). Although every paediatric cancer center in the Netherlands has an adult survivor clinic and survivors are usually transitioned around 18 years of age, some clinics remain in the paediatric setting. A disadvantage of staying in the paediatric setting, is that young people are always reminded of the period they would rather like to leave behind because they want to move forward. So, not only is the paediatric setting not developmentally appropriate, it is also a setting that they perhaps would like to move away from. This will be a challenge for the new late effects clinic of the new national paediatric cancer center, the Prinsess Máxima Center. Therefore we have setup the new late effects clinic in close contact with the survivors themselves, through representation by VOX, the Dutch survivor organization. The late effect clinic will be in the same building, but in a separate unit, close to the entrance hall, and adult survivors will be seen by adult professionals. Furthermore, we will transition survivors to their general practitioner whenever possible".

Transition programmes are needed to enhance personal growth and increase control and independence by promoting skills in communication, decision-making and self-management. There is however no 'one-size fits all model of transition' [30]. That approach may be inappropriate, as it may not consider variation in the young people themselves, or their preferred style of engagement [31]. Personalized planning for transition seems more appropriate, where young people's preferences, combined with the knowledge healthcare professionals have of their patient population, could lead to more effective and efficient engagement with adult care. Certainly, reflecting on a comment made by Allen and Gregory in 2009 [32] might help us, as professionals, when we are thinking about transitional care: "rather than asking how best to manage transition, we might ask how best to meet the needs of young people with (a long-term condition) at this stage of their life course".

There is a significant and ever growing evidence base for the need for transitional care. Formal transition of follow-up care has been described as a standard of practice for young people [33]. What is limited is the corresponding evidence for how transitional care should be delivered until a young person is established within adult services [34]. Despite this current lack of evidence, it is possible to discern from the literature key elements for transitional care. We are now witness to many programmes being developed:

> "The goal in Sweden is to follow the PanCare definition of transition. In 2016 national guidelines for follow up after paediatric cancer were published in Sweden. The guidelines are now slowly being implemented in the six paediatric cancer-centres and county hospitals. Specialists both from paediatric oncology and adult oncology were involved in the work with the guidelines and most specialities in adult medical care were consulted. International guidelines and medical publications were used and as far as possible data were evidence based by the GRADE system. The first chapter in the guidelines concerns: Life after treatment, follow up and rehabilitation. This includes psychological/mental health, physical activity, diet/weight, lifestyle like sunburn, smoking and tobacco, alcohol, other drugs, sexuality and fertility. The information should be individualized and age-related".

Seamless continuity of care is the aim of transitional care. It is necessary for young people to assume responsibility for their ongoing care or chronic care management, a gradual process, a process that is more complex than a simple transfer of care from one service to another. For health care professionals, there is a need to deliver 'youth-friendly care,' care that is respectful of and responsive to the preferences of young people, their needs, values, consistent with the level of development, capacity and interest: and this rests upon meaningful participation, underpinned by, for example, staff attitude, communication, and age appropriate environments [35].

7.4 Key Elements for Transitional Care

Consensus statements are emerging, as are best practice statements that reflect the varying nature of healthcare delivery in our various countries. This section aims to draw on some of these and the body of published work, to offer to the reader, irrespective of geography, health insurance, and healthcare provider roles, core principles to underpin transitional care. To structure this chapter 'Benchmarks for Transition' have been used here to illustrate their universal potential as indicators for transitional care (Fig. 7.1) [20, 21].

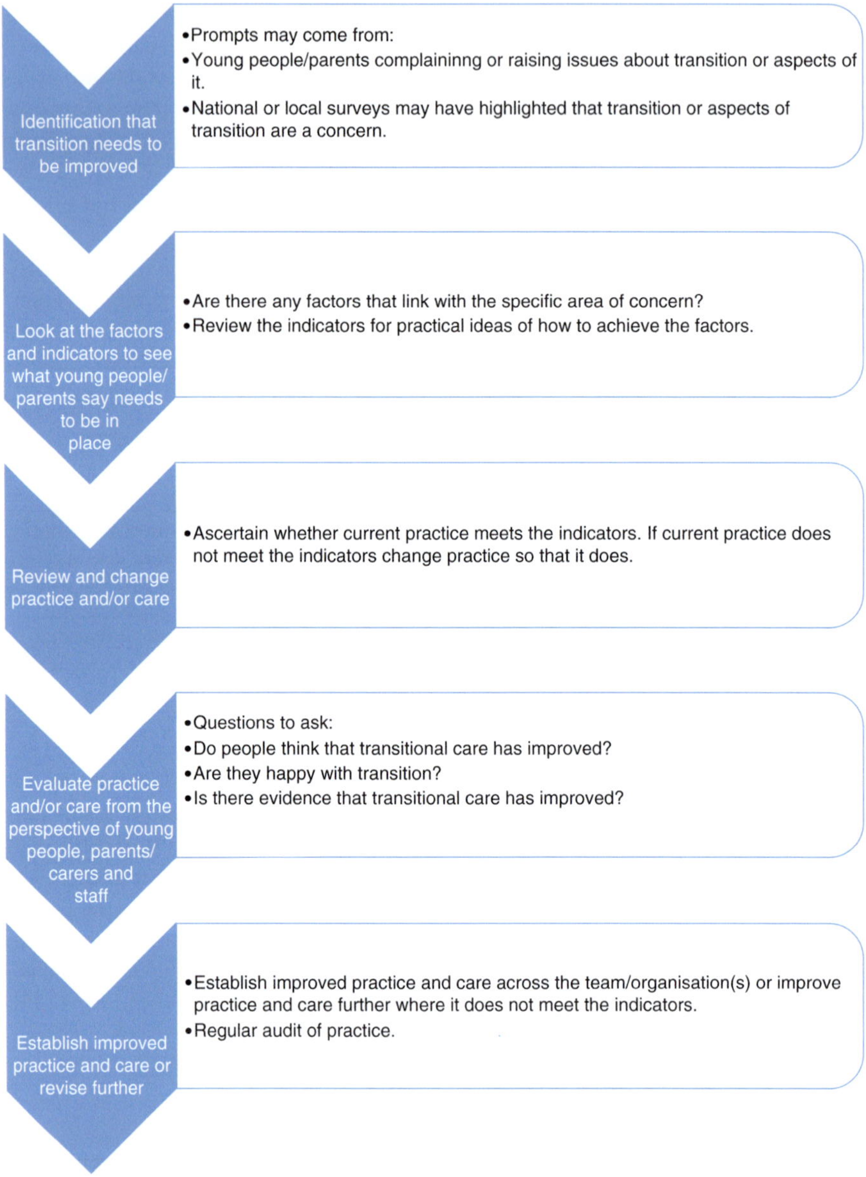

Fig. 7.1 Using the benchmarks for transition from child to adult health services. Adapted from: Department of Health. How to Use Essence of Care (2010) The Stationery Office https://www.gov.uk/government/uploads/system/uploads/attachment_data/file/216690/dh_119970.pdf

The opinion of three discrete groups of experts was sought in the development of the benchmarks: (1) group of professionals involved in either researching transitional care or influencing policy and practice; (2) healthcare professionals involved in the delivery of transition programmes; (3) young people aged 13–21 with a long-term health

Table 7.1 Benchmarks for transition: factors and statements of best practice

Factor	Best practice
Factor 1: Moving to manage a health condition as an adult	Young people are offered advice and information in a clear and concise manner about how to manage their health condition as an adult
Factor 2: Support for gradual transition	The young person as they progress through the transition process is gradually prepared and provided with personally understandable information and support
Factor 3: Co-ordinated child and adult teams	The young person is supported through a smooth transition by knowledgeable and coordinated child and adult teams
Factor 4: Services 'young people friendly'	Young people are provided with care and in an environment that recognises and respects that they are a 'young person', not a child or adult
Factor 5: Written documentation	Concise, consistent and clear written document containing all relevant information about the young person's transition is provided to the teams involved in the transition process
Factor 6: Parents	Parents are included in the transition process gradually transferring responsibility for health to the young person
Factor 7: Assessment of 'readiness'	The young person's readiness for transition to adult care is assessed
Factor 8: Involvement of the GP	The young person's GP is informed of the plan for transition and is able to liaise with other relevant teams to facilitate services requested/needed by the young person

condition and their parents. The eight factors and their associated statements of best practice, which were included in the final document, can be seen in Table 7.1. The complete benchmarks document is available from www.transitionstudy.co.uk. Each factor is considered along with supporting text and examples of practice from published sources and where appropriate practical examples described by healthcare professionals and young people in our study are included in the Benchmark document [20].

7.4.1 Factor 1 Moving to Manage a Health Condition as an Adult

Self-management is essential prior to transfer to adult services. There are however documented concerns regarding young people's knowledge and risk of serious cancer-related health problems [36, 37], and the possible association with non-adherence to recommended follow-up care [38], that suggests self-management can be difficult for some. Self-management requires a young person to manage their symptoms, treatment, lifestyle, and the physical and psychological consequences of living with a chronic health condition. These skills have been shown to increase with age, with females performing better than males, and some evidence that family structures impact on the development of these skills [39]. Fundamental is the need to understand their health condition, including what happened when they were younger and how it may affect them now and in the future: ongoing education, and timely discussions with young people to check their understanding and knowledge must be maintained through transition, transfer and beyond [40]:

> "So, from a survivor's perspective (age-) appropriate information and education is of utmost importance in order to take responsibility for our health in our own hands. Health care professionals should not be afraid of giving too much information, however they should be aware of HOW the information is delivered and about HOW they can educate survivors about late-effects, follow-up and health prevention, rather than just explaining what might happen and then send them home. In my opinion, this kind of education and communication of cancer related information is one major issue in the transitioning-process that starts during follow-up in paediatrics".

There are many elements to self-management, some more practical than others, such as the knowledge of how to access support, how to order prescriptions, and how to book and cancel appointments. But the young person must also learn to effectively communicate their needs, to be able to accurately describe their own healthcare needs: gaining confidence in talking with healthcare professionals that know them before they need to do this with adult focussed professionals is a further essential skill to learn. Split consultations for parents and the young person may be an appropriate intervention also. More complex, and maybe more concerning for the young person is the need to make decisions about their own health management, such as lifestyle choices around smoking and drinking, with some evidence suggesting that young people may have unhealthy lifestyles [41]. Transitional care will both inform and shape the development of these skills. It can take time and for those more dependent on their parents/significant other they might be particularly challenged. Self-management does not mean 'going it alone' [38]: hence the need to transition parent's/family members and the young person gradually to reduce overdependency and hand-over autonomy [41]:

> "This knowledge will make them involved and give them increased opportunities to live autonomously. Through this knowledge, the survivor may get a better quality of life".

7.4.2 Factor 2 Support for Gradual Transition

Starting to plan transition at an early age is consistently mentioned in best practice statements. Age of course always presents an initial hurdle; services will always be provided differently across the age range, which is why rigidity to an age threshold may not be helpful. In the UK, services refer to two transitional points, transition to young adult services, and much later transition to adult services [42]. However, much will depend on the availability of services. Agreed general principles are that planning for adulthood from age 13–14 establishes preparation early; the transfer of care is influenced by transition to adulthood [43]; transfer of care requires skills development and an individualized approach [44]:

> "Only that one day we are too old for the paediatric clinic we were treated at—so the tricky part for survivors often begins after paediatric care is no longer in charge. Sooner or later many survivors will be faced by the question of where to turn to with their somatic and/or psychosocial late effects, whom to ask for advice and how to coordinate the necessary long-

term follow-up. In order to take on that responsibility in terms of self-management, survivors must be informed and educated about the risk of possible late effects, necessary check-ups and about the necessity of long-term follow-up. Many survivors report that they didn't know about late-effects until they occurred. One major topic here is the fertility issue: during follow-up the effects that treatments can cause, like premature menopause, are often not discussed with the survivors. The same applies for psychosocial late-effects like depression, fatigue and anxiety-issues: If you don't know what could occur due to your previous cancer experience and treatments, you might not pin certain symptoms to your cancer history and thus not get the appropriate care you need for your condition".

One generic programme for young people with long-term conditions that is both structured and adaptable is a transition programme called 'Ready Steady Go' (http://www.uhs.nhs.uk/Ourservices/Childhealth/TransitiontoadultcareReadySteadyGo/Transitiontoadultcare.aspx). Empowering young people is a key principle of this particular programme. Young people move through this programme, starting at about 11 years of age, every stage is documented, each young person has a 'health passport' and training to prepare them, as well as their parents, for the eventual transfer [45]. This programme also helps young people to reflect on what they might need, and can help them to distinguish between self-management and where they might need help from other people or health professionals. But this is not the only model, there are many examples reported in the literature to aid this gradual transition. Similarly, in cancer care models are beginning to emerge (see for example [37, 46]): however, PanCare have endorsed the use of Ready to Steady Go with young people who have cancer. Although elements may vary, there are some practical suggestions and these include: young people being introduced to an adult service, having a chance to visit the adult team and look around the adult clinic environment; enabling appropriate disengagement from a long-term patient/provider relationship; use of websites, leaflets and other preparatory materials; health passport to document the timeline. Transition clinics, joint clinics (staffed by professionals from both the child and adult care teams), and the availability of young adult services are all useful approaches to ensure gradual transition. Consistently mentioned is the need for everyone to understand the process, to be clear on the timeline, what needs to be done and when to ensure a young person has the knowledge they need to assume responsibility for their own long-term care. Transfer to adult services does not represent the end of transition, support for the young person should continue after the move to adult care has taken place.

7.4.3 Factor 3 Co-ordinated Child and Adult Teams

Assuring good coordination, that is predicated by good communication, is essential. Transition by its very nature will involve different teams of healthcare professionals, and for some young people this will be further complicated if they have multiple health problems needing to be overseen by different specialists. Communication between the various teams must begin early, and this will be supported best by the young person holding a survivorship passport [47]:

> "a survivorship-passport, addressing the individual risk for late-effects and including recommendations based on follow-up guidelines will be an essential tool to support both health care professionals in communicating late-effects as well as survivors in terms of empowerment and self-management".

Also, the healthcare teams need to share relevant documentation and use a treatment summary and survivorship care plan to inform care going forward [38]. Relevant and accurate documentation helps everyone. In Sweden for example:

> "The survivorship passport is an important 'tool' for transition. We have now the possibility to print a survivorship passport from the National registry of paediatric cancer. The focus is now to provide all survivors with a survivorship passport at the age of 18. This means during the last visit to the paediatric clinic, the paediatric oncologist sums up all facts and gives an explanation of the diagnosis, treatment and need of follow up. Lifestyle factors are also discussed. The parents are mostly present during this clinic visit, but it is important that the teenager is also given time alone with the physician. In some paediatric centres the transition can be multidisciplinary e.g. endocrinology. The patient will get a copy of the survivorship passport and it can also be sent to the GP and different specialists the patient needs to have contact with. It is difficult to estimate the number of patients who actually do receive the survivorship passport and adequate information, today. All paediatric oncology centres in Sweden are aware about this and the number of individuals who receive the survivorship passport are increasing".

Why is the passport so important? Young people we know are frustrated when asked to repeat their history time and time again, and healthcare providers who are not cancer specialists might also feel unprepared when faced with limited information. The widespread adoption of online technology by young people and health care providers will hopefully be soon maximised through cancer portals, transition 'apps,' and interactive websites that support education, communication and advocacy [48]. In addition to these 'tools' a named person, key worker or care navigator has also been described as helpful in coordinating care, liaising with the various members of the multi-professional team and delivering transitional support [49]. Transition clinics, 'meet the new team' events, joint clinics, clear and shared policies can all support a smooth, co-ordinated and timely transition: see Youtube for examples of young people talking about their transition experiences, such as https://www.youtube.com/watch?v=FcNAvGLyGFo, https://www.youtube.com/watch?v=y9qIHCc4B9E The foundation of co-ordinated care rests on the skills, knowledge, and competence of the healthcare professionals involved in this care. Young people speak of their appreciation of being valued, listened to and kept at the centre of health care encounters [35]. Effective educational initiatives, training and the development of communities who deliver transitional care will help to harness the expertise across child and adult services. Promoting continuity of contact between these two services could reduce the risk of early disengagement from care.

7.4.4 Factor 4 Services 'Young People Friendly'

Age sensitive care or age appropriate care has been accepted as the only way to care for young people: this approach is also relevant to transitional care. Young people require information that is honest, accessible and that incrementally builds to increase knowledge germane to their health needs, enabling decision-making and health choices. To do this requires knowledge of 'adolescence,' 'adolescents' and the delivery of developmentally appropriate care that recognises the dynamic relationship between young people and their parents [41]. One known barrier to young people accessing services is where their perception was that they have not been spoken to as an 'adult,' their views not sought, with conversations held between parents and professionals rather than with them directly [50]. There is a particular skill set required to successfully communicate with young people, here again training and education has a role to play across all clinical teams. Appropriately skilled professionals delivering care is but one aspect for services to consider but an appropriate environment is also required [51]. Privacy that enables communication and the delivery of extra emotional support is also necessary. For some young people, it can be the environment that is an immediate and mitigating barrier, for example the presence of elderly patients in an all-adult waiting room and the loss of the familiar 'child-centred surroundings.' For some, adjustment comes easily but for others less so [4]. The loss of what has become 'familiar' also requires transitioning, being prepared for what lies ahead, and being prepared for a change in culture and in relationships must also feature to avoid young people feeling 'abandoned, dumped or shuffled around' ([4] p131). Informing young people about the differences between child and adult settings will also help foster the development of realistic expectations [52].

7.4.5 Factor 5 Written Documentation

Having a written transition protocol/plan available to the healthcare team, young person and their parents is critical to success. It has been suggested in the UK NICE Guidance that co-production of written policies and strategies is a good place to start [53]. Written plans, treatment summary and survivorship care plans have already been mentioned as important elements of transitional care. Timelines for transition/transfer need to be included so that everyone knows what to expect and when. It must also be stressed that keeping these documents 'live' is important, regular reviews and updates are needed if information is to remain current and responsive to changes in health need. Web-based resources endorsed by healthcare professionals have been described by young people as essential, and will assist in filling the knowledge deficit [50]. Having a healthcare plan is known to be an effective communication 'tool', and can help young people advocate for what they need [54].

7.4.6 Factor 6 Parents

As young people move into adulthood, responsibility for health needs to shift from the parent to the young person [55]. Facilitating this transfer of responsibility for health to the young person is an issue often faced by healthcare professionals, but also by young people and parents.

> "For me as a survivor, a well-functioning transitioning-programme should start with proper education of parents and survivors in an early stage of follow-up (if not already during treatment). It should teach parents, survivors and also their paediatricians how to slowly and in an age appropriate way shift health-management from doctors' and parents' side to survivors' side, so that they can acquire all the knowledge and competences they will need to manage their own long-term follow-up once they are discharged from the paediatric clinic and transferred into adult health care. In a well-functioning transitioning-programme, parents and survivors are made aware of late-effects and the importance of follow-up and they have a constant contact person who they know in person and who they can confide in. As soon as discharge from child setting is approaching, survivors and maybe also parents should be acquainted with their future-key-workers who will be in charge for survivors' long-term follow-up in adult health care. At the end of a functioning transition-programme, survivors are transferred to one facility, one place where they have a key-worker, where they get all the information about what medical and psychosocial specialists, institutes and organizations they should/can turn to and where all results from check-ups are collected and reported back to the survivor".

Healthcare professionals have described how they aim to make this a gradual process, starting early, using checklists to monitor progress and give young people targets to work towards, such as making their own appointments [45]. Having time alone with a doctor or nurse is seen as a vital step for young people to take to prepare them for the adult service and allow discussion of issues they may not wish to raise with their parents present (such as sexual health). One practical solution is offering a room and refreshments in clinic for parents to meet and speak together while young people are seen in another consulting room. This can also enable peer support and offer the young people time away from parents during the clinic. It is important to work with both the young person and parent together and recognize parents also need preparation for transition; this can sometimes be viewed as more challenging with the possibility to impede a young person's ability to manage their own health care [56]. Previous research has reported that young people and parents do not always have the same views concerning transition [57], parents may be reluctant to relinquish their role, due to their own concerns, worries and fear, often related to the fear of long term complications [58]. Ten reasons why mothers attend follow-up clinic with a young person (in decreasing order of frequency) were derived in a qualitative study by Doshi et al. [56]: (1) Concern for Child's Health and Well-Being, (2) Practical Support, (3) Transportation, (4) Familial Experience, (5) General Support, (6) Companionship, (7) Personal Interest in Follow-up Care, (8) Characteristics of their Child, (9) Emotional Support, and (10) Parental Duty. These indicate the complexity of reasons for continuing to attend, the need to fully understand these reasons and to be inclusive of all stakeholders, including parents, in transitional care plans. With an incremental process and progression towards self-management, parents in that particular study generally viewed transition positively, and were able to provide scaffolding and support for the young person. Reassuring for parents is the availability of a transition plan, clear written information, and a full understanding of how the adult service works: enabling them to embrace their role as that of 'partner' as a bridge to full independence, while maintaining their investment in their child's health care.

7.4.7 Factor 7 Assessment of 'Readiness'

Many of the clinical guidelines refer to transition readiness assessments as contributing towards development of transition care plans [59]. To enable an individualised approach to transitional care, assessment of readiness can be the first step. Readiness that involves patients, parents and healthcare providers has been recommended [60]. Structured transition readiness assessments have been developed to assess behaviours that would indicate a young person is 'ready for transition' (see for example [61]). Goals are agreed and plans made, young people are helped to fill gaps in terms of skills, knowledge, and the confidence needed to manage their health. Transition readiness is associated with factors such as age, responsibility for healthcare, parental involvement and disease severity: however, all of these have been shown to be variable, with self-management being the best indicator of readiness, and reinforce the need for an individual approach and evaluation of approaches [62]. The lack of an individualised approach in such 'tools' is a concern for some:

> "Perhaps I am the only one who is not a fan of transition readiness assessments because they do not seem focussed on developing self-management skills, but rather to put the YP to the test. We asked YP how they felt about doing an "exam" about their illness before moving to AC and they really hated the idea. Therefore, I do not agree with your sentence: "To enable an individualized approach to transitional care, assessment of readiness is the first step". Most transition readiness assessments such as TRAQ (http://www.etsu.edu/com/pediatrics/traq/) are not individualized, are they?"

7.4.8 Factor 8 Involvement of the General Practitioner

Informing a young person's primary practitioner, such as a paediatrician, general practitioner (GP), nurse practitioner or advanced practice nurse is key to the transition process. Indeed, in some countries the primary care model of survivorship care has become increasingly important. Three important elements of this model are noted to be: awareness of long-term needs of adolescent cancer survivors; opportunities for ongoing education in survivorship care; and a secure health record [63]. Each of these three elements has been mentioned already. The GP is an important link to other services, such as university/college health teams, as such if not the main provider of survivorship care a transition plan can be shared with a GP. Certainly, keeping primary care in the loop, notifying where a young person has failed to keep appointments and requires follow-up is essential.

7.5 Using the Benchmarks for Transition

The benchmark model is one way for an organization to learn about its own practices, discover the practices of others, and make changes that will enable the organization to reach its goals: not intended to be only a general measurement of one organization (or part of an organization) against another, but it also includes the study and transfer of exemplary practice [64]. The basic principle of benchmarking is that a point for comparison is identified (a benchmark) against which all can compare [65]. At the local level benchmarking also encompasses: regularly comparing indicators; identifying differences in outcomes through inter-organizational visits; seeking out new approaches in order to make improvements that will have the greatest impact on outcomes; and monitoring indicators [66]: supporting the attainment of patient focused outcomes [67]. Our study was concerned with the development of a clinical practice-benchmark 'tool'; a 'tool' that would combine evidence from research and policy, informing the points of comparison that would be used as the benchmark to facilitate transitional care [20]. Used here, cancer specific literature has been threaded throughout to support the universal use of the benchmarks, that can be aligned closely with published consensus statements, and guidelines developed for use in individual countries.

But it's not the only approach, and other guidance is available:

> "Based on our research On Your Own Feet (2004–2008), we developed the 'Ten Commandments of Transition'. There is an important overlap with your benchmarks:

1. Plan and start the transfer early.
2. *Place young people at the center.*
3. *Involve the family/parents.*
4. *Prepare young people for self-management and responsibility for their own care.*
5. *Prepare young people for the differences between pediatric and adult care.*
6. *Pay attention to other life transitions as well (social participation).*
7. *Ensure continuity of care.*
8. *Collaborate with adult care.*
9. *Provide support and resources during transition.*
10. *Work in multidisciplinary teams.*

The benchmarks may offer a starting point, but as suggested here they may need to be adapted and individualised to populations, and 'owned' by teams so that they can work with young people more effectively, through treatment and beyond:

> "Because we will have to live with late-effects like cardiologic issues, fears of recurrence, risk of second malignancies, endocrine issues or neuropsychological issues for the rest of our lives, we need to be followed up for the rest of our lives".

7.6 In conclusion

These benchmarks can take a significant role in shaping transitional care. Better-tailored approaches to transition is key if we are to bridge the "care-gap" between child and adult services described in the literature: interventions that teach life skills and self-management need to be evaluated; strategies that improve collaboration between services and enhance a shared understanding of approaches to care must be

Table 7.2 Consensus indicators for transitional care (from Suris et al. [68])

Indicator	Statement
1	Patient not lost to follow-up
2	Attending scheduled visits in adult care
3	Patient building a trusting relationship with adult provider
4	Continuing attention for self-management
5	Patients first visit in adult care no later than 3–6 months after transfer
6	Number of emergency room (accident and emergency) for regular care in the past year
7	Patient and family satisfaction with transfer of care
8	Maintain/improvement of standard for disease control evaluation

described and made known; different models of transitional care need to be examined and finally, we need to know more from the populations we care for about their experiences of services and care in order to shape services as we move forward. Top of the priority list, is the need to learn from others, as there is much that can be shared across populations of young people irrespective of their chronic illness. We must continue to seek feedback from those who receive our care, and that feedback must inform either change or sustainability in the services we provide. The perspectives of young people are evidenced in the literature, and there is consistency in what they are reporting. We might now be confident in knowing what young people want to assist them across these transitional points, *into adulthood* and *into adult services*, we now need to take action with this knowledge. The benchmarks are just one 'tool' that can help support the delivery of transitional care, but there are others, not dissimilar, that can aid action without the need to start at the very beginning: 're-inventing the wheel'. There are also additional indicators to assess whether transitional care has been successful, for example Suris et al. [68]: see Table 7.2. Good partnerships underpin many elements of transitional care. Relationships between young people, parents, and healthcare professionals, where there is clarity of roles, and responsibilities, can enable transitional care. Holistic transition programmes are however required, and maybe now that is where our energy and resources need to be placed.

Acknowledgements Thank you to those who offered real examples from practice, and from their own care, as well as offering comment on the benchmarks for transition: (1) **Maria Olsson**, Nurse consultant Pediatric Oncology PhD student, Gothernburg, Sweden. (2) **Kirsti Pekkanen,** Clinical Nurse Specialist, Pediatric Oncology and late Effects, Gothernburg, Sweden. (3) **Marianne Jarfelt**, Senior Consultant Pediatric Oncology, Gothernburg, Sweden. (4) **Carina Schneider**, Psychologist, Childhood Cancer Survivor, Patient Advocate, Vienna, Austria. (5) **AnneLoes van Staa,** Professor Transitions in Care, Rotterdam University of Applied Sciences, the Netherlands. (6) **Helena van der Pal,** Medical Oncologist, Late Effects Clinic Princess Máxima Center, Utrecht, the Netherlands. Thank you also to Susie Aldiss for her critical reading of this chapter.

References

1. Arnett JJ. Emerging adulthood. 2nd ed. New York: Oxford University Press; 2015.
2. van Staa AL. On your own feet: preferences and competencies for care of adolescents with chronic conditions. Dissertation Erasmus University Rotterdam, The Netherlands. 2012.

3. Van Staa AL, Sattoe JNT. Young adults' experiences and satisfaction with the transfer of care. J Adolesc Health. 2014;55:796–803.
4. Fegran L, Hall E, Uhrenfeldt L, Aagaard H, Ludvigsen M. Adolescents' and young adults' transition experiences when transferring from paediatric to adult care: a qualitative metasynthesis. Int J Nurs Stud. 2014;51:123–35.
5. Van Staa AL, Sattoe JNT, Strating MMH. Experiences with and outcomes of two interventions to maximise engagement of chronically ill adolescents during hospital consultations: a mixed methods study. J Pediatr Nurs. 2015;30:757–75.
6. Howard AF, Goddard K, Tan de Bibiana J, Pritchard S, Olson R, Kazanjian A. Adult childhood cancer survivors' narratives of managing their health: the unexpected and the unresolved. J Cancer Surviv. 2016;10:711–25.
7. Zebrack BJ. Psychological, social, and behavioural issues for young adults with cancer. Cancer. 2011;15:2289–94.
8. Patterson P, Millar B, Desille N, McDonald F. The unmet needs of emerging adults with cancer. Cancer Nurs. 2012;35:e32–40.
9. Millar B, Patterson P, Desille N. Emerging adulthood and cancer: how unmet needs vary with time-since-treatment. Palliat Support Care. 2010;8:151–8.
10. Zebrack BJ, Block R, Hayes-Lattin B, Embry L, Aguilar C, Meeske KA, Butler M, Cole S. Psychosocial service use and unmet need among recently diagnosed adolescent and young adult cancer patients. Cancer. 2013;119:201–14.
11. Galan S, De La Vega R, Thome Pires C, Racine M, Sole E, Jensen MP, Miro J. What are the needs of adolescents and young adults after a cancer treatment? A Delphi study. Eur J Cancer. 2016;26 https://doi.org/10.1111/ecc.12488.
12. Hilgers MV, Slater ME, Sadak KT. Location, location, location: does it matter for childhood cancer survivors considering pediatric vs. adult care settings. Pediatr Blood Cancer. 2016;64:e26426. https://doi.org/10.1002/pbc.26426.
13. van Laar M, Glaser Z, Phillips RS, Feltbower RG, Stark DR. The impact of a managed transition of care upon psychosocial characteristics and patient satisfaction in a cohort of adult survivors of childhood cancer. Psychooncology. 2013;22:2039–45.
14. Berg C, Stratton E, Esiashvilli N, Mertens A, Vanderpool RC. Providers' perspectives of survivorship care for young adult survivors of childhood cancer. J Cancer Educ. 2016;31:31–8.
15. Berg C, Stratton E, Esiashvilli N, Mertens A. Young adult cancer survivors' experiences with cancer treatment and follow-up care and perceptions of barriers to engaging in recommended care. J Cancer Educ. 2016;31:430–42.
16. Smits-Seemann RR, Kaul S, Zamora ER, Wu YP, Kirchoff AC. Barriers to follow-up care among survivors of adolescent and young adult cancer. J Cancer Surviv. 2016;11:126–32.
17. Hugh-Yeun K, Kumar D, Moghaddamjou A, Ruan JY, Cheung WY. Young adult cancer survivors' follow-up care expectations of oncologists and primary care physicians. J Cancer Surviv. 2017;11:295–301. https://doi.org/10.1007/s11764-016-0587-7.
18. McCann L, Kearney N, Wengstrom Y. "It's just going to a new hospital … that's it." Or is it? An experiential perspective on moving from pediatric to adult cancer services. Cancer Nurs. 2014;37:23–31.
19. Sawyer SM, Ambresin AE, Bennett K, Patton GC. A measurement framework for quality health care for adolescents in hospital. J Adolesc Health. 2014;14:570–6.
20. Aldiss S, Cass H, Ellis J, McCutcheon D, Rose L, Gibson F. Transition from child to adult care-'its not a one-off event': development of benchmarks to improve experience. J Pediatr Nurs. 2015;30:638–47.
21. Aldiss S, Cass H, Ellis J, Gibson F. 'We sometimes hold on to ours' – professionals' views on factors and facilitators that delay transition. Front Pediatr. 2016;4:125. https://doi.org/10.3389/fped.2016.00125.
22. Blum R, Garell D, Hodgman C, Jorissen T, Okinow N, Orr D, Slap G. Transition from child-centred to adult health-care systems for adolescents with chronic conditions: a position paper of the Society for Adolescent Medicine. J Adolesc Health. 1993;14:570–6.

23. Ladores S. Concept analysis of health care transition in adolescents with chronic conditions. J Pediatr Nurs. 2015;30:e19–129.
24. Mulder RL, van der Pal HJH, Levitt GA, Skinner R, Kremer LCM, Brown MC, Windsor R, Michel G, Frey E. Transition guidelines: an important step in the future care for childhood cancer survivors. A comprehensive definition as groundwork. Eur J Cancer. 2016;54:64–8.
25. Svedberg P, Einberg EL, Warnestal P, Stigmar J, Castor A, Enskar K, Nygren JM. Support from healthcare services during transition to adulthood-experiences of young adult survivors of pediatric cancer. Eur J Oncol Nurs. 2016;21:105–12.
26. Gleeson H, Turner G. Transition to adult services. Arch Dis Child Educ Pract Ed. 2012;97:86–92.
27. Kenney LB, Melvin P, Fishman LN, O'Sullivan-Oliveira J, Sawicki GS, Ziniel S, Diller L, Fernandes SM. Transition and transfer of childhood cancer survivors to adult care: a national survey of pediatric oncologists. Pediatr Blood Cancer. 2017;64:346–52.
28. Quillen J, Bradley H, Calamaro C. Identifying barriers among childhood cancer survivors transitioning to adult health care. J Pediatr Oncol Nurs. 2017;34:20–7. pii: 1043454216631953.
29. Royal College of Nursing. Lost in Transition; Moving young people between child and adult health services. 2013. http://wwwrcnorguk/__data/assets/pdf_file/0010/157879/003227_WEBpdf. Accessed Feb 2017.
30. Betz CL, Smith KA, Van Speybroeck A, Hernandez FV, Jacobs RA. Movin' on up: an innovative nurse-led interdisciplinary health care transition program. J Pediatr Health Care. 2016;30:323–38.
31. Hislop J, Mason H, Paar J, Vale L, Colver A. Views of young people with chronic conditions on transition from pediatric to adult health services. J Adolesc Health. 2016;59:345–53. https://doi.org/10.1016/j.jadohealth.2016.04.004.
32. Allen D, Gregory J. The transition from children's to adult diabetes services: understanding the 'problem'. Diabet Med. 2009;26:162–6.
33. Freyer DR. Transition of care for young adult survivors of childhood and adolescent cancer: rationale and approaches. J Clin Oncol. 2010;28:4810–8.
34. Campbell F, Biggs K, Aldiss S, O'Neill PM, While A, Clowes M, McDonagh J, Gibson F. Transition of care for adolescents from paediatric services to adult services. Cochrane Database Syst Rev. 2016;4:CD009794. https://doi.org/10.1002/14651858.CD009794.pub2. Review
35. Ambresin AE, Bennett K, Patton GC, Sanci LA, Sawyer SM. Assessment of youth friendly health care: a systematic review of indicators drawn from young people's perspectives. J Adolesc Health. 2013;52:670–81.
36. Syed IA, Klassen AF, Barr R, Wang R, Dix D, Nelson M, Rosenberg-Yunger ZR, Nathan PC. Factors associated with childhood cancer survivors' knowledge about their diagnosis, treatment, and risk for late effects. J Cancer Surviv. 2016;10:363–74.
37. Ganju RG, Nanda RH, Esiashvilli N, Swichenko JM, Wasilewski-Masker K, Marchak JG. The effect of transition clinics on knowledge of diagnosis and perception of risk in young adult survivors of childhood cancer. J Pediatr Hematol Oncol. 2016;38:197–201.
38. Syed IA, Nathan PC, Barr R, Zahava RS, Rosenberg-Yunger ZR, D'Agostino NM, Klassen AF. Examining factors associated with self-management skills in teenage survivors of cancer. J Cancer Surviv. 2016;10:686–91.
39. Ford JS, Chou JF, Sklar CA. Attendance at a survivorship clinic: impact on knowledge and psychosocial adjustment. J Cancer Surviv. 2013;7:535–43.
40. Warner EL, Kent EE, Trevino KM, Parsons HM, Zebrack BJ, Kirchoff AC. Social well-being among adolescents and young adults with cancer: a systematic review. Cancer. 2016;122:1029–37.
41. Docherty SL, Kayle M, Maslow GR, Santacroce SJ. The adolescent and young adult with cancer: a developmental life course perspective. Semin Oncol Nurs. 2015;31:186–96.
42. Glaser A, Levitt G, Morris P, Tapp J, Gibson F. Enhanced quality and productivity of long-term aftercare of cancer in young people. Archiv Dis Child. 2013;98:818–24.
43. Sattoe JNT, Hilberink SR, van Staa A. How to define successful transition? An exploration of consensus indicators and outcomes in young adults with chronic conditions. Child Care Health Dev. 2017; https://doi.org/10.1111/cch.123436. [Epub ahead of print].

44. Sawicki GS, Kelemen S, Weltzman ER. Ready, set, stop: mismatch between self-care beliefs, transition readiness skills, and transition planning among adolescents, young adults, and parents. Clin Pediatr. 2014;53:1062–8.
45. Nagra A, McGinnity P, Davis N, Salmon A. Implementing transition: ready steady go. Arch Dis Child Educ Pract Ed. 2015;100:313–20.
46. McClellan W, Fulbright JM, Doolittle GC, Alsman K, Klemp JR, Nelson EL, Stegenga K, Krebill H, AL-Hihi EM, Schuetz N, Heiman A, Lowry B. A collaborative step-wise process to implementing an innovative clinic for adult survivors of childhood cancer. J Pediatr Nurs. 2015;30:e147–55.
47. Beishon M. Passport to the future: improving life for survivors of childhood cancer. Cancer World. 2014;59:46–9.
48. Williamson R, Meecham L, Cherven B, Hassen-Schilling L, Edwards P, Palgon M, Espinoza S, Mertens A. Predictors of successful use of a web-based healthcare document storage and sharing system for pediatric cancer survivors: cancer SurvivorLink™. J Cancer Surviv. 2015;8:355–63.
49. Martins A, Aldiss A, Gibson F. Specialist nurse key worker role development in children's cancer care: professionals' perspectives on the core characteristics of the role. Eur J Oncol Nurs. 2016;24:70–8. https://doi.org/10.1016/j.ejon.2016.08.009.
50. Frederick NN, Bober SL, Berwick L, Tower M, Kenney LB. Preparing childhood cancer survivors for transition to adult care: the young adult perspective. Pediatr Blood Cancer. 2017; https://doi.org/10.1002/pbc.26544. [Epub ahead of print].
51. Hargreaves DS, McDonagh JE, Viner RM. Validation of you're welcome quality criteria for adolescent health services using data from national inpatient surveys in England. J Adolesc Health. 2013;52:50–7.
52. Lugasi T, Achille M, Stevenson M. Patients' perspectives on factors that facilitate transition from child-centred to adult-centred health care: a theory integrated meta summary of quantitative and qualitative studies. J Adolesc Health. 2011;48:429–40.
53. National Institute for Health and Care Excellence. Transition from children's to adults' services for young people using health or social care services. 2016. https://www.nice.org.uk/guidance/ng43. Accessed Feb 2017.
54. Poplack DG, Fordis M, Landier W, Bhatia S, Hudson MM, Horowitz ME. Childhood cancer survivor care: development of the Passport for Care. Nat Rev Clin Oncol. 2014;11:740–50.
55. While A, Forbes A, Ullman R, Lewis S, Mathes L, Griffiths P. Good practices that address continuity during transition from child to adult care: synthesis of the evidence. Child Care Health Dev. 2004;30:439–52.
56. Doshi K, Kazk AE, Hocking MC, DeRosa BW, Schwartz LS, Hobbie WL, Ginsberg JP, Deatrick J. Why mothers accompany adolescent and young adult childhood cancer survivors to follow-up clinic visits. J Pediatr Oncol Nurs. 2014;31:51–7.
57. Fair C, Goldstein B, Dizney R. Congruence of transition perspectives between adolescents with perinatally-acquired HIV and their guardians: an Exploratory Qualitative Study. J. Pediatr Nurs. 2015;30:684–90.
58. Heath G, Farre A, Shaw K. Parenting a child with chronic illness as they transition into adulthood: a systematic review and thematic synthesis of parents' experiences. Patient Educ Couns. 2017;100:76–92.
59. Sawicki GS, Garvey KC, Toomey SL, Williams KA, Chen Y, Hargraves JL, Leblanc J, Schuster MA, Finkelstein JA. Development and validation of the adolescent assessment of preparation for transition: a novel patient experience measure. J Adolesc Health. 2015;57:282–7.
60. Schwartz LA, Tuchman LK, Hobbie WL, Ginsberg JP. A social-ecological model of readiness for transition to adult-oriented care for adolescents and young adults with chronic health conditions. Child Care Health Dev. 2011;37:883–95.
61. National Child and Maternal Health Intelligence Network. http://www.chimat.org.uk/tranistions/prof/checklist. Accessed Feb 2017.
62. Speller-Brown B, Patterson Kelly K, VanGraafeiland B, Feetham S, Sill A, Darbari D, Meier ER. Measuring transition readiness: a correlational study of perceptions of parent and adolescents and young adults with sickle cell disease. J Pediatr Nurs. 2015;30:788–96.

63. Meacham LR, Edwards PJ, Cherven BO, Palgon M, Espinoza S, Hassen-Schilling L, Mertens AC. Primary care providers as partners in long-term follow-up of pediatric cancer survivors. J Cancer Surviv. 2012;6:270–7.
64. Jones C. Towards benchmarking in British acute hospitals. Health Serv Manage Res. 2001;14:125–38.
65. Codling S. Best practice benchmarking. Cambridge: Gower; 2000.
66. Ettocrhi-Tardy A, Levif M, Michel P. Benchmarking: a method for continuous quality improvement in health. Health Policy. 2012;7(4):e101–19.
67. Ellis J. Sharing the evidence: clinical practice benchmarking to improve continuously the quality of care. J Adv Nurs. 2000;32:215–25.
68. Suris J, Akre C. Key elements for and indicators of, a successful transition: an international Delphi study. J Adolesc Health. 2015;56:612–8.

8 Fertility in the Adolescent and Young Adult Patient with Cancer

Nivedita Reddy, Caroline L. Furness, and Melanie C. Davies

8.1 Background

Survival in adolescent and young adult (AYA) patients with cancer is improving [1] and there is increasing recognition embedded within national guidance [2–4] that high quality care for this age group should aim to minimise the late effects of cancer treatment including effects on fertility. AYA patients require multidisciplinary support to allow timely and appropriate information provision about risk of infertility and enable decisions regarding fertility preservation (FP) where practicable. Even if there is urgency to initiate chemotherapy, discussion of these issues remains key and is recommended by international and national guidelines [4, 5]. Compliance with the recommendation to discuss oncofertility early in the cancer treatment pathway is improving [6] but remains variable and is influenced by factors such as physician knowledge and regional access to fertility preservation programmes [7–9]. In the UK, physicians identified that the main barriers to initiating discussions about FP were lack of time, knowledge, perceived low success rates of FP and poor patient prognosis [7]. The provision of AYA-focused care within specialized principal treatment centres in the UK will hopefully lead to an improvement in these statistics, but there remains a need for development of oncofertility networks and appropriate referral pathways to fertility specialists in a timely fashion at diagnosis.

N. Reddy (✉)
Guy's and St. Thomas NHS Foundation Trust, London, UK
e-mail: Nivedita.Reddy@gstt.nhs.uk

C.L. Furness
University Hospitals Bristol NHS Foundation Trust, Bristol, UK
e-mail: carolinefurness@nhs.net

M.C. Davies
University College London Hospitals (UCLH) NHS Foundation Trust, London, UK
e-mail: melanie.davies@uclh.nhs.uk

J. Chisholm et al. (eds.), *A Practical Approach to the Care of Adolescents and Young Adults with Cancer*, https://doi.org/10.1007/978-3-319-66173-5_8

This chapter sets out the perceived contribution of the AYA physician to the oncofertility pathway, and considers the effects of different oncological treatment modalities on fertility with reference to published ASCO guidance for chemotherapy regimens [5]. Established available fertility preservation methods are described as well considering the developing research in this area. We consider how fertility discussions should be incorporated in the late effects/survivorship post-treatment pathway, and consider available options for menstrual suppression in this age group as well as the medical issues surrounding AYA sexuality.

8.2 Role of the Oncology Team in Preparing for Fertility Consultation

Assessment of the likely effect of the treatment regimen on fertility should form part of the informed consent process for all patients, as well as an assessment of whether fertility preservation measures are appropriate, and whether the treating physician deems that this will result in unacceptable delay to initiation of therapy. The risk balance should be discussed with the patient, and early referral made to fertility services to contribute to these decisions. An outline of what a consultation with a fertility specialist is likely to involve, including the practicalities of semen cryopreservation, can help the patient and family to prepare for their consultation. Even if clinical urgency to start chemotherapy means that it will not be possible for the (usually female) patient to undergo a fertility preservation procedure, then a timely referral to fertility services should still be offered so that the patient may be fully informed about likely impact on future fertility and potential for reassessment. Input from a fertility specialist for females may also be useful from a practical point of view for consideration of menstrual suppression options. Patients should be counselled about the possibility of early menopause as well as infertility and this should also form part of 'late effects' follow-up.

Paediatric oncologists will need to assess whether it is appropriate to refer for sperm banking and may need to formally assess pubertal status in young males who are peri-pubertal, in order to assess whether spermatogenesis has commenced or if ejaculation is possible. Sperm can be detected in the urine at a median age of 13.4 years (range, 11.7–15.3 years) [10] with up to 20% of boys aged 11–12.5 years having detectable sperm in the urine [11]. Studies suggest that almost 80% of boys over the age of 13 can collect semen by self-stimulation [12] and boys who have established secondary sexual characteristics or who have a testicular volume 10–12 mL should be encouraged to do so [13–15].

8.3 Fertility in the Male AYA Patient

8.3.1 Male Reproductive System

The adult testis has two major functions: the production of sperm and synthesis of hormones. The bulk of the testis is made up of seminiferous tubules containing the sperm-producing germ cells and the Sertoli or supporting cells. The Leydig cells

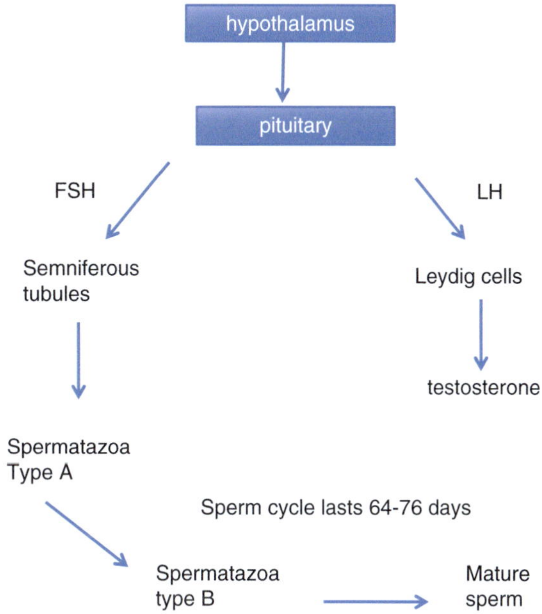

Fig. 8.1 Spermatogenesis. The germ cells (spermatogonia) are of two types, A and B. The type A spermatogonia divide to replenish the stem cell pool and to form type B spermatogonia which undergo differentiation to form mature sperm. Figure reproduced from open access article 2010 Wallace, Kelsey, Human ovarian reserve from conception to the menopause [63]

between the tubules synthesise testosterone, responsible for secondary sexual characteristics. The production of LH and FSH from the pituitary at the onset of puberty triggers the maturation of germ cells and testosterone production by the Leydig cells to initiate spermatogenesis (Fig. 8.1).

Type A spermatogonia are relatively resistant to external insults such as chemoradiotherapy and when damage occurs can undergo mitosis to replenish the differentiating sperm which are highly radio- and chemo-sensitive. More toxic treatment modalities can result in complete type A spermatogonia destruction leading to an irreversible loss of spermatogenesis (Fig. 8.2).

The Leydig cells are more resistant to chemo-radiotherapy and hormone production is unlikely to be affected even if spermatogenesis is lost. Thus young adults who have completed puberty before cancer treatment are not likely to require testosterone replacement therapy. Cancer therapy before or during puberty may not affect the progress of development of sexual maturity even if spermatogenesis is compromised or absent [16]. Ablative treatments such as testicular radiation which destroy Leydig cell function mean that hormone therapy will be required.

8.3.2 Effects of Cancer and Its Therapy on Male Fertility

All oncological treatment modalities may affect male fertility and cancer itself can affect semen quality [17] although the aetiology of this is unclear. Systemic and autoimmune effects of the cancer, local effects of the tumour, endocrine changes, and pre-existing defects in germ cells have been suggested [18]. Certain disease groups e.g. testicular cancer may be at higher risk [19, 20].

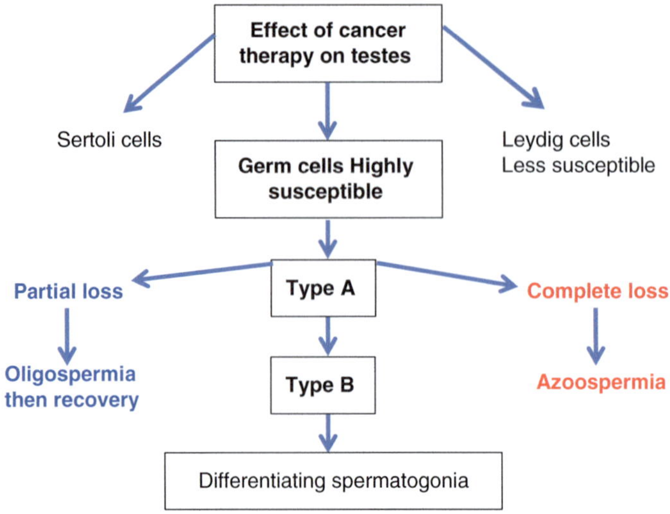

Fig. 8.2 Effect of cancer therapy on spermatogenesis: Partial loss of spermatogonial stem cells (A) leads to a decline and then recovery. Complete loss results in permanent azoospermia

8.3.2.1 Effects of Surgery

Oncological surgery to reproductive organs will have a direct effect on fertility with up to 50% reduction in sperm density reported after orchidectomy [21]. However secondary complications of surgery e.g. nerve or blood vessel damage from pelvic surgery for other types of cancer may also impair reproduction through effects on erection and ejaculation.

8.3.2.2 Effects of Chemotherapy

Effects of chemotherapy can be transient or permanent [22, 23] and as the majority of treatments involve multi-modality regimens it can be difficult to evaluate the toxicity of individual drugs. The early rapidly differentiating spermatogonia are most susceptible and first to be lost. The surviving later stage spermatocytes and spermatids are less sensitive and continue differentiation. However lack of replacement leads to a progressive loss of mature sperm, accounting for the declining numbers of sperm after commencing chemotherapy/radiotherapy. Subsequent recovery will depend upon the degree of toxicity of the drug regimen used, and the survival and function of the spermatogonial stem cells.

The majority of chemotherapeutic agents can impair gonadal function but the alkylating agents including busulfan, melphalan, high dose cyclophosphamide, procarbazine and total body irradiation for bone marrow transplant are associated with the highest risk of gonadal failure. A comprehensive tabular summary of the effect of commonly used chemotherapy and radiotherapy regimens on sperm production is available as data supplement to the 2013 ASCO guideline [5] available online at http://www.asco.org/sites/new-www.asco.org/files/content-files/practice-and-guidelines/documents/2014-fp-data-supplements.pdf (data supplement five, last viewed by authors July 2017). However even in lower risk regimens males should be encouraged to sperm bank where possible given this is not likely to lead to delays in treatment and unforeseen factors such as relapse or need for treatment escalation may impact risk at a later stage. One such example is the response-directed approach currently taken in the management of Hodgkin's lymphoma, escalating from the lower risk ABVD regimen to BEACOPP where interim PET demonstrates a poor response to initial therapy. BEACOPP is associated with a high likelihood of infertility when used for >6 cycles [24] and published rates of azoospermia approaching 90% [25]. Patient counselling in this scenario may also reflect a degree of uncertainty as follow up data emerges for modified regimens using BEACOPP for a limited number of cycles (2) [26]. Hormonal profiling data and assessment of spermatogenesis suggest that although recovery can occur this may be prolonged and deleterious effects on semen quality may persist [24, 26].

8.3.2.3 Mutagenic Effects of Cancer Therapy

Initial data about the mutagenic changes on germ cells due to chemotherapy was initially obtained from animal studies where it is possible to study individual drugs [27, 28]. Studies in human subjects undergoing chemotherapy confirm the presence of treatment-related sperm aneuploidies and chromosomal aberrations [29, 30] that can be seen soon after chemotherapy [31]. Martin et al. [32] used FISH (fluorescent in-situ hybridization) to demonstrate chromosomal abnormalities in men with testicular cancer before, during and after BEP (bleomycin, etopside and cisplatin) therapy [32]. More recent studies of BEP in testicular cancer observed a peak in abnormalities at 6–12 months with about 60% of patients recovering their pre treatment levels of aneuploidy 2 years after the end of treatment [24, 33]. Other studies have shown persistence of aneuploidy for up to 3 years [34–36]. These observations would lead us to avoid sperm banking after commencement of chemotherapy and it is recommended to postpone conception for at least one to 3 years after completion of chemotherapy depending upon the regimen used [35].

8.3.2.4 Gonadal Dysfunction After Radiotherapy

The extent of testicular dysfunction is influenced by the field of exposure, the total dose, and the fractionation schedule [31]. Testicular damage can occur as a consequence of scattered irradiation, for example to para-aortic or pelvic nodes for Hodgkin's disease and testicular cancer or direct exposure as occurs in leukaemias with testicular involvement. The time to recovery of spermatogenesis is related to absorbed testicular dose, pre-treatment sperm count, age, and any additional chemotherapy [37].

The testis is a highly radiosensitive tissue. Spermatogenesis can be temporarily impaired with doses as low as 0.1 Gy. Reduced sperm count or azoospermia can occur at a dose below 1 Gy, with effects lasting 9–18 months, and doses of 2–3 Gy up to 30 months; doses of 4–6 Gy resulted in azoospermia for 5 years or remained permanent [38–40]. Higher doses of radiation are likely to kill all spermatogonial stem cells resulting in permanent azoospermia.

Fractionation of radiotherapy is associated with increased toxicity, with greater delay in sperm recovery [31], as the repeated injury does not allow the surviving stem cell population to repair and regenerate. A total gonadal dose of 2.5 Gy administered in fractionated doses generally produces permanent azoospermia, whereas >6GY is required to produce azoosperrmia if given as a single dose [41]. Total body irradiation given with concomitant chemotherapy caused azoospermia in 85% of men (41/48) and oligospermia in the remaining 15% [38, 42] with recovery in only 18% of men (81/463) after median follow up of 20 years. Only 1% (5) men achieved pregnancy [42].

Radiation induces DNA damage, and the differentiating spermatogonia are most susceptible. With a complete spermatogenic cycle lasting approximately 60–90 days, men are advised to avoid conception during treatment and after completion of treatment until all mature sperm have been depleted, for at least a year to be safe. This is of particular relevance when assisted reproduction may be undertaken with low semen parameters or azoospermia. The androgen-secreting Leydig cells are more resistant to radiation than the germ cells. Increased levels of LH and reduced testosterone levels were noted with exposure to 15–20 Gy and persisted for >5 years [16, 43]. High doses of 24 Gy for testicular leukaemia will cause gonadal failure that requires androgen replacement therapy [44, 45].

Cranial irradiation, and particularly targeted pituitary irradiation, can disrupt the hypothalamic–pituitary axis, impair gonadotropin production and indirectly result in infertility. As the testes remain unaffected (unless additional treatments are given), these patients will respond to gonadotropin therapy to achieve pregnancy [46].

8.3.3 Fertility Preservation in the Male

8.3.3.1 Semen Cryopreservation

Cryopreservation of sperm was first performed in the 1950s [47] and banking for cancer patients since the 1970s. It is strongly recommended that sperm are collected prior to initiation of treatment because the quality of the sample and sperm DNA integrity may be compromised even after a single treatment session [29]. In patients with testicular cancer the most appropriate time to cryopreserve sperm is prior to surgery, as quality may deteriorate after orchidectomy [17]. Preliminary analysis of semen samples may indicate reduced quality of semen in cancer patients (and commonly in adolescents) [48] and the process of cryopreservation and subsequent thawing can further impair quality. Nevertheless, sperm banking should be encouraged even when semen parameters are suboptimal, as the subsequent use of assisted reproduction techniques including intracytoplasmic sperm injection (ICSI) can achieve fertilisation and pregnancy. Ideally men are encouraged to produce one to three samples, with an interval of at least 48 h in between. Clinical urgency to start therapy may be a limiting factor in some cases. The collection of multiple samples, if suitable quality, may mean that subsequent fertility treatment could involve the less invasive method of intrauterine insemination to achieve a pregnancy. Production of sperm by masturbation is achieved by most adults. However, in some cases, the patient may be unwell or under considerable stress and unable to do so in which case adjuncts should be offered (Table 8.1). If no sperm sample is obtained, or if the

Table 8.1 Options for fertility preservation in males

Procedure	Patient population
Sperm cryopreservation (includes use of self stimulation, vibrator, drugs, phosphodiesterase type 5 inhibitors)	Post pubertal
Gonadal shielding	Pre and post pubertal
Surgical sperm retrieval (ONCO TESE, PESA, TESA)	Post pubertal
Testicular tissue cryopreservation	Pre pubertal (currently experimental)

Key: *ONCO TESE* testicular sperm extraction for fertility preservation, *PESA* percutaneous epidydimal sperm aspiration, *TESA* testicular sperm aspiration

analysis reveals azoospermia, it is important that the patient receives appropriate counselling from a fertility specialist to discuss alternatives and future fertility options.

8.3.3.2 Surgical Sperm Retrieval

Semen analysis and hormone profile (FSH, LH, testosterone and tumour markers) are assessed at the initial presentation of all patients. For the young person unable to provide a semen sample, sperm aspiration from the epididymis or testes may be attempted. Where there is azoospermia in the semen sample, a biopsy from the testes can be taken and any sperm recovered may be frozen. Onco-TESE (testicular sperm extraction for fertility preservation) may be appropriate for young men with testicular cancer who are found to be severely oligospermic or azoospermic at their initial assessment, as the sperm extraction can be performed at the same time as their orchiectomy. A coordinated pathway between the urologist and the fertility team has enabled this to be achieved and there are reports of later use resulting in clinical pregnancy and live birth [49]. Although the process of storing testicular tissue has advanced, transplantation of the tissue and recovery of fertility has not yet been achieved in humans and is still considered experimental [50]

8.3.3.3 Special Considerations for Sperm Banking

Providing a sperm sample may be a particular problem with the young adolescent who is already distressed by their diagnosis or quite unwell. Some may be unclear about what the semen sample is or how they are expected to provide one. Age-appropriate language must be used and specially written information may be available. There may be cultural or religious barriers to self-stimulation or providing aids to produce a sample. For the underage male, parents must be included in the discussion, although with their permission it is often useful to have a separate session with the patient. However any aids to provide a sample, either visual or medical, must be given with prior parental consent in these cases. Many hospitals do not have private facilities to provide samples, which can add to the stress of a young adolescent and can be avoided by a referral to a fertility centre.

8.3.4 Follow-Up and Assessment of Fertility After Cancer Treatment

Young men should be encouraged to return for post-treatment evaluation of their fertility status, with a semen analysis one to 2 years after completion of their cancer therapy. Patients can be advised regarding their future fertility prospects and the need for contraception, or may be advised to continue monitoring as spermatogenesis may take longer to recover in some men. If the analysis shows azoospermia, hormone assay of FSH, LH and testosterone levels are assessed. A lack of libido is often encountered after cancer therapy which is likely to be multifactorial, and does not always correlate with the levels of testosterone [51]. Hormone replacement therapy is not indicated except in testosterone deficiency.

8.3.5 Male Fertility After Cancer

Recovery of spermatogenesis is variable, and time taken can range from months to years, depending upon the type and dose of cancer therapy [52, 53] and fertility status prior to treatment. There is reduced paternity and increased use of androgen replacement therapy (ART) in AYA male cancer survivors [54] although survivors of testicular cancer were more successful than those with haematological and other cancers in achieving a pregnancy following low-dose chemotherapy or radiation therapy [55]. There does not appear to be an increase in the incidence of birth abnormalities following spontaneous conception compared with the normal population [56–58]. The use of ICSI can achieve fertilisation even when there are DNA abnormalities in the sperm, and natural selection of healthy sperm is circumvented. These procedures must be undertaken with caution and patients counselled regarding the potential theoretical risk of genetic damage [59]. In the presence of poor or absent sperm in the ejaculate, the use of cryopreserved sperm should be discussed. The live birth rate using assisted reproductive technologies among these patients is at least comparable to that of the non-cancer population [60]. Testicular sperm extraction after chemotherapy can be attempted in men who are azoospermic after cancer treatment with successful sperm retrieval reported in 37% patients in a single study [61]. Although the numbers are small and patients heterogeneous, the patients with testicular cancer had the highest retrieval rate, and those exposed to alkylating agents had lower retrieval rates.

8.3.6 Uptake of Cryopreserved Sperm

Recent publications suggest less than 10% of men return to use cryopreserved sperm although of the remainder, it is not known how many chose not to have a family and how many have fathered children naturally or with the use of assisted reproduction. A postal survey to assess the fertility outcome of men who had cryopreserved sperm prior to chemotherapy was more encouraging [62]: it was completed by 43% of whom 60% (133) attempted conception. Natural conception was achieved by 35% (47) and 45%

(60) underwent assisted conception using previously cryopreserved sperm resulting in a successful outcome in 43% of those treated. A higher number of spontaneous pregnancies were seen than previously reported, particularly in those diagnosed with testicular cancer. Available data suggest that numbers proceeding to ART where fertility has been compromised by cancer therapy could be improved and reasons behind failure to utilize available therapies and uptake cryopreserved sperm should be explored.

8.4 Fertility in the Female AYA Patient

8.4.1 Female Reproductive System

Natural conception requires a functioning ovary with adequate reserve, a healthy uterus, and intact hypothalamic-pituitary-ovarian axis. It is currently accepted that females have a fixed number of primordial follicles that cannot be replaced (Fig. 8.3). At about 20 weeks gestation the number is as high as 6–7 million when a massive process of depletion of follicles by apoptosis begins. At birth the number is estimated to be about a million, decreasing to 4–500,000 by puberty [64]. During a woman's reproductive lifespan, approximately 400–500 mature follicles will ovulate. Meanwhile oocyte loss continues until there are about 10,000 follicles remaining and the woman attains menopause. The rate of loss of follicles can be influenced by genetics, external insults or may be idiopathic. The remaining pool of oocytes will determine the 'ovarian reserve' or 'fertility potential' of the woman. Differences in ovarian reserve influence the degree to which ovarian function may be affected consequent to cancer therapy.

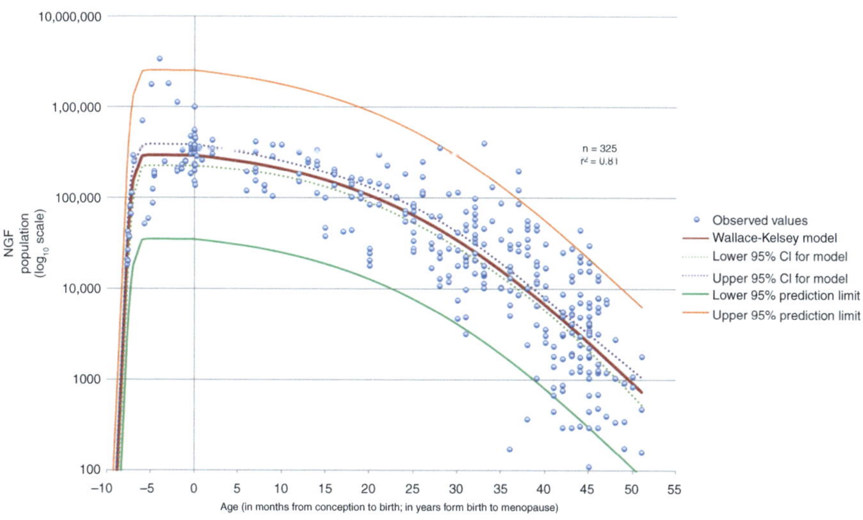

Fig. 8.3 Decline in ovarian function with age as assessed by NGF (non-growing follicles) population versus age until menopause as described by an ADC model published by [63], figure reproduced from open access article 2010 Wallace, Kelsey, Human ovarian reserve from conception to menopause [63]

8.4.2 Effects of Cancer and Its Therapy on Female Fertility

The risk of gonadal failure will vary according to the age of the patient, the type and dose of chemotherapy drug used, the radiation dose and field, and pre-treatment ovarian reserve. Even where there is not a noticeable immediate loss of fertility, there may be an increased risk of early menopause, with hormonal production affected in synchrony.

8.4.2.1 Effects of Chemotherapy

Chemotherapy will largely affect oocytes in the process of maturation, and the proliferating somatic cells that support the oocyte, resulting in disruption or cessation of the menstrual cycle. Where the residual ovarian reserve is adequate, following an interval to recover from the external insult, ovarian function and menstruation will resume. However, the diminished ovarian reserve will determine the length of time for which the ovary will continue to function and the increased risk of an early menopause (Fig. 8.4a). The variability of ovarian reserve in different women makes it difficult to predict the degree to

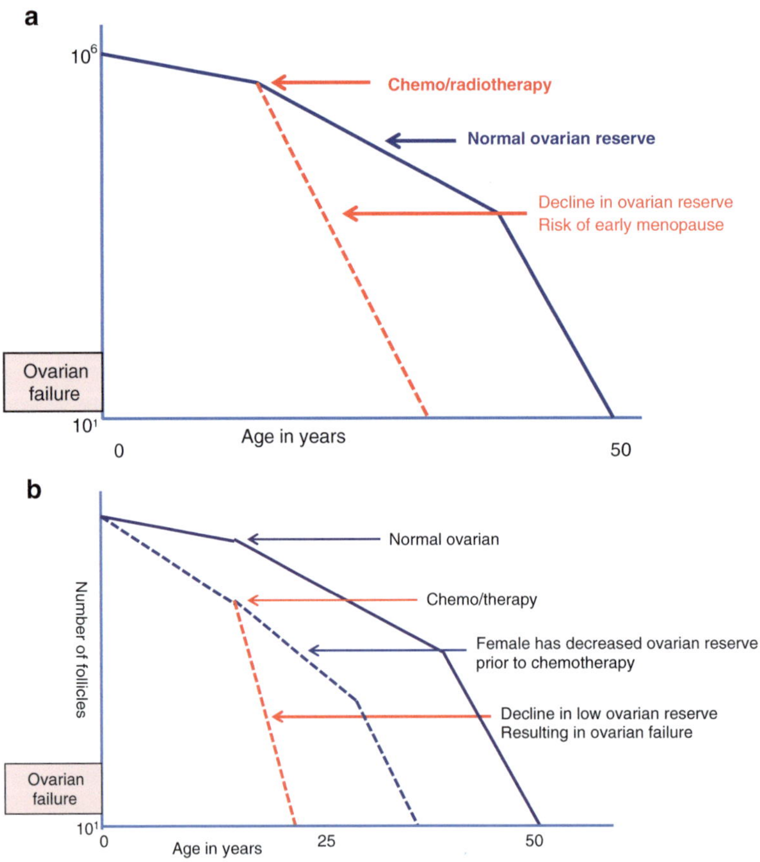

Fig. 8.4 (**a**) Effect of chemo/radiotherapy in female with a normal ovarian reserve. (**b**) Effect of chemo/radiotherapy in female who has a decreased ovarian reserve prior to treatment resulting in ovarian failure at the end of treatment

which ovarian function may be affected consequent to cancer therapy. Commonly used chemotherapy regimens may be classified as carrying a low (<30%), medium (30–70%), or high (>70%) risk of post-treatment amenorrhoea as per the 2013 ASCO guidance (Loren et al., [5]). A young woman with a prior low ovarian reserve is at increased risk of devloping ovarian failure even with low risk regimes (Fig. 8.4b). As for males a comprehensive tabular summary of the effect of commonly used chemotherapy and radiotherapy regimens on menstrual function is available as data supplement to the 2013 ASCO guideline [5] available online at http://www.asco.org/sites/new-www.asco.org/files/content-files/practice-and-guidelines/documents/2014-fp-data-supplements.pdf (data supplement 6, last viewed by authors July 2017). Similar to the discussion in males, counselling should include a discussion of the potential for treatment escalation during treatment e.g. ABVD to BEACOPP and fertility preservation if practical should be considered upfront although time constraints will often preclude this in female patients. Again with treatment protocol modifications a degree of uncertainty in patient counselling exists e.g. with reference to the male example given earlier initial results from use of limited cycles of BEACOPP (2) suggest a reduction in rates of amenorrhoea [26] compared to use of 6 cycles. However the longer term effects on pregnancy rates and fertility remain to be determined.

8.4.2.2 Effects of Radiotherapy

The effect of irradiation on the ovaries, uterus, or hypothalamic-pituitary axis may affect fertility. As in males, the degree of impairment is dependent upon the dose, field of exposure and the fractionation schedule. Pelvic irradiation leads to follicular atresia and atrophy of the ovarian cortex. Not only are developing follicles affected, but there is also a depletion of the resting pool, making radiotherapy the most significant risk factor in developing ovarian failure. Faddy et al. [65] provided a model that showed the depletion of primordial follicles after radiotherapy is proportional to the size of the oocyte pool - therefore for a given dose of radiation, the younger the patient the later the onset of menopause. Wallace et al. [66] refined the model to predict the age at which ovarian failure is likely to develop for a given dose of radiation to the ovaries, which may help in counselling a young woman about the window of reproduction after radiotherapy. The sterilising dose at birth is 20.3 Gy, reducing to 16.5 Gy by the age of 20.

Exposure to abdominal irradiation will compromise the uterine musculature and blood vessels leading to impaired uterine function. A study by Bath et al. [67] demonstrated that development of the uterus to adult size and function is not achieved when there is pre-pubertal exposure to irradiation. Uterine size is comparable with the age at which the patient was treated, and subsequently the pregnancy outcome is poor. Total body irradiation for stem cell transplant has the poorest outcome for future pregnancy. The ovaries and uterus are affected and the concomitant chemotherapy increases the risk of gonadal failure [42, 68]. Direct radiation, for example, for cancer of the cervix, will result in complete loss of uterine function, necessitating the use of a surrogate for future pregnancy.

Disruption of the hypothalamic-pituitary-ovarian axis is an established complication of cranial irradiation for brain tumours. Hormonal evaluation suggested a primary hypothalamic rather than pituitary dysfunction with doses of 39.6–70.2 Gy [69]. Young women considering future fertility should be followed up, for evidence of endocrinopathy. However these women will respond to gonadotrophin therapy to achieve a pregnancy if there is no concomitant treatment given that has compromised ovarian reserve.

Table 8.2 Options for fertility preservation in females

FP option	Specific use	Procedure and timing	Other comment
Ovarian Transposition	Planned radiotherapy	Requires laparoscopy	Ovarian function variable 18–80%
Fertility sparing surgery	Early gynaecological cancers		Variable pregnancy rate 50–60%
GnRH analogue	Efficacy debated	Given through chemotherapy	
Oocyte cryopreservation	Accepted method of FP	Takes 10–14 days	
Embryo cryopreservation	Accepted method of FP	Takes 10–14 days	Requires partner and consent
Ovarian tissue cryopreservation	Considered experimental at present	Requires laparoscopy, chemotherapy can be started within 24 h	

8.4.3 Fertility Preservation in the Female

A summary of the fertility preservation options are listed in Table 8.2.

8.4.3.1 Ovarian Transposition/Oophoropexy

When radiotherapy fields encompass the pelvic organs and the dose of radiation is expected to exceed the sterilizing dose for ovaries, repositioning of the ovaries can be considered to minimize the risk of ovarian failure. The procedure is performed laparoscopically with the ovary generally being placed laterally, ideally at least 3 cm away from the field of radiation. Current modified technique permits a simple procedure to restore the position of the ovaries in the pelvis after completion of radiotherapy. Though natural conception is documented after oophropexy without repositioning, leaving the ovaries makes them difficult to access for egg harvest if required at a later date. There also appears to be a tendency to cyst formation which may complicate follow-up. Where the radiotherapy can affect uterine function the patient should be suitably counselled that even if oophropexy is performed in an attempt to retain ovarian function, the patient will still require a surrogate for any future pregnancy. Though there appears to be a renewed interest in these techniques, the lack of long-term data on ovarian function questions its benefit.

8.4.3.2 Fertility-Sparing Surgery

Cervical cancer incidence is low in the AYA group. With early detection for lesions under 2 cms without parametrial and nodal involvement, radical trachelectomy (removal of the cervix and retention of the body of the uterus) combined with laparoscopic lymphadenectomy may be performed to preserve fertility. There are encouraging pregnancy rates after this procedure [70, 71] but it carries an increased risk of preterm labour [72]. Similarly for early stage cancer of the ovary or borderline ovarian tumours in young women, a conservative approach is adopted where the affected ovary alone is removed. Long-term surveillance however is important and further surgery that may result in loss of fertility may be required.

8.4.3.3 Oocyte and Embryo Cryopreservation

Oocyte and embryo cryopreservation are the two established methods of fertility preservation currently available for young women. If cancer therapy can be deferred safely for 2–3 weeks, controlled ovarian stimulation and recovery of mature oocytes for cryopreservation can be undertaken. Laboratory techniques have improved considerably since oocyte freezing was first attempted in the 1980s, with current freeze thaw survival rates of 90% [73, 74]. Later fertilization requires sperm injection into the eggs, and pregnancy rates now reported are close to those with fresh oocytes used for IVF [75].

Both the American Society of Reproductive Medicine, (ASRM) American Society of Clinical Oncology (ASCO) and National Institute of Health & Care Excellence (NICE) have included oocyte freezing with the process of vitrification in their recommendations for fertility preservation as it is no longer deemed experimental. This has transformed care for young women without a partner who previously had to consider the use of donor sperm for embryo cryopreservation. It should be noted that most of the data on outcomes of oocyte freezing are obtained from egg donation cycles, using eggs retrieved from healthy young donors, and not from women with a diagnosis of cancer so patient should be counselled that data on pregnancies from eggs cryopreserved before oncology treatment are limited although live births are now reported [76, 77]. Additional follow-up will be needed to determine long-term success of this procedure in the oncology setting.

If the woman has a partner and is in a stable relationship, the oocytes can be fertilized with the partner's sperm and the resulting embryos frozen. However, couple must be counselled about the future use of their embryos. Written consent is required from both partners at the time the embryos are created, and again when the embryos are replaced. Should there be a change in circumstances and the partners are no longer in a relationship, or either partner withdraws consent, the embryos cannot be transferred (HFEA [78], test case Evans versus UK). Where a good number of oocytes are likely to be recovered, couples can elect to freeze both eggs and embryos.

8.4.3.4 Ovarian Stimulation Protocols

Ovarian stimulation protocols for fertility preservation are similar to those used in conventional IVF. Gonadotrophin injections are commenced on day 2–3 of the menstrual cycle. Serial ultrasound monitoring and assessment of serum estradiol levels is performed during the course of stimulation. GnRH antagonist is administered when the leading follicle is 14 mm. When three of the follicles are greater than 18 mm in size, oocyte maturation is triggered with hCG and 36 hours later the oocyte retrieval is performed under intravenous sedation or anaesthesia. Data are conflicting on whether patients with cancer show a lower response to stimulation than expected [79].

Previously it was standard practice to commence stimulation at the start of the menstrual cycle, to optimize clinical outcome. Postponement of chemotherapy may not be acceptable, so several strategies are now used in IVF protocols to minimise delay. Where women are on the oral contraceptive pill (OCP) at diagnosis, and there is no contraindication, they are best advised to continue it whilst discussing fertility preservation; the OCP can then be stopped and ovarian stimulation commenced as soon as the decision is made. The introduction of 'random start' protocols in which ovarian stimulation can be commenced at any stage in the cycle minimises the interval before commencing oncotherapy. Reported data on the response to stimulation with random start protocols suggest similar numbers of mature oocytes are harvested compared with conventional protocols [80]. However luteal phase stimulations are slightly longer and require higher dosage of gonadotrophins for ovarian stimulation.

8.4.3.5 Ovarian Stimulation in the Adolescent

Although sexually mature, the adolescent ovary does not always respond in the same way as in the adult. In the peripubertal female the hypothalamic-pituitary axis may be immature, resulting in anovulatory cycles. Assessment of ovarian reserve may be inaccurate as the level of anti-mullerian hormone (AMH) usually peaks in the mid-20s. Though conventionally stimulation with FSH alone is adequate to elicit a good ovarian response, the adolescent may benefit from a combination of FSH and LH for ovarian stimulation.

8.4.3.6 Ovarian Tissue Cryopreservation (OTC)

Ovarian tissue cryopreservation is the only method of fertility preservation for the pre-pubertal female patient at high risk of ovarian failure after cancer treatment. It can also be performed in selected cases, when time constraints will not permit ovarian stimulation for oocyte/ embryo freezing. At the current time this procedure is deemed experimental rather than established, because of the lack of large case series and long-term follow-up. Availability of ovarian tissue freezing varies widely in different countries; in the UK it is undertaken in selected cases using eligibility criteria under the auspices of a research programme in a small number of centres.

The ovarian cortex contains the primordial follicles in varying stages of maturation. Thin layers of the cortex are separated from the underlying medulla and prepared in small strips, enabling many thousands of follicles to be stored. It may therefore be an option to consider even after initial mild chemotherapy in young patients. The patient has to undergo a laparoscopy under general anaesthesia, when several samples of ovarian tissue or a whole ovary are removed depending upon the risk of developing ovarian failure. When cancer therapy is completed and the patient is free of disease, a further laparoscopy is performed and using a microsurgical technique the tissue is thawed and re transplanted into the remaining ovary or ovarian fossa, or in some cases replaced in a heterotopic site in the abdomen or forearm. Re-establishing a blood supply is critical to the return of function of the newly grafted tissue. During the initial period of ischaemia before revascularisation, a large number of follicles will be lost, and will determine the duration and viability of the graft. After re-implantation endocrine function returns after a delay usually 3–6 months and ovarian activity resumption resumes in up to 93% cases. Although the procedure is still deemed experimental live births are reported [81, 82]. with the most recent report documenting 86 successful live births [83]. Future studies will need to address how to overcome concerns that regrafting of ovarian tissue may carry a possible risk of contamination with malignant cells and therefore a risk of recurrence of the cancer.

8.4.3.7 *In Vitro* Maturation of Oocytes

Immature oocyte retrieval with in vitro maturation of oocytes has also been undertaken in some young women where there was insufficient time or it is contraindicated to undergo ovarian stimulation for cryopreservation of mature oocytes. The procedure has been performed both in the follicular and luteal phase of the menstrual cycle with oocytes showing no significant differences in the maturation rate [84]. The number of oocytes and embryos is low, with few reported live births at present [85] probably because many of these are young women who have not returned to attempt pregnancy. To maximize fertility preservation options there are reports of combining in vitro maturation and vitrification of immature oocytes retrieved from ovarian tissue taken for cryopreservation [86].

8.4.3.8 GnRH Analogues

The principle of suppression of the hypothalamic–pituitary–ovarian axis during chemotherapy to reduce the risk of ovarian failure has been debated for more than a decade. The use of a GnRH analogue (GnRH-a) for chemo-protection of the ovaries has been common in clinical practice, usually as a monthly depot injection concomitantly throughout the course of chemotherapy. Initial studies suggested that administration was beneficial with reduction in rates of premature ovarian failure (POF). However emerging evidence has been conflicting [56, 87–89]. Meta-analysis demonstrated a positive effect in breast cancer patients but not confirmed in other groups such as lymphoma and ovarian cancer [90]. Longer term follow-up data seems to suggest that although premature ovarian failure may be reduced this does not necessarily translate in to a statistically significant improvement in pregnancy rates [87, 91, 92]. GnRH-a may provide an effective means of menstrual suppression as discussed below but it remains unclear whether it should be used as a fertility preservation measure in view of the conflicting evidence base.

8.4.3.9 Special Considerations in Female Fertility Preservation

Monitoring for ovarian stimulation is usually undertaken by transvaginal ultrasound scanning to obtain concise information on follicular development, which may cause anxiety for young adolescent females who have not been sexually active. Where this is an issue it is possible to monitor treatment using transabdominal scanning (although this impacts on accuracy) followed by oocyte recovery via transvaginal approach under sedation having obtained suitable consent. In the event that cultural barriers do not allow this despite discussion, then transabdominal oocyte recovery can be performed, although the number of oocytes collected is usually reduced due to access limitations. The patient should be counselled appropriately.

Fertility preservation when chemotherapy has already been given e.g. prior to treatment escalation poses a difficult ethical dilemma in view of potential mutagenic effects of chemotherapy and this is discussed in earlier sections with regard to Hodgkin's lymphoma. Appropriate counselling and informed involvement of the patient in the decision-making process is key.

8.4.3.10 Safety in Female Fertility Preservation Procedures

Interventional procedures carry risks which need to be balanced against potential benefits, taking into account prognosis, risk of being rendered infertile and future chance of achieving pregnancy. Laparoscopy for ovarian transposition or ovarian tissue cryopreservation is considered a minimally invasive surgical procedure but factors specific to the underlying cancer that may influence risk e.g. mediastinal mass complicating anaesthesia, pancytopenia requiring transfusion product support should be carefully considered. Ovarian stimulation and egg harvest is normally a low-risk procedure with a 1% risk of bleeding or infection; the risk of ovarian hyperstimulation has become almost negligible with the introduction of the GnRH analogue to trigger ovulation. Ovarian stimulation causes a substantial rise in oestradiol levels; although transient, this will predispose to thrombosis and oncology patients often have other prothrombotic risk factors, so appropriate thromboprophylaxis is advised.

Women with cervical cancer are at a theoretical risk of increased bleeding and risk of dissemination from egg harvest, and may require a transabdominal approach to reduce risk. Following stimulation, the ovaries will be enlarged for a few days after egg retrieval, and if subsequent pelvic irradiation is planned, the oncologist should be aware that the mapping of the field of radiation can change and may be inaccurate. Pelvic surgery immediately after egg retrieval, when the ovaries are enlarged and vascular, significantly increases the risk of bleeding. It is important that a constant dialogue be maintained with the oncology team to ensure that supervision is continued and treatment planned safely with a multidisciplinary approach. It is good practice to assess the young patient after completion of fertility procedures to ensure that it is safe to proceed with cancer treatment and provide advice for future follow-up.

8.4.4 Follow-Up and Assessment of Fertility After Cancer Treatment

Recovery of ovarian function after cancer therapy is variable and may fall in to one of the following categories:

1. Little or no menstrual disturbance during treatment
2. Menstruation ceases during treatment followed by return to regular or irregular cycles after completion of treatment (menstrual suppression therapy may place patients in this category)
3. Menstrual cycles cease with no recovery after treatment

Regular menstrual cycles are usually indicative of ovulation and therefore fertility (although pregnancy may occur even with infrequent menses or before return of menses in young women). Despite the presence of menstrual cycles and apparently normal ovarian function, ovarian reserve will be reduced following gonadotoxic therapy, with an increased risk of premature ovarian failure. Patients should be made aware that there may be a limited window of reproductive opportunity. It is therefore advisable for a fertility assessment to be included in the follow-up of young cancer survivors 6–12 months after completion of therapy, unless symptoms of ovarian failure warrant earlier referral.

Further follow-up can be planned according to the patient's age, cancer treatment and risks of late effects. Assessment may include gynaecological history, hormone assays (if FSH, LH, Oestradiol are measured this should be in the first few days of the menstrual cycle; AMH is stable through the cycle); ultrasound assessment of the pelvis and ovaries including an antral follicle count. Even if the ovarian reserve is very low, in the presence of menstruation natural conception is still possible.

In women experiencing menopausal symptoms, hormone replacement therapy (HRT) should be instituted after suitable assessment. Monitoring is still required in these women, as some will recover ovarian function at a later time. Patients with prolonged amenorrhoea should be investigated for ovarian failure with FSH and oestradiol, and assessed with bone mineral densitometry. Some patients may experience significant effects of hypoestrogenism and may require earlier referral. Patients receiving therapy likely to be severely gonadotoxic would benefit from seeing a gynaecologist (preferably with a special interest in cancer-related ovarian insufficiency) soon after completion of therapy. This would enable assessment of ovarian function and institution of hormone replacement therapy (HRT) if required. Women who did not see a fertility specialist prior to cancer treatment or who were unable to undergo FP would also benefit from seeing a fertility specialist to discuss their fertility options.

Women undergoing bone marrow transplant (BMT) have a high risk of ovarian failure and often experience significant menopausal symptoms soon after treatment. It is advisable to refer these patients as early 6–8 weeks after the transplant as most will have ovarian failure and appropriate HRT can be commenced before they develop the unpleasant side-effects of acute oestrogen deprivation. In patients at risk, it also facilitates assessment and advice regarding early detection of genital graft-versus-host disease. There is an increased risk of cervical dysplasia in long-term survivors of allogenic stem cell transplantation [93] and an association of cervical abnormalities is also noted with chronic vulvo-vaginal graft-versus-host disease and presence of HPV. Regular surveillance for cervical dysplasia is therefore important in these patients. The advent of HPV vaccination may impact on this risk.

8.4.5 Uptake of Cryopreserved Oocytes and Embryos After Fertility Preservation

It will be several years before sufficient data accumulates on the uptake of fertility treatment using stored embryos and eggs in oncology patients; the usage of ovarian tissue is unknown as in contrast to sperm banking, these are relatively new techniques. Current data on fertility outcomes, as discussed above, are encouraging.

8.4.5.1 Consent for Fertility Preservation

Fertility interventions are highly regulated in the UK; the Human Fertilisation & Embryology Act [94] controls the procurement, storage, and use of gametes and embryos. Storage is illegal without the patient's consent, and proxy consent is not allowed for egg/sperm storage, so a young person must have the capacity to understand and give informed consent. Consent for use is specific to a named partner, and posthumous use is allowed but again only with a named partner. It is therefore crucial for patients with stored samples to be aware that they should update their consent forms when their circumstances change. Taking consent in young patients can present ethical issues if the wishes of the young person differ from that of their parents, in which case an assessment of Gillick competence must be clearly demonstrated.

8.4.5.2 Pregnancy After Cancer

Conception after cancer will depend upon whether there is a return of gonadal function after treatment. Women are generally advised not to try to conceive for a minimum of 6 months after completion of chemotherapy as there is a theoretical risk that oocytes with damaged DNA may give rise to an affected pregnancy. Depending upon the diagnosis and treatment, patients may be advised by their oncologist to wait for at least 1–2 years in follow-up, to ensure that they are in sustained remission. There is no evidence that pregnancy will induce cancer recurrence, even in hormone-receptor-positive breast cancer, but any recurrence is more likely in the earlier years. Recurrence during pregnancy is a complex clinical situation, which may lead to termination of pregnancy, elective early delivery, and in some cases limited use of chemotherapy from the mid-trimester of pregnancy until the fetus is viable and delivery can be safely achieved.

In considering pregnancy risks, the patient's cardiac status should be considered – risk factors for abnormal cardiac function include use of cardiotoxic chemotherapeutic agents (predominantly anthracyclines) and exposure to mantle or mediastinal radiotherapy. Cardiac function assessment should be undertaken on cancer survivors before embarking on a pregnancy to avoid complications from the increased demands on the heart associated the physiological changes in pregnancy. Specialist advice from a cardiologist may be required. Renal function may also warrant pre-pregnancy assessment and review by a renal physician. Obstetric care should be managed as 'high risk' pregnancies. In particular, women who have received abdominal/pelvic irradiation are at increased risk of miscarriage, preterm birth and low birth weight babies, and should be monitored during pregnancy in a specialist obstetric (fetal medicine) unit.

8.4.5.3 Menstrual Suppression in Adolescent Females Undergoing Chemotherapy

Myelosuppresive treatment can induce severe thrombocytopenia and cause significant problems with vaginal bleeding. Menstrual suppression may be offered and should be maintained for the duration of the risk of thrombocytopenia. Use of the oral contraceptive pill, progestogens and GnRH analogues (GnRH-a) can be considered, taking into account the potential for liver toxicity and thromboembolic risk (in many situations the combined oral contraceptive pill will be be contra-indicated in view of thrombosis risk).

Norethisterone is the most common progestogen therapy in use, administered orally in higher doses than used for contraception (e.g. 5 mg three times daily). This is an established method of menstrual suppression. However, caution is required when considering use in patients with abnormal liver function or those at high risk of thromboembolism as Norethisterone is partly metabolised to ethinylestradiol. GnRH-a may be more appropriate in such patients where reliable menstrual suppression is required. If GnRH analogue is used to prevent menstruation, pituitary suppression is not achieved straightaway, depending upon the point of administration within the menstrual cycle,and a vaginal bleed may occur after the first administration. If given just prior to chemotherapy, the development of thrombocytopenia may coincide with vaginal bleeding. The timing of the first dose of the analogue should ideally be at least 2 weeks prior to myelosuppression, but this is not always practical. Vaginal bleeding may need to be managed with other supportive methods including platelet transfusion and tranexamic acid if no contra-indication. GnRH-a acts via the pituitary gland to decrease FSH secretion, resulting in cessation of cyclical ovarian activity, decline in levels of oestrogen and amenorrhoea, which is reversible on withdrawal of the drug. Hot flushes as a result of the decline of oestrogen levels may be troublesome. The suppression should be maintained for the duration of the chemotherapy or throughout the risk of severe thrombocytopenia (Note in ALL chemotherapy which lasts for >2 years GnRHa administration is not required in maintenance and should be discontinued after intensive phases of the protocol are completed).

8.4.5.4 Issues Surrounding Sexuality in AYA Patients

Sexuality is a significant issue for many AYA patients: for some sexuality may be emergent whereas others already may be in sexual partnerships at the time of diagnosis. The impacts of a cancer diagnosis and treatment on sexuality are both psychosocial (briefly covered in Chap. 4 and reviewed with recommendations for dealing with issues including body image, intimacy and overall sexual satisfaction in [95]) and medical. Here we touch on the potential medical issues surrounding sexuality.

8.4.5.5 Contraception

An unintended pregnancy at the time of cancer diagnosis will result in delay to the start of therapy, the risk of teratogenic exposure, and pregnancy termination adding to the distress of the recent diagnosis. Any plan to undergo fertility preservation will have to be deferred and subsequent attempts are likely to be suboptimal. Contraception should be continued where there is no contra-indication (note earlier discussed caveats regarding thrombo-embolic risk and contraceptive pill). If both contraception and menstrual suppression are required the use of the progestogen-only pill could be considered rendering patients anovulatory although there may be episodes of breakthrough bleeding which require additional intervention. When there is persistent amenorrhoea post therapy, presumed infertility may also lead to an unplanned pregnancy. Contraception should be actively discussed during and after cancer therapy with advice tailored to the individual [96].

8.4.5.6 Sexual Dysfunction

Sexual dysfunction after cancer therapy is multifactorial [97]. Physical effects of chemotherapy, surgery and radiotherapy resulting in ovarian failure, loss of fertility and negative body self image can affect patients' ability to establish and maintain sexual relationships. The abrupt fall in oestrogen levels due to treatment can lead to marked menopausal symptoms, and dyspareunia secondary to vaginal dryness. This may be further exacerbated by pelvic radiotherapy causing vaginal stenosis. Whilst women attend cancer services these problems are often not volunteered. A follow-up assessment with the gynaecologist or fertility specialist soon after completion of chemotherapy is an opportunity to address these issues or they should be routinely incorporated in to clinical assessment during 'late effects' follow-up.

Genital graft-versus-host disease can be seen in association with chronic GvHD following allogenic stem cell transplant. Topical therapy and treatment of systemic GVHD may be required. The presenting symptom is commonly dyspareunia. However in the young patient who is not sexually active the condition may go unnoticed, until the development of significant vaginal or cervical stenosis requiring surgical intervention.

8.4.5.7 Summary

Fertility and sexuality issues should form part of the multi-disciplinary care of all adolescent and young adult patients. Oncofertility is an emerging discipline that provides both short- and long-term care and management of gonadal dysfunction in patients with cancer. It requires a multidisciplinary approach to provide a seamless path for the patient in negotiating complex decision pathways. Service provision varies both within and between countries. Oncofertility centres have been set up in association with some of the larger cancer units in the UK, which provide rapid access and dedicated pathways for referral. Even in the absence of such a service local oncologists and haematologists can identify the local fertility centre and become familiar with this service to allow close dialogue and prompt referral where indicated. Having named members of the oncology and fertility teams with a special interest in Oncofertility facilitates meaningful discussions that may require a decision in a limited period of time. Provision of written information before or after fertility consultation can be extremely helpful. Referral to reproductive specialists can enable more patients to take advantage of optimal fertility preservation methods (i.e. sperm banking with up to three collections time permitting, or ovarian stimulation with egg or embryo freezing requiring 2–3 weeks). Timely referral is invaluable in giving the patient the best chance to avail of fertility preservation and minimizing delays to initiation of therapy. Subsequent gynaecological care, preferably in a multidisciplinary 'late effects' service, can pre-empt and treat long-term complications of cancer therapy which impacts on sexuality, fertility, and hormone function.

References

1. O'Hara C, Moran A, Whelan JS, Hough RE, Stiller CA, Stevens MC, Stark DP, Feltbower RG, McCabe MG. Trends in survival for teenagers and young adults with cancer in the UK 1992-2006. Eur J Cancer. 2015;51(14):2039–48.
2. CRUK, R. o. t. i. c. t. Achieving world class cancer outcomes—a strategy for england 2015–2020. 2015. http://www.cancerresearchuk.org/sites/default/files/achieving_world-class_cancer_outcomes_-_a_strategy_for_england_2015-2020.pdf.
3. NHSEngland. NHS standard contract for cancer: teenagers and young adults. 2013. https://www.england.nhs.uk/wp-content/uploads/2013/09/b17.pdf.
4. NICE, c. g.-. (2013). "Fertility: assessment and treatment for people with fertility problems." NICE Clinical Guideline 156 guidance.nice.org.uk/cg156.
5. Loren AW, Mangu PB, Beck LN, Brennan L, Magdalinski AJ, Partridge AH, Quinn G, Wallace WH, Oktay K, American Society of Clinical. Fertility preservation for patients with cancer: American Society of Clinical Oncology clinical practice guideline update. J Clin Oncol. 2013;31(19):2500–10.
6. Salsman JM, Yanez B, Smith KN, Beaumont JL, Snyder MA, Barnes K, Clayman ML. Documentation of fertility preservation discussions for young adults with cancer: examining compliance with treatment guidelines. J Natl Compr Canc Netw. 2016;14(3):301–9.
7. Adams E, Hill E, Watson E. Fertility preservation in cancer survivors: a national survey of oncologists' current knowledge, practice and attitudes. Br J Cancer. 2013;108(8):1602–15.
8. Ben-Aharon I, Abir R, Perl G, Stein J, Gilad G, Toledano H, Elitzur S, Avrahami G, Ben-Haroush A, Oron G, Freud E, Kravarusic D, Ben-Arush M, Herzel G, Yaniv I, Stemmer SM, Fisch B, Ash S. Optimizing the process of fertility preservation in pediatric female cancer patients - a multidisciplinary program. BMC Cancer. 2016;16:620.
9. Louwe LA, Stiggelbout AM, Overbeek A, Hilders CG, van den Berg MH, Wendel E, van Dulmen-den Broeder E, Ter Kuile MM. Factors associated with frequency of discussion of or referral for counselling about fertility issues in female cancer patients. Eur J Cancer Care (Engl). 2016.
10. Nielsen CT, Skakkebaek NE, Richardson DW, Darling JA, Hunter WM, Jorgensen M, Nielsen A, Ingerslev O, Keiding N, Muller J. Onset of the release of spermatozoa (spermarche) in boys in relation to age, testicular growth, pubic hair, and height. J Clin Endocrinol Metab. 1986;62(3):532–5.
11. Schaefer F, Marr J, Seidel C, Tilgen W, Scharer K. Assessment of gonadal maturation by evaluation of spermaturia. Arch Dis Child. 1990;65(11):1205–7.
12. Keene DJ, Sajjad Y, Makin G, Cervellione RM. Sperm banking in the United Kingdom is feasible in patients 13 years or older with cancer. J Urol. 2012;188(2):594–7.
13. Bahadur G, Ling KL, Hart R, Ralph D, Wafa R, Ashraf A, Jaman N, Mahmud S, Oyede AW. Semen quality and cryopreservation in adolescent cancer patients. Hum Reprod. 2002;17(12):3157–61.
14. Hagenas I, Jorgensen N, Rechnitzer C, Sommer P, Holm M, Schmiegelow K, Daugaard G, Jacobsen N, Juul A. Clinical and biochemical correlates of successful semen collection for cryopreservation from 12-18-year-old patients: a single-center study of 86 adolescents. Hum Reprod. 2010;25(8):2031–8.
15. Kamischke A, Jurgens H, Hertle L, Berdel WE, Nieschlag E. Cryopreservation of sperm from adolescents and adults with malignancies. J Androl. 2004;25(4):586–92.
16. Rowley MJ, Leach DR, Warner GA, Heller CG. Effect of graded doses of ionizing radiation on the human testis. Radiat Res. 1974;59(3):665–78.

17. Petersen PM, Skakkebaek NE, Vistisen K, Rorth M, Giwercman A. Semen quality and reproductive hormones before orchiectomy in men with testicular cancer. J Clin Oncol. 1999;17(3):941–7.
18. Agarwal A, Allamaneni SS. Disruption of spermatogenesis by the cancer disease process. J Natl Cancer Inst Monogr. 2005;34:9–12.
19. Rueffer U, Breuer K, Josting A, Lathan B, Sieber M, Manzke O, Grotenhermen FJ, Tesch H, Bredenfeld H, Koch P, Nisters-Backes H, Wolf J, Engert A, Diehl V. Male gonadal dysfunction in patients with Hodgkin's disease prior to treatment. Ann Oncol. 2001;12(9):1307–11.
20. Williams DH t, Karpman E, Sander JC, Spiess PE, Pisters LL, Lipshultz LI. Pretreatment semen parameters in men with cancer. J Urol. 2009;181(2):736–40.
21. Ferreira U, Netto Junior NR, Esteves SC, Rivero MA, Schirren C. Comparative study of the fertility potential of men with only one testis. Scand J Urol Nephrol. 1991;25(4):255–9.
22. Apperley JF, Reddy N. Mechanism and management of treatment-related gonadal failure in recipients of high dose chemoradiotherapy. Blood Rev. 1995;9(2):93–116.
23. Colpi GM, Contalbi GF, Nerva F, Sagone P, Piediferro G. Testicular function following chemoradiotherapy. Eur J Obstet Gynecol Reprod Biol. 2004;113(Suppl 1):S2–6.
24. Paoli D, Rizzo F, Fiore G, Pallotti F, Pulsoni A, Annechini G, Lombardo F, Lenzi A, Gandini L. Spermatogenesis in Hodgkin's lymphoma patients: spermatogenesis in Hodgkin's lymphoma patientsa retrospective study of semen quality before and after different chemotherapy regimens. Hum Reprod. 2016;31(2):263–72.
25. Sieniawski M, Reineke T, Nogova L, Josting A, Pfistner B, Diehl V, Engert A. Fertility in male patients with advanced Hodgkin lymphoma treated with BEACOPP: a report of the German Hodgkin study group (GHSG). Blood. 2008;111(1):71–6.
26. Behringer K, Mueller H, Goergen H, Thielen I, Eibl AD, Stumpf V, Wessels C, Wiehlputz M, Rosenbrock J, Halbsguth T, Reiners KS, Schober T, Renno JH, von Wollff M, van der Ven K, Huehr M, Fuchs M, Diehl V, Engert A, Borchmann P. Gonadal function and fertility in survivors after Hodgkin lymphoma treatment within the German Hodgkin Study Group HD13 to HD15 trials. J Clin Oncol. 2013;31(2):231–9.
27. Choudhury RC, Jagdale MB, Misra S. Cytogenetic toxicity of cisplatin in bone marrow cells of Swiss mice. J Chemother. 2000a;12(2):173–82.
28. Choudhury RC, Jagdale MB, Misra S. Potential transmission of the cytogenetic effects of cisplatin in the male germline cells of Swiss mice. J Chemother. 2000b;12(4):352–9.
29. Frias S, Van Hummelen P, Meistrich ML, Lowe XR, Hagemeister FB, Shelby MD, Bishop JB, Wyrobek AJ. NOVP chemotherapy for Hodgkin's disease transiently induces sperm aneuploidies associated with the major clinical aneuploidy syndromes involving chromosomes X, Y, 18, and 21. Cancer Res. 2003;63(1):44–51.
30. Robbins WA, Meistrich ML, Moore D, Hagemeister FB, Weier HU, Cassel MJ, Wilson G, Eskenazi B, Wyrobek AJ. Chemotherapy induces transient sex chromosomal and autosomal aneuploidy in human sperm. Nat Genet. 1997;16(1):74–8.
31. Meistrich ML. Effects of chemotherapy and radiotherapy on spermatogenesis in humans. Fertil Steril. 2013;100(5):1180–6.
32. Martin RH, Ernst S, Rademaker A, Barclay L, Ko E, Summers N. Analysis of sperm chromosome complements before, during, and after chemotherapy. Cancer Genet Cytogenet. 1999;108(2):133–6.
33. Rives N, Walschaerts M, Setif V, Hennebicq S, Saias J, Brugnon F, Auger J, Berthaut I, Szerman E, Daudin M, Bujan L. Sperm aneuploidy after testicular cancer treatment: data from a prospective multicentre study performed within the French Centre d'Etude et de conservation des Oeufs et du Sperme network. Fertil Steril. 2017;107(3):580–8.
34. Brandriff BF, Meistrich ML, Gordon LA, Carrano AV, Liang JC. Chromosomal damage in sperm of patients surviving Hodgkin's disease following MOPP (nitrogen mustard, vincristine, procarbazine, and prednisone) therapy with and without radiotherapy. Hum Genet. 1994;93(3):295–9.
35. Martinez G, Walschaerts M, Le Mitouard M, Borye R, Thomas C, Auger J, Berthaut I, Brugnon F, Daudin M, Moinard N, Ravel C, Saias J, Szerman E, Rives N, Hennebicq S, Bujan L. Impact of Hodgkin or non-Hodgkin lymphoma and their treatments on sperm aneuploidy: a prospec-

tive study by the French CECOS network. Fertil Steril. 2017;107(2):341–350.e5. https://doi.org/10.1016/j.fertnstert.2016.10.001. Epub 2016 Oct 31
36. Tempest HG, Ko E, Chan P, Robaire B, Rademaker A, Martin RH. Sperm aneuploidy frequencies analysed before and after chemotherapy in testicular cancer and Hodgkin's lymphoma patients. Hum Reprod. 2008;23(2):251–8.
37. Hansen PV, Trykker H, Svennekjaer IL, Hvolby J. Long term recovery of spermatogenesis after radiotherapy in patients with testicular cancer. Radiother Oncol. 1990;18(2):117–25.
38. Anserini P, Chiodi S, Spinelli S, Costa M, Conte N, Copello F, Bacigalupo A. Semen analysis following allogeneic bone marrow transplantation. Additional data for evidence-based counselling. Bone Marrow Transplant. 2002;30(7):447–51.
39. Centola GM, Keller JW, Henzler M, Rubin P. Effect of low-dose testicular irradiation on sperm count and fertility in patients with testicular seminoma. J Androl. 1994;15(6):608–13.
40. Kinsella TJ, Trivette G, Rowland J, Sorace R, Miller R, Fraass B, Steinberg SM, Glatstein E, Sherins RJ. Long-term follow-up of testicular function following radiation therapy for early-stage Hodgkin's disease. J Clin Oncol. 1989;7(6):718–24.
41. Sandeman TF. The effects of x irradiation on male human fertility. Br J Radiol. 1966;39(468):901–7.
42. Sanders JE, Hawley J, Levy W, Gooley T, Buckner CD, Deeg HJ, Doney K, Storb R, Sullivan K, Witherspoon R, Appelbaum FR. Pregnancies following high-dose cyclophosphamide with or without high-dose busulfan or total-body irradiation and bone marrow transplantation. Blood. 1996;87(7):3045–52.
43. Petersen PM, Giwercman A, Daugaard G, Rørth M, Petersen JH, Skakkeaek NE, Hansen SW, von der Maase H. Effect of graded testicular doses of radiotherapy in patients treated for carcinoma-in-situ in the testis. J Clin Oncol. 2002;20(6):1537–43.
44. Brauner R, et al. Leydig cell function in children after direct testicular irradiation for acute lymphoblastc leukaemia. N Engl J Med. 1983;309:25–8.
45. Sklar CA, Robison LL, Nesbit ME, Sather HN, Meadows AT, Ortega JA, Kim TH, Hammond GD. Effects of radiation on testicular function in long-term survivors of childhood acute lymphoblastic leukemia: a report from the Children Cancer Study Group. J Clin Oncol. 1990;8(12):1981–7.
46. Wang JH, Muller CH, Lin K. Optimizing fertility preservation for pre- and postpubertal males with cancer. Semin Reprod Med. 2013;31(4):274–85.
47. Bunge RG, Sherman JK. Fertilizing capacity of frozen human spermatozoa. Nature. 1953;172(4382):767–8.
48. Ragni G, Somigliana E, Restelli L, Salvi R, Arnoldi M, Paffoni A. Sperm banking and rate of assisted conception treatment indights from a 15 year cryopreservation programme for male cancer patients. Cancer. 2003;97:1624–9.
49. Roque M, Sampaio M, Salles PG, Geber S. Onco-testicular sperm extraction: Birth of a healthy baby after fertility preservation in synchronous bilateral testicular cancer and azoospermia. Andrologia. 2015;47(4):482–5.
50. Onofre J, Baert Y, Faes K, Goossens E. Cryopreservation of testicular tissue or testicular cell suspensions: a pivotal step in fertility preservation. Hum Reprod Update. 2016;22(6):744–61.
51. Wallace EM, Groome NP, Riley SC, Parker AC, Wu FC. Effects of chemotherapy-induced testicular damage on inhibin, gonadotropin, and testosterone secretion: a prospective longitudinal study. J Clin Endocrinol Metab. 1997;82(9):3111–5.
52. Gandini L, Lombardo F, Lenzi A, Spano M, Dondero F. Cryopreservation and sperm DNA integrity. Cell Tissue Bank. 2006;7(2):91–8.
53. Spermon JR, Ramos L, Wetzels AM, Sweep CG, Braat DD, Kiemeney LA, Witjes JA. Sperm integrity pre- and post-chemotherapy in men with testicular germ cell cancer. Hum Reprod. 2006;21(7):1781–6.
54. Gunnes MW, Lie RT, Bjorge T, Ghaderi S, Ruud E, Syse A, Moster D. Reproduction and marriage among male survivors of cancer in childhood, adolescence and young adulthood: a national cohort study. Br J Cancer. 2016;114(3):348–56.
55. Huddart RA, Norman A, Moynihan C, Horwich A, Parker C, Nicholls E, Dearnaley DP. Fertility, gonadal and sexual function in survivors of testicular cancer. Br J Cancer. 2005;93(2):200–7.

56. Clowse ME, Behera MA, Anders CK, Copland S, Coffman CJ, Leppert PC, Bastian LA. Ovarian preservation by GnRH agonists during chemotherapy: a meta-analysis. J Womens Health (Larchmt). 2009;18(3):311–9.
57. Schrader M, Muller M, Straub B, Miller K. The impact of chemotherapy on male fertility: a survey of the biologic basis and clinical aspects. Reprod Toxicol. 2001;15(6):611–7.
58. Green DM, Fiorello A, Zevon MA, Hall B, Seigelstein N. Birth defects and childhood cancer in offspring of survivors of childhood cancer. Arch Pediatr Adolesc Med. 1997;151(4):379–83.
59. Hassold T, Abruzzo M, Adkins K, Griffin D, Merrill M, Millie E, Saker D, Shen J, Zaragoza M. Human aneuploidy: incidence, origin, and etiology. Environ Mol Mutagen. 1996;28(3):167–75.
60. Garcia A, Herrero MB, Holzer H, Tulandi T, Chan P. Assisted reproductive outcomes of male cancer survivors. J Cancer Surviv. 2015;9(2):208–14.
61. Hsiao W, Stahl PJ, Osterberg EC, Nejat E, Palermo GD, Rosenwaks Z, Schlegel PN. Successful treatment of postchemotherapy azoospermia with microsurgical testicular sperm extraction: the Weill Cornell experience. J Clin Oncol. 2011;29(12):1607–11.
62. Kopeika J, Khalaf Y, Reddy N. ESHRE poster 2014. http://www.posters2view.eu/eshre2014/view.php?nu=282
63. Wallace WH, Kelsey TW. Human ovarian reserve from conception to the menopause. PLoS One. 2010;5(1):e8772.
64. Faddy M, Gosden R. Numbers of ovarian follicles and testing germ line renewal in the postnatal ovary: facts and fallacies. Cell Cycle. 2007;6(15):1951–2.
65. Faddy MJ, Gosden RG, Gougeon A, Richardson SJ, Nelson JF. Accelerated disappearance of ovarian follicles in mid-life: implications for forecasting menopause. Hum Reprod. 1992;7(10):1342–6.
66. Wallace WH, Thomson AB, Saran F, Kelsey TW. Predicting age of ovarian failure after radiation to a field that includes the ovaries. Int J Radiat Oncol Biol Phys. 2005;62(3):738–44.
67. Bath LE, Critchley HO, Chambers SE, et al. Ovarian and uterine characteristics after total body irradiation in childhood and adolescence : responses to sex steroid replacement. Br J Obstet Gynaecol. 1999;106:1265–72.
68. Salooja N, Szydlo RM, Socie G, Rio B, Chaterjee R, Ljungman P, Late eddects working party of the European group for Blood and Marrow transplantation, et al. Pregnancy outcomes after peripheral blood or bone marrow transplantation: a retrospective survey. Lancet. 2001;358(9278):271–6.
69. Constine LS, Woolf PD, Cann D, Mick G, McCormick K, Raubertas RF, Rubin P. Hypothalamic pituitary dysfunction after radiotherapy for brain tumours. N Engl J Med. 1993;328(2):87–94.
70. Arbyn M, Simoens C, Goffin F, Noehr B, Bruinsma F. Treatment of cervical cancer precursors: influence of age, completeness of excision and cone depth on therapeutic failure, and on adverse obstetric outcomes. BJOG. 2011;118(10):1274–5. author reply 1275-1276
71. Schneider A, Erdemoglu E, Chiantera V, Reed N, Morice P, Rodolakis A, Denschlag D, Kesic V. Clinical recommendation radical trachelectomy for fertility preservation in patients with early stage cervical cancer. Inj J Gynaecol Cancer. 2012;33(4):659–66.
72. Bruinsma FJ, Quinn MA. The risk of preterm birth following treatment for precancerous changes in the cervix: a systematic review and meta-analysis. BJOG. 2011;118(9):1031–41.
73. Cobo A, Garrido N, Pellicer A, Remohi J. Six years' experience in ovum donation using vitrified oocytes: report of cumulative outcomes, impact of storage time, and development of a predictive model for oocyte survival rate. Fertil Steril. 2015;104(6):1426–34. e1421–1428
74. Doyle JO, Richter KS, Lim J, Stillman RJ, Graham JR, Tucker MJ. Successful elective and medically indicated oocyte vitrification and warming for autologous in vitro fertilization, with predicted birth probablities for fertility preservation according to number of cryopreserved oocytes and age at retrieval. Fertil Steril. 2016;105(2):459–66.
75. Argyle CE, Harper JC, Davies MC. Oocyte cryopreservation: where are we now. Hum Reprod Update. 2016;22(4):440–9.
76. Druckenmiller S, Goldman KN, Labella PA, Fino ME, Bazzocchi A, Noyes N. Successful oocyte cryopreservation in reproductive aged cancer survivors. Obstet Gynecol. 2016;127(3):474–80.

77. Porcu E, Bazzocchi A, Notarangelo L, Paradisi R, Landolfo C, Venturoli S. Human oocyte cryopreservation in infertility and oncology. Curr Opin Endocrinol Diabetes Obes. 2008;15:529–35.
78. HFEA – Human Fertilisation and Embryology (1990) European Court of Human Rights judgment is http://hudoc.echr.coe.int/eng?i=001-80046
79. Friedler S, Koc O, Gidoni Y, Raziel A. Ovarian response to stimulation for fertility preservation in women with malignant disease: a systematic review and meta-analysis.Fertil. Steril. 2012;97(1):125–33.
80. Cakmak H, Rosen MP. Random-start ovarian stimulation in patients with cancer. Curr Opin Obstet Gynecol. 2015;27(3):215–21.
81. Donnez J, Dolmans MM. Ovarian cortex transplantation: 60 reported live births brings the success and worldwide expansion of the technique towards routine clinical practice. J Assist Reprod Genet. 2015;32(8):1167–70.
82. Rodriguez-Wallberg KA, Tanbo T, Tinkanen H, Thurin-Kjellberg A, Nedstrand E, Kitlinski ML, Macklon KT, Ernst E, Fedder J, Tiitinen A, Morin-Papunen L, Einarsson S, Jokimaa V, Hippeläinen M, Lood M, Gudmundsson J, Olofsson JI, Andersen CY. Ovarian tissue cryopreservation and transplantation among alternatives for fertility preservation in the Nordic countries- compliation of 20 years of multicenter experience. Acta Obstet Gynecol Scand. 2016;95(9):1015–26.
83. Jensen AK, Macklon KT, Fedder J, Ernst E, Humaidan P, Andersen CY. 86 successful births and 9 ongoing pregnancies worlwide in women transplanted with frozen thawed ovarian tissue: focus on birth and perinatal outcomes in 40 of these children. J Assist Reprod Genet. 2016;34(3):325–36.
84. Creux H, Monier P, Son WY, Tulandi T, Buckett W. Immature oocyte retrieval and in vitro oocyte maturation at different phases of the menstual cycle in women with cancer who require urgent gonadotoxic treamtent.Fertil. Steril. 2017;107(1):198–204.
85. Uzelac PS, Delaney AA, Christensen GL, Bohler HC, Nakajima ST. (2015) liver birth following in vitro maturation of oocytes retrieved from extracorporeal ovarian tissue aspiration and embryocryopreservation for 5 years. Fertil Steril. 2015 Nov;104(5):1258–60.
86. Yin H, Jiang H, Kristensen SG, Andersen CY. Vitrification of in vitro matured oocytes collected from surplus ovarian medulla tissue resulting from fertility preservation of ovarian cortex tissue. J Assist Reprod Genet. 2016;33(6):741–6.
87. Chen H, Li J, Cui T, Hu L. Adjuvant gonadotropin-releasing hormone analogues for the prevention of chemotherapy induced premature ovarian failure in premenopausal women. Cochrane Database Syst Rev. 2011;9(11):CD008018.
88. Del Mastro L, Boni L, Michelotti A, Gamucci T, Olmeo N, Gori S, Giordano M, Garrone O, Pronzato P, Bighin C, Levaggi A, Giraudi S, Cresti N, Magnolfi E, Scotto T, Vecchio C, Venturini M. Effect of the gonadotropin-releasing hormone analogue triptorelin on the occurrence of chemotherapy-induced early menopause in premenopausal women with breast cancer: a randomized trial. JAMA. 2011;306(3):269–76.
89. Shen YW, Zhang XM, Lv M, Chen L, Qin TJ, Wang F, Yang J, Liu PJ, Yang J. Utility of gonadotropin-releasing hormone agonists for prevention of chemotherapy-induced ovarian damage in premenopausal women with breast cancer: a systematic review and meta-analysis. Onco Targets Ther. 2015;8:3349–59.
90. Del Mastro L, Ceppi M, Poggio F, Bighin C, Peccatori F, Demeestere I, Levaggi A, Giraudi S, Lambertini M, D'Alonzo A, Canavese G, Pronzato P, Bruzzi P. Gonadotropin-releasing hormone analogues for the prevention of chemotherapy-induced premature ovarian failure in cancer women: systematic review and meta-analysis of randomized trials. Cancer Treat Rev. 2014;40(5):675–83.
91. Munhoz RR, Pereira AA, Sasse AD, Hoff PM, Traina TA, Hudis CA, Marques RJ. Gonadotropin-releasing hormone agonists for ovarian function preservation in premenopausal women undergoing chemotherapy for early-stage breast cancer: a systematic review and meta-analysis. JAMA Oncol. 2016;2(1):65–73.
92. Demeestere I, Brice P, Peccatori FA, Kentos A, Dupuis J, Zachee P, Casasnovas O, Van Den Neste E, Dechene J, De Maertelaer V, Bron D, Englert Y. No evidence for the benefit of gonad-

otropin-releasing hormone agonist in preserving ovarian function and fertility in lymphoma survivors treated with chemotherapy: final long-term report of a prospective randomized trial. J Clin Oncol. 2016;34(22):2568–74. https://doi.org/10.1200/JCO.2015.65.8864. Epub 2016 May 23
93. Negri G, Herz M, Deola S, Piccin A, Casini M, Babich B, Tauber M, Messini S, Marucci MR, Vittadello F. Abnormal cervical cytology after allogeneic bone marrow transplantation. Am J Clin Pathol. 2014;142(2):222–6.
94. HFEA ACT (1990) https://embryo.asu.edu/pages/human-fertilisation-and-embryology-act-199
95. Barbera L, Zwaal C, Elterman D, McPherson K, Wolfman W, Katz A, Matthew A. Interventions to address sexual problems in people with cancer. Curr Oncol. 2017;24(3):192–200.
96. Quinn MM, Letourneau JM, Rosen MP. Contraception after cancer treatment: describing methods, counseling, and unintended pregnancy risk. Contraception. 2014;89(5):466–71.
97. Soanes L, White ID. Sexual consequences of cancer and its treatment in adolescents and young adults. In cancer in adolescents and young adults. Springer International Publishing 2017, pp. 603–631.

9 Palliative Care in Adolescents and Young Adults

Anna-Karenia Anderson

9.1 Introduction

Despite cancer continuing to be the third leading [1] cause of death in adolescents and young adult (AYA), palliative care is often only considered towards end of life [2]. The majority of AYAs with progressing or relapsing disease continue to die in hospital receiving cancer-directed therapies [3]. With access to more clinical trials and further lines of therapies, the AYA may live longer, burdened with increasingly complex symptoms, as a result of their cancer or its treatment. This, and the recent evidence [4] of early palliative care input having a life prolonging effect even in the face of less cancer-directed therapy and active intervention at end of life, supports its early introduction, from either diagnosis or first relapse.

For the health professional, an AYA facing the diminishing odds of cure is a unique challenge with their searing astute opinions, changing balance of power in decision making, their effortless altruism and an ability to give 'life to days' through a desire to maintain hope even when in facing death [5]. They may face death with a worldly savvy wit and sharp astute reflections on everything, from the professionals they encounter to the care they receive. Their honesty, if listened to, can often be the panacea for a service, enabling it to improve and respond.

A.-K. Anderson
Royal Marsden Hospital, Sutton, UK
e-mail: annakarenia.anderson@rmh.nhs.uk

J. Chisholm et al. (eds.), *A Practical Approach to the Care of Adolescents and Young Adults with Cancer*, https://doi.org/10.1007/978-3-319-66173-5_9

9.2 Principles of Palliative Care

9.2.1 The AYA

'You know when you go and visit someone old in hospital and they are really sick.
You sit there for a bit and talk to them and then you, like, leave.
As soon as you shut the door, you think….mmm…
'What will I have for lunch?'
People are doing that about me now.'
(patient, 17 years)

The AYA receiving palliative care wants to be viewed as a young person first and as being unwell as a secondary consideration. They want to live until they die, capturing new life experiences, for life to have meaning and for them to be remembered. They prefer to be informed even when prognosis is poor [5–7] and have an altruistic desire to help others by participating in research [8]. They will seek to remain in control over their bodies rather than medication controlling them and to be respected in the decisions they make.

9.2.2 Services

'I have two words for you… Travel lodge….I ain't dying in no Travel lodge'

AYAs usually receive care from either a paediatric or adult palliative care service. Both have unique benefits. In practice, coordination of services around the AYA to meet the individual's current and anticipated needs is ideal [7]. There are some dedicated AYA services and hospices developing but their experience with specific tumour types may be limited and requires on-going engagement and links with oncology services for symptom advice and support. Services across regions cater for differing age group demarcations. For example in the UK some paediatric services stop at 16 years of age with adult services starting at 18 years [7] leaving a gap in service provision for 16–17 year olds.

When looking at services, be realistic with AYA and their family about the provision of services, level of care provided and needed at each phase of illness [9] delivered in each care setting. It is important to identify as early as possible the potential places of care and death and also to consider the anticipated symptoms and practical needs of the AYA now and as their condition deteriorates. Specialist cancer centres should have access to a palliative care service. A lead palliative service should be identified for each individual that coordinates with other services. Often a clinical nurse specialist (CNS) in symptom or palliative care can lead the coordination of the service, providing an outreach or a linking role between hospital and community settings. If flexibility is built in and a relationship between Adult and Paediatric palliative services is developed, it may enable cross working in the AYA group to achieve the best care outcome for the individual. For example, a young adult with a diffuse intrinsic pontine glioma (more common in the paediatric population), may require a nasogastric tube since their appetite is maintained despite the increasing loss of physical functioning including the ability to safely swallow. Often their symptoms are managed with steroids contributing to the sensation of hunger. Paediatric services can provide support in placing and maintaining nasogastric tubes but adult services may be better resourced to provide the practical support in daily cares including moving and handling.

9.2.2.1 Place of Care

AYAs should be offered choice in where to receive palliative and end of life care [10] whether it is in the same or a different setting: hospital [7], at home or in a hospice. For example they may want to remain in hospital to receive a further course of cancer-directed therapy but desire to die at home. Flexibility and realistic possibilities of place of care and death should be explored early. Perception that dying at home equates to an excellent service delivered, does not reflect the complexity and needs of this population but it should be acknowledged that most AYAs want to die at home [11]. Dying well in the AYA's preferred place of care and death, where possible, should be considered the best outcome. On occasion the place of care will be dictated by the provision of care needed for the AYA, for example, an AYA with a brain tumour with slow neurological deterioration may benefit from the practical support a hospice can provide. Consistent policies and practices adaptable to local services should be in place across all care settings including an approach to rapid transfers from hospital to home or hospice.

9.2.2.2 Hospice Care

The AYA patient may have the choice of a children's or adult hospice depending upon the hospice's age criteria. AYA and their family should be offered the opportunity to look around a hospice before making any decisions about care. Each hospice's service will vary but may include in-hospice bed, community outreach services, outpatient clinics and joint hospice/hospital services. Their psychosocial support, complementary services, allied health team and bereavement programs may vary but are often tailored to the specific needs of the local population. All hospices are expert in supporting people reaching the end of their life.

9.2.2.3 Transition

AYA may, during the course or at the end of their cancer treatment, be transitioned to adult cancer services, depending on local pathways of care. An AYA receiving palliative care will usually remain with their existing palliative care service. However for some, transitioning to adult palliative services is a positive step and may enable access to local support and services that were prohibited before. The main aspects of transition are identifying the new lead service, clear communication [7] and handover, and ensuring advance care plans are in place throughout the process. The decision to transfer should be based on overall benefit to the AYA in meeting their needs. The transition can be complex, for example with only a community and hospice service transitioning to an adult service whilst the specialist cancer service is unchanged especially with the advent of AYA specialist oncology units.

9.2.2.4 Referral to Palliative Care Service

Early referral is the mantra in palliative care. Many AYAs continue to receive cancer treatment in the last weeks of life [2]. For some this prohibits a much longed for chance to accomplish activities, visit loved ones and special places, or for a slice of normality, even for a little while, such as attending school. For some AYAs, receiving on-going cancer directed therapy promotes hope and, depending upon the treatment, may give very little toxicity and side effects. Early referral to palliative care should be a dual approach to care [12], providing both oncology and palliative care in parallel. When on-going cancer-directed therapy is offered in advanced cancer there should be clear communication about the anticipated outcome (for example: improvement in symptoms, disease-holding or slowing the disease progression). Goals of care, time frames, parallel planning and even discussions around symptoms at end of life and place of death should take place. For example, AYA with metastatic lung disease can remain relatively well with only mildly intrusive symptoms until their disease process tips them into irreversible respiratory failure with a rapid end of life phase. Lack of communication around anticipated symptoms with AYA and their families can lead to inappropriate and futile interventions including intensive care and other invasive procedures that ultimately do no alter the outcome. An integrated palliative care service with early engagement can start to tackle anticipated challenging symptoms, provide information and open discussions around advance care planning in manageable pieces and set to the pace of the AYA and their family.

9.2.2.5 Phases of Illness

The phases of illness describes the distinct stages in a patient receiving palliative care [9]. The phases consist of stable, unstable, deteriorating, dying and deceased. They are classified according to the care needs of the patient and give an indication of the suitability of the current care plan. This enables services and symptom plans to be reviewed or adapted as the patient moves in and out of different phases. In some places phases of illness are used to identify and allocate resources and funding and support outcome measures.

9.2.2.6 Multidisciplinary Team

The multidisciplinary team (MDT) provides a holistic approach to palliation and end of life care encompassing psychological, social, spiritual and educational elements [3]. Each role is valuable in maintaining and supporting the wellbeing of the AYA. Access to services, advance and end of life care planning, physical and psychological symptom assessments and interventions, and communication and decision-making should be addressed by the MDT. Allied health professionals can provide practical support and adaptions within the AYA's home and school to promote safe independence. School and teacher's involvement can enable the AYA to attend school, in limited capacity if needed, and support them through exams, if wished. Some AYAs are very keen to complete their school exams giving a great sense of accomplishment and normalisation with peers. The MDT should also support professionals in maintaining professional boundaries with the AYA and their families.

Components of an Advance care plan
Demographics on AYA
Information of family and involved health professionals
Statement about who has responsibility for consent
Summary of medical condition
Record of significant discussions
Regular planned reviews
Service coordination and provision
Planning for place of care and death
Agree treatment plans and objectives
Management of life - threatening events
Emergency care including DNR orders and ambulance directive
Wishes and memory making
Organ and Tissue donation
Symptom management plans

Fig. 9.1 Advanced care plans

9.2.2.7 Advance Care Plans

An Advance care plan (ACP) is a voluntary process, enabling better planning and provision of care [13] and helping AYAs to live and die in the place and the manner of their choosing [14] ACP enable families to understand and honour the AYA's wishes [15]. According to AYAs, the introduction of ACP should not be when they are first ill or hospitalized but early on in diagnosis or when dying [16]. An ACP can help AYA make decisions about their care and how they wish to be remembered after their death. Examples of ACPs include Voicing My CHOICES (recently developed age-appropriate North American guide) [17] and the West Midlands Palliative Care toolkit (commonly used UK based under 18 years of age) [18]. Figure 9.1 shows the important components of an ACP.

9.2.2.8 Difficult Discussions

> *'I can't take back and undo anything I hear. I will leave the room but I want my parents to listen and tell me later at home.' (patient, 18 years)*

Timing of introduction and discussion on ACP should ideally occur at a time when AYA is relatively well and they and their family are willing to engage in discussions about future treatments, or lack thereof. The discussion should be initiated and tailored to the individual needs of the AYA and their family. Introduction of the ACP should ideally be done by a health professional they 'click with' or trust. The professional should talk frankly about end of life care without it being portrayed as a loss of hope [5, 19]. The discussion should focus on issues that are meaningful to the AYA rather than 'filling the form'. Often AYA concerns about palliative and end of life care are very different from those of professionals and parents. It should be acknowledged that there may be a difference in views between adolescents and adults on 'wanting to know if I am dying' [11]. AYA may focus on when they can go home, see friends, if they will be in pain, who gets their room and their stuff, where they will die and how they wish to be remembered rather than resuscitation status and further treatment options.

It has been noted that 'clinicians still find it difficult to speak with AYAs about death'. As a result, AYAs are less likely to develop a clear understanding of their illness and there may be a disconnection between clinicians and parents about prognosis. Insufficient communication and poor understanding may increase the risk of AYAs feeling isolated, mistrustful and anxious, and deprive them of a role model who can communicate about painful issues or share difficult feelings. [20].

Adult Europeans, when asked if they would like to be informed in the scenario of having a serious illness such as cancer with less than a year to live, a minority (21%) did not want such information unless they ask, or at all [21]. This concurs with the views of AYAs [5–7]. However, while all AYAs deserve the opportunity to prepare and consider the realities of advancing disease, not everyone desires to do so. The relationship built and approach to communication paved, may go some way in guiding the clinician in how an individual AYA wants difficult news to be shared. Clinicians should provide an open and honest communication style, paced to the individual AYA's needs. Stopping frequently and answering only the questions the AYA asked whilst providing open questions for AYAs to explore, reframe and ask further questions, if they wish, is a starting point in sharing difficult news.

9.2.2.9 Managing Conflict in Decision-Making

The AYA has, in being diagnosed and treated for cancer, experienced first-hand the impact on their life including their physical wellbeing, body image, confidence, education, friendships and family life. They are uniquely aware of the 'cost' of taking on, or not, further treatment including experimental early phase trials. Navigating the choice between 'maintaining hope' through further cancer-directed therapy or focusing on life away from hospitals and professionals -even for a brief period is an immense decision. The AYA may, having conformed and endured various therapeutic options, choose to forgo the diminishing odds of further therapeutic interventions. This decision may bring them into direct conflict with their parents. The professional is best placed to guide the AYA and their parents on the realistic options available to them, on the impact of further treatments including less intensive options or palliation alone. The professional must ensure that the AYA is fully informed of their options and aware of the outcome and impact of the decision made. The professional should support and share the burden of the decision with the AYA whilst navigating the distress and concerns that may arise from the AYA's parents who maybe in conflict with the AYA's decision.

9.2.2.10 Wishes and Memory Making

Many AYAs want to ensure their life had meaning, was worthwhile and that they would be remembered [22]. Memory making and exploring wishes with the AYA [23], for example what to do with precious cherished possessions or any money saved, may help them, their partner, friends, siblings [24] and parents start to prepare for the AYA's death and enable the AYA to feel they have left a meaningful legacy. Some AYA may even plan their funeral. Professionals are in an ideal position to provide guidance to the AYA and their families about starting conversations enabling closure for the AYA and guidance for their family on fulfilling the AYA's expressed wishes. Without engaging the AYA, important facets of their wishes at end of life may not be known by their family [11].

9.2.2.11 Do Not Resuscitate (DNR) Orders

Three quarters of AYAs with cancer believed it was appropriate to discuss end of life decisions early and only 12% were not comfortable discussing death [11]. Yet do-not-resuscitate (DNR) orders are frequently written only when death appeared imminent [2]. Broaching end of life is challenging for all professionals. A consistent clear message of agreed goals of care across the MDT can support the AYA and their family at this difficult time. Perceptions from parents and clinicians, fearing that raising end of life and DNR discussions will send a message to the AYA and the team caring for them that they are 'giving up', should be expunged. In some countries, DNR orders have expanded into more detailed documents called Emergency health (resuscitation) care plans [25]. These are a detailed stepwise approach to escalating levels of medical intervention from airway positioning, oxygen, rescue breaths through to cardiopulmonary resuscitation, intubation and ventilation and other advanced life support measures. Rather than completing a 'Do not' document, the process is more about what will and can provide benefit. AND (Allow Natural death) documents [26, 27]) have the same philosophical approach. Involving AYAs in end of life planning can help parents and professionals make informed decisions, alleviate distress, avoid decisional regret, and, perhaps, improve the patient's quality of life by respecting their values, beliefs, and preferences [28].

Ambulance directives are succinct distilled information for ambulance crews attending an AYA's home on the level of medical intervention agreed.

9.2.2.12 Tissue and Organ Donation

'When I die I want to give my body to science' (patient, 22 years)

AYAs with cancer in some circumstances may be able to donate, tissue or, in rare cases, organs. Donation should be part the Advance Care Plan discussions. AYAs have also asked about 'if they could donate their bodies to science so that they might help someone with the same disease in the future' [22] Donation for human transplant, scientific research or education may give some AYAs and their families a sense of altruism and meaning.

9.3 Symptoms and Their Management

Pain and symptom management in the AYA population requires an holistic approach utilising pharmacological, complementary interventions and therapies dependent on the needs of the individual. Robust studies are lacking in most areas of pain and symptom management with approaches extrapolated from adult and some paediatric research, clinical experience and historical practice.

In patients under 18 years of age prescribed medications are either on a weight-based measurement or in weight or age grouping. A cautious approach for a small AYA should be taken where weights of less than 50 kg may require a weight-based dosing schedule to reduce the side effect profile. The dichotomy of dosing means for some patients a marked sensitivity to the side effects of medication at start doses, whereas, others require higher doses to gain symptom control. Some AYAs consciously choose to have less medication than prescribed due to the side effect profile and to tolerate the symptoms they experience.

9.3.1 Compliance

> *"I take the drugs (prophylactic anticonvulsants), most of the time...when I remember..... when my left arm starts to shake. I definitely take it then." (patient, 19 years)*

63% of AYA cancer patients do not adhere to their treatment regimens [29]. AYAs are more frequently non-adherent than adults in chronic conditions [30]. Motivation, persistence, collaboration, mindfulness, cognitive capacity, flexibility and active participation are considered good indicators of adherence. The perceived value of adherence and identifying the consequences, may lead to improved adherence [31]. Similarly in palliative care setting, AYAs will continue to take medication if they perceive that the medication provides more benefit than side effects.

9.3.2 Symptom Management Plans

Symptom management plans consider and address anticipated symptoms providing pharmacological and non-pharmacological approaches to managing anticipated symptoms.

9.3.3 Pain and Symptom Assessment

A holistic assessment and management plan should occur separately but contemporaneously to the treatment and management of the AYA's cancer. The assessment should incorporate the biological, psychological and social aspects of their symptoms. For example, for pain assessment, the biological aspects should include site, description, temporal features, intensity, radiation, precipitants and the relieving factors of pain. Mood, sleep, anxiety and cognitive understanding are some of the psychological aspects that affect the AYA's perception of their pain and other symptoms. The attribution of meaning of the pain or symptom may have a powerful impact on how the AYA expresses and experiences that symptom. Social functioning (friendships and love relationships), educational issues and attendance and parental behaviours (for example catastrophising or minimizing of symptom experience) and their relationship with the AYA can influence the perceptions of their symptoms and how effective an intervention maybe.

9.4 Pain

9.4.1 Pain Tool

The numerical pain assessment scale is the commonest pain assessment tool used in the AYA population. A numerical scale should be introduced and clearly explained. For each pain episode, the scale should be used prior and after an intervention. The severity rating, mild (1–3), moderate (4–6) and severe (7–10), enables decision-making about the choice of analgesic or non-pharmacological approach. Staff should have appropriate training on the numerical scale. However, scales are only one part of a pain assessment.

9.4.2 Concepts and Definitions of Pain

Persisting Pain is cancer related pain, including treatment-related pain, but excludes procedure or investigation related pain (4).

Breakthrough pain is a sudden or rapid onset, occurring for short periods of time, and is usually severe. Typically, breakthrough dosing is 5–10% of total daily opioid requirement. In practice, increment of the breakthrough dose can occur separately to the background dose.

Incident pain is a specific breakthrough pain related to an activity or movement.

End of dose pain occurs before the next long-acting opiate is due.

9.4.3 Pain Ladder

The most significant change to AYA pain management is the change in the WHO (4) pain ladder from a 3-step to 2-step approach. Correct use of analgesics, dosing at regular intervals, using the appropriate route of administration and adapting treatment to the individual AYA is unchanged. Step one is simple non-opioid analgesics, for example Acetaminophen. If pain is moderate to severe, or poorly controlled, despite step 1, then move to strong opiates (step 2). Weak opiates are not recommended for persisting pain. Low dose strong opiates should be used and titrated with clinical effect. Adjuvant analgesics may be used.

9.5 **Medication** (Table 9.1)

9.5.1 Non-opioid Analgesics

Acetaminophen is a simple and effective form of pain relief. In neutropenic patients there is concern around masking fevers. Local guidance on temperature monitoring and Acetaminophen use should be followed. In the palliative care setting, the

Table 9.1 Analgesic medications

Analgesic medication			
WHO ladder for persisting pain		Adjuvants: To use in addition to WHO ladder	
Step 1: For mild to moderate pain		*Bone pain*	
Drug and route	**Cautions**	**Drug and route**	**Cautions**
Acetaminophen	Masks fever; caution in neutropenic patients	**NSAIDS**	Regular use with gastric protection
PO; PR;IV		PO;Topical; IV (some)	
Regular and/or PRN dosing		IR and MR preparations	
Non-steroidal anti-inflammatory (NSAIDS)	Masks fever; caution in neutropenic patients	**Bisphosphonates: Pamidronate**	Intravenous infusion
PO;Topical; IV (some)	Risk of effect on platelets	**Zolondronic acid**	Several infusions needed before possible clinical benefit
IR and MR preparations	Consider gastric protection in prolong use	IV	Side effect: Flu-like illness, hypocalcaemia, osteonecrosis (not reported in <18 years)
		PO (not considered effective in this context)	
Step 2: For moderate to severe pain		*Neuropathic agents*	
Morphine	Recommended first line opiate	**Antiepileptic classification**	
PO;PR;SC;IV	Where opioid substitution or rotation occurs: OME (Oral morphine equivalent) is used		
IR and MR preparations			
Oxycodone	Combination with naloxone available to reduce peripheral opiate effect including opiate-induced constipation	**Gabapentin**	Slow titration to reduce mild initial sedative and dizziness effects
PO;SC;IV		PO	
IR and MR preparations		Three times a day dosing	
Fentanyl	For IR preparations start at lowest dose and titrate.	**Pregabalin**	Compliance better due to twice daily dosing
Bu; SL; IN; SC;IV;TD	Convenient transdermal patch	PO	
IR and MR preparations	Rapid onset formulations for incidental or sudden pain	Twice times a day dosing	
	Opiate of use in renal failure		
Hydromorphine	Wide inter-individual variation	**Antidepressant classification**	
PO;IV;SC			
IR and MR preparation			

Table 9.1 (continued)

Analgesic medication			
WHO ladder for persisting pain		Adjuvants: To use in addition to WHO ladder	
Diamorphine	Only available in UK	**Amitriptyline**	Improvements in sleep and appetite may precede analgesic effect
Bu; IN; SC;IV	Potency enables reduced infusion volumes in syringe driver	PO	Anticholenergic side effects
	Suitable for subcutaneous and buccal administration due to solubility	Once to twice daily dosing	
Buprenorphine	Opiate agonist and antagonist properties	**Other adjuvant**	
SL;TD	Sublingual action 6–8 h	**Ketamine**	NMDA antagonist
IR and MR preparations	Some patches with 7 day application length		Higher doses as an anaesthetic
			Small risk of urinary symptoms
Methadone	Indications include:	Oral, PR-Rectal IV- Intravenous; SC-Subcutaneous, IM- intramuscular; SL-Sublingual; TD-Transdermal; IN-Intranasal; Bu-Buccal	
PO;IV;SC	Neuropathic pain	IR-immediate release preparation; MR-modified release preparation; NMDA- N-methyl-D- aspartate	
	Poorly responsive or uncontrolled pain		
	Specialist use only with various titration methods		
	Complex pharmacokinetics with long and variable half life with second peak phenomenon		

balance of controlling tumour related fever and mild pain to provide comfort outweighs the risk of potentially masking an infection.

Non-Steroidal Anti-Inflammatory Drugs *(NSAIDs)* are not recommended during treatment except for specific indications, for example, bone tumours. However, NSAIDs provide benefit in palliative care in bony pain and pleuritic chest pain. There is a small risk of increased bleeding and bruising with low platelet counts. Gastric protection with a proton-pump inhibitor is recommended if NSAIDs are given regularly.

9.5.2 Opioid Analgesics

Weak opioids are not recommended for persisting pain in adolescences (4). They can be considered for short-term acute pain, for example, post procedures and those AYAs over 18 years of age.

The choice of a *strong opioid* should be based on local practice. Morphine is recommended as first-line by WHO (4) for under 18 years of age. AYAs should be, where possible, offered a choice in the route of administration. Opiate switching should only occur if the AYA develops opioid tolerance, intrusive side effects or, rarely, opioid-induced hyper-analgesia.

9.5.3 Immediate Release (IR) Opioids for Breakthrough Pain

When commenced on an IR opiate, regular use provides around the clock effective pain relief. In practice, the IR opiate is often taken as required by the AYA due to compliance and concerns over side effects. Decision-making about the type of IR used is dependent on the rapidity of pain onset and ability to absorb and tolerate oral medications. Usually oral IR opiate formulations are used but other formulations, including buccal, intranasal and sublingual, are available in some countries. These ultra-rapid IR opiate formulations (buccal, intranasal and sublingual), provide a quicker onset and shorter duration of action. Due the nature of these products concerns about addiction are high; though, may be less relevant in this population. Recommendations on limiting the total number used per day and the appropriate indication of use should be clearly documented and explained to the AYA. Patient controlled analgesia (PCA) in the palliative care setting can be useful in some cases for severe, frequent, rapid onset pain and in patients with enteral absorption issues, for example, bowel obstruction. Community PCA [32] is available in some centres.

9.5.4 Modified Release (MR) Opioids for Background Pain

After a minimum of 48 h the IR requirement is averaged for each 24 h period and then converted into a modified release (sustained release) form (MR). Break through doses of IR preparations should continue to be prescribed as required. Increases in the MR should be based on the preceding days breakthrough doses. Discuss with the AYA about the timing to convert to MR formulation since some AYA prefer to remain on IR for a prolonged period before converting. Information about tolerance, dependency and addiction should be provided and appropriate reassurances given.

9.5.4.1 Morphine

Morphine is often the first line opiate in severe cancer pain. The morphine IR onset of action is 20 min with peak effect at 60 min and an average length of action of 4 h In the AYA population the length of effect can be shorter. Decisions about increasing the dose or more frequent prescribing, for example, 3 h, requires consideration of response to the dose and side effects experienced. Titration of breakthrough doses is usually by 10–25% on the previous dose. Morphine MR is available as 12 and 24 h formulations. Usual practice is 12 h preparations. Some AYA experience end of dose failure with need to increase the MR dose accordingly. There is a marked dichotomy of response by AYA to morphine (and other opiates), with some AYA being very sensitive to very small doses and other requiring rapid titration to high doses to control pain. A common-sense approach is starting low and reassess frequently. AYA describe a sense of 'spaced out' or 'removed from the situation' sensation as being very intrusive; this often leads to discontinuation of the opiates early on. Reassurance that this sensation usually settles is important to explore up front. Low start doses and low dose titrations maybe needed.

9.5.4.2 Fentanyl

Fentanyl is a well tolerated, first line in renal impairment and a good option in AYA's with bowel obstruction. Fentanyl has various routes of administration making it a popular choice. It has a rapid onset of action and is absorbed transdermally and buccally. There are now Fentanyl products available for buccal, sublingual and intranasal use. These preparations have a 5–15 min onset of action. Owing to the lack of published data in the AYA group, it is recommended to follow initial guidance to start at the lowest possible dose and titrate accordingly observing caution in the opiate-naïve patient. Fentanyl IR productions should be considered only once the patient has been exposed to at least an oral morphine equivalent of 30–60 mg/day. Due to the rapid onset of action they have a high risk of abuse and only up to 4 doses per day should be prescribed.

Fentanyl transdermal preparations (MR opioid) may improve compliance due to ease of use. The 72 h matrix transdermal fentanyl formulation can be cut enabling smaller dose increases. In some AYAs, the 72 h patches require changing every 48 h due to reports of increased breakthrough pain on day 3. On application, sedation increases initially, itching (25%) and erythema (15%) occurs but with no other significant side are reported [33].

Oxycodone

Oxycodone is considered to have a cleaner side effect profile and is often well tolerated in the AYA population. It is often second line to Morphine when used enterally. Anecdotally it is preferentially used in the presence of metastatic bone disease and other related bone pain in some centres due to its perceived benefit compared to Morphine. It has both IR and MR formulations.

9.5.4.3 Hydromorphine

Hydromorphine is an alternative opioid analgesic for severe pain and is antitussive. It has both enteral (IR and MR) and parenteral formulations. There is a wide potency ratio and inter-patient variability.

Buprenorphine

Buprenorphine has opiate agonist and antagonist properties and is used in moderate to severe pain with both sublingual and transdermal [34] routes available. Due to the strong receptor affinity, standard doses of Naloxone will not reverse the respiratory effects of Buprenorphine. This opiate is often used in stable persisting cancer. Compared to other opiates, Buprenorphine, over the long term, may have a lesser impact on endocrine dysfunction [35].

9.5.4.4 Methadone

Methadone is indicated for severe intractable pain, complex neuropathic pain or as an opiate switch due to intolerable undesirable effects. It has a wide inter-patient variability in the drug's absorption, metabolism, relative analgesic potency and duration of action with repeated doses having an accumulative effect. Therefore, it should only be utilised by a specialist with experience in its use. At a clinically effective analgesic dose, methadone dosage and duration were not correlated with QTc prolongation, even in the presence of other risk factors, suggesting that methadone use may be safe in the under 18 year age group [36]. Methadone can be used for complex neuropathic pain and should be seen as a part of the armamentarium against cancer-related pain with few side effects reported [37].

9.6 Managing Opiate Side Effects

9.6.1 Constipation

Opiate induced constipation is a well-known side effect. Standard local constipation guidance should be used including diet advice, fluid intake and exercise. Osmotic laxatives are often first line with stimulants added if there is no clinical response. Peripheral acting opioid antagonist preparations are available, such as methylnaltrexone, which can be administered subcutaneously or intravenously, and PEGylated naloxol as an oral preparation taken daily. Some MR opiate preparations have naloxone incorporated into the formulation. Compliance with laxative medication is a significant issue in the AYA population and AYAs may often present with significant abdominal pain secondary to constipation, compounded by taking further opiates to alleviate the abdominal pain. Education and shared agreement on a palatable laxative for the individual AYA may improve compliance.

9.6.2 Nausea and Vomiting

Cyclizine is the standard antiemetic prescribed for opioid induced nausea. However AYAs have a wealth of experience related to the personal effects of individual antiemetics, having often been exposed to emetogenic therapies. $5HT_3$ antagonists are commonly continued in palliation due to the experience of the patient and on-going cancer directed therapy. However $5HT_3$ antagonists are constipating and may, therefore, contribute to gastrointestinal upset; encouragement of laxative or consideration of switching antiemetics should be explored.

9.6.3 Somnolance and Sedation

Opiate induced sedation is a common. Daytime somnolence or sedation often settles once a stable opiate dose is reached. Initially a reduction in the opiate dose may be required followed by a slower titration to a clinically effective dose, which may support the AYA in gaining some tolerance to this unwanted side effect. Switching to an alternative opiate or adding an adjuvant may limit the opiate dose, hence limiting the sedation effects. Methylphenidate (psychostimulant) may be useful for daytime somnolence with an AYA taking a dose prior to a planned event, providing a period of increased wakefulness for 4 h.

9.6.4 Adjuvant

9.6.4.1 Ketamine

Ketamine is a NMDA receptor antagonist, used in severe neuropathic intractable pain, adjuvant for severe pain and for reducing high opiate requirements. Oral bioavailability is low but it can be given buccally. There are no randomized, controlled trials on the use of Ketamine in the under 18 years old population with cancer pain. However a few studies report safety data [38, 39] and consider it as an option for refractory cancer pain in both adults and children [38, 39]. The psychotomimetic effects are common, which can be treated with haloperidol or a benzodiazepine.

9.6.4.2 Steroids

Officially corticosteroids are not recommended [40] in the management of cancer pain for adolescence. There are no studies in this age group to support adjuvant use and the well-known adverse effects, particularly with chronic use are well known. Corticosteroids are indicated in the management of specific conditions, which secondarily improve the symptom of pain. Raised intracranial pressure, peritumour oedema, nerve or spinal cord compression may all respond to a course of steroids and hence improve pain. A systematic review [41] in adults suggested that corticosteroids may have a moderate analgesic effect in cancer patients. They were well tolerated in medium doses for up to 7 days with serious toxicity and higher mortality rates with high doses over 8 weeks. The paucity of relevant studies was striking with evidence graded as "very low."

Muscle relaxants including benzodiazepines and baclofen may provide benefit in managing pain related to muscle spasms.

9.6.4.3 Bisphosphonates

Bisphosphonates are used to reduce anticipated pain secondary to bony metastases, with clinical effects taking up to several months to be realised. The AYA may not tolerate the flu-like symptoms experienced with the initial few infusions. To date, there have been no reports of jaw osteonecrosis associated with bisphosphonate use in the under 18 years age group.

9.6.5 Neuropathic Pain

Neuropathic pain is the abnormal processing of pain signals by the brain and spinal cord in the peripheral or central nervous system resulting in pain persisting without on-going stimuli. It can be caused by structural damage and/or nerve cell dysfunction (both peripheral and central nervous system).

There are various options in managing neuropathic pain including neuropathic agents, local anaesthetics or other modalities or interventions. In isolated nerve pain, local or regional nerve blocks may be used in specific cases. A steroid pulse or radiotherapy to a local tumour causing direct nerve compression may be appropriate. The use of neuropathic agents is commonplace, titrating to a clinically effective dose and sometimes requiring drug combinations to gain control. Opiates may provide a partial short-term role only in relieving severe neuropathic pain, especially in a mixed pain presentation.

For complex mixed pain cases approaches including the use of Opiates (including methadone), Ketamine, neuropathic agents and a benzodiazepine maybe indicated. Benzodiazepines may provide benefit in sleep and anxiety-enhanced pain.

9.6.6 Neuropathic Agents

Gabapentin is used in adolescents [42] with **Pregabalin** as a viable alternative [43] especially in compliance-challenging adolescents due to its twice daily dosing. Both are well tolerated with a low incidence of adverse effects. Low dose **Amytriptyline** may improve sleep and appetite, preceding an analgesic effect but its side effect profile (constipation, drowsiness and dry mouth) may limit its use. Other antidepressants may have neuropathic analgesic benefits but specialist psychiatric advice should be taken combined with psychosocial support, due to the increased risk of suicide in the adolescent population taking certain antidepressants. Lidocaine patches [44], a topical local anaesthetic and Menthol and Capsaicin creams (variable concentrations) may provide a local cooling or anaesthetic effect to manage local topical areas of neuropathic pain.

9.7 Non-pharmacological Pain Management

Effective pain management requires a holistic approach; just as in drug therapy, there are many non-drug therapies available but finding the most effective for the individual AYA may require some trial and error.

Psychological approaches that can be used include multicomponent cognitive behavioural therapy, hypnosis, biofeedback and pacing. With pacing, there is a learning to balance time spent on activity and rest to achieve increased function and participation in meaningful activity. Behavioural and physical interventions are offered by Occupational therapists and physiotherapists, and can include relaxation techniques, such as progressive and passive muscular relaxation, guided visualization and psycho-education (eg mantras and desensitisation). TENS and cold and heat therapy aides may provide effective relief. Complementary therapy including reflexology, massage and acupuncture may be available in some centres and provide benefit to some. *Sleep* is an integral part of pain management. Adolescents should have their sleep assessed (clinical review, sleep diary or standardized sleep measures) and treated [45]. Sleep disorders have been associated with pain, fatigue, medication and hospitalisation in adolescents suffering from cancer [46].

9.8 Symptom Management

9.8.1 Anorexia and Fatigue

Anorexia and fatigue are significant problems in palliative and end of life care. The causes are usually multifactorial and 'treatable' issues should be addressed. For example, nausea and vomiting in anorexic cases and fatigue secondary to anaemia are potentially responsive to intervention. The effective management of other symptoms, in particular, pain and breathlessness may also improve fatigue and improve appetite.

The use of steroids has shown some clinical benefits [41, 47] with no clear guidance on the most effective corticosteroid drug, dose, or duration of treatment [48]. For the AYA the impact of steroids on their physical appearance may minimize their use. Other agents including methylphenidate for fatigue and cannaboids for appetite may be considered, depending on local prescribing practice and guidance.

Moderate exercise, pacing, avoiding daytime naps, improving nighttime sleeping may be more important in improving fatigue than pharmacological management. Similarly, with the support of a dietician, use of small meals sizes, snacking and effective management of other gastrointestinal symptoms may improve cancer-related anorexia.

9.8.2 Anxiety and Agitation

Anxiety is often considered a psychological issue with agitation being either the physical manifestation of anxiety or resulting from a somatic cause. The AYA's anxiety should be explored and addressed. Assessment of psychological wellbeing including sleep disorders, depression and other anxiety related mental health conditions should be considered. Exploration around facing one's own mortality alongside the transition from childhood to adulthood, managing family, relationships, one's own identity and friendships may require talking therapy or practical support. Referral to a psychologist may be beneficial. Complementary and alternative therapies, including relaxation and guided visualization techniques, may be of benefit. Provision of short-term anxiolytics, for example sublingual Lorazepam, to be used for anxiety inducing events, may be of benefit.

Agitation may manifest towards end of life. There are a plethora of possible causes including unexpressed fears, potentially reversible medical causes, other symptoms inadequately managed and the need to address basic care. A systematic approach is required to address reversible conditions and enable concerns and fears to be expressed. As the AYA enters end of life, agitation may increase. Consider the environment,; a quiet and calm atmosphere may be of benefit, although for some, a noisy household brings comfort and familiarity. Reduce triggers of agitation by providing visual clues to place and time, for example, curtains open and closed representing day and night time. If the agitation is pronounced then medication may be required. A short-acting benzodiazepine may be used. Antipsychotic medication, for example, haloperidol, may be useful for AYAs experiencing disinhibition or hallucinatory elements to their agitation. In some cases, a combination of medications is required. Levomepromazine may be needed to provide increased level of sedation in severe agitation. If the AYA continues to be agitated, they may benefit from regular antipsychotic or long acting benzodiazepine or an infusion can be started. Both haloperidol and Levomepromazine have an additional antiemetic benefit. Risperidone and Olanzepine can also be considered but often at an earlier stage.

Terminal agitation occurs at end of life and is a diagnosis of exclusion with the cause poorly understood. The AYA may insist on getting up, despite being very weak, constantly changing position and complaining they are not comfortable. They may become very angry, restless or unable to be comforted. They may experience hallucinations and have fluctuating conscious levels. Benzodiazepines, Haloperidol or Levomepromazine can be used. The route of administration may be parenteral rather than oral to gain rapid relief from symptoms.

9.8.3 Breathlessness

Besides pain, breathlessness is one of the most frequently observed symptoms [3]. Breathlessness is a subjective experience of breathing discomfort that consists of qualitatively distinct sensations that can vary in intensity. Often an objective assessment is made with the rate and intensity of breathing rather than the subjective experience of the AYA. Management should focus on the AYA's perception of any intervention providing a subjective improvement. Simple numerical rating scale (0–10) on the AYA's subjective level of breathlessness can be used serially to determine clinical benefit for any interventions. A holistic approach is needed to maximise symptom relief. Reversible, or partially reversible conditions should be considered and managed accordingly including bronchospasm, retained secretions, infection, anxiety and fluid overload. Simple measures, including fans and resting in areas providing cross ventilation, can enable a subjective feeling of increased air being present. Support from occupational therapy and physiotherapy are vital in providing the AYA a choice in techniques for managing breathless episodes including positioning, mirroring of breathing, pacing of activities and relaxation techniques. Anxiety can trigger or exacerbate breathlessness and vice versa and management of both is required. Complementary therapies, including massage, for relaxation and deep breathing, and acupuncture including self-needling techniques and beads, may also provide perceived benefit.

The role of oxygen for breathlessness, while it is contentious, should be considered if it provides subjective relief to the AYA. Air may be as effective in relieving breathlessness. Oxygen should be humidified and heroic doses avoided. On-going saturation monitoring is a poor predictor of clinical relief from breathlessness and is better to ask the AYA. An awareness and understanding of the risk of hypercapnia in some patients and the risk of increasing oxygen should be well understood. Other measures, including saline nebulisers, may provide support to dry mucosal membranes and help clear thickened retained secretions.

Anxiolytic medication and low dose opiates may be needed if the measures mentioned above do not control the on-going symptoms of breathlessness. Opioid receptors are distributed throughout the respiratory system and, when used, reduce the sensation of breathlessness. Low dose (commonly quoted as 30–50% of the pain dose) IR opiates can be used initially and then MR opiates prescribed if appropriate. For patients who are already on opioids for pain control, it is reasonable to offer as required doses of 25–50% less than those being used for breakthrough pain.

Benzodiazepines are used to reduce the anxiety associated with breathlessness but other interventions should be tried first due to their sedating profile. Levomepromazine is an alternative when sedation is needed in severe breathlessness.

Terminal breathlessness has a severe sudden onset, often moving from breathlessness on exertion to at rest. When this occurs, it is often a terminal event. The goal of care is to settle and make the AYA as comfortable as possible as quickly as possible. Both a short acting benzodiazepine and opiate IR should be used; given 15–30 mins apart. They may be repeated to gain rapid relief from symptoms. An infusion of both benzodiazepine and opiate may be required.

9.8.4 Cough

Cough is an intrusive irritant. The underlying cause needs to be considered including local disease, reflux, secretions, aspiration, hiccups, bronchospasm and pneumonia. Initial management should relate to the underlying cause. Further measures can include humidified oxygen, nebulised salbutamol or saline, physiotherapy or cough suppressants including low dose morphine.

9.8.5 Seizures

In identified at risk patients, including primary brain tumour and brain metastases, intracranial bleed or biochemical imbalances, provide AYAs and their families with information on how to recognise and manage a seizure including acute rescue medication. The use of prophylactic anticonvulsants may be appropriate. Levetiracetam is a commonly used prophylactic anticonvulsant in the brain tumour population.

Breakthrough seizures can be managed with rescue medication, often a short acting benzodiazepine that can be repeated. Second line rescue medication may include paraldehyde, phenytoin or a phenobarbitone loading dose or an alternative benzodiazepine. Choice of medication should depend on local policy and/or national guidelines. Regular anticonvulsants may then require increasing.

Status epilepticus can occur and, on occasions, be a terminal event. This is defined as seizures occurring so frequently that one has not recovered from the coma produced by one seizure, before the next seizure supervenes. Ultimately, if the seizure is not controlled, it becomes continuous leading to hypoxia, brain damage and death. Decision-making about the level of intervention, including admission to intensive care for airway support and sedation, requires consideration of the reversibility of the seizure and the appropriateness for the individual AYAs at the time of presentation. Terminal seizures have increasing seizure frequency in the end of life phase even when they do not merge into a continuous seizure as in status epilepticus. Palliative care management for both types are similar, involving a stepwise approach using rescue medication, usually a short acting benzodiazepine that can be repeated. Infusions may be required to abate or continue to control the recalcitrant or recurrent seizures. On-going rescue medication will inform increments in the background infusion to gain seizure control. Medications used usually include benzodiazepine and phenobarbitone. In the brain tumour population low dose benzodiazepine infusions are usually enough. Phenobaritone is used when the seizures are partially, or completely, unresponsive to increments in benzodiazepines. Midazolam can be mixed with other syringe driver medication and phenobarbitone must be given as a separate infusion as it cannot be mixed with other medication.

9.9 Neurological Deterioration

Managing the neurological deterioration often seen in AYA with brain tumours, requires complex coordinated support. The AYA experiences their body beginning to fail them whilst often maintaining their cognition and sense of self. The emotive and physical impact to the AYA and their loved ones cannot be underestimated. Effects on independence, mobility, self care [49], communication and eating are seen and each area should be addressed in turn with the support of the MDT.

Particular areas of contention include the use of mobility equipment; AYAs may often resist support unless it enables them some sense of real independence. Nasogastric tubes or planned gastrostomy insertion to support nutrition and reduce hunger, particularly experienced with steroids, should be explored early. Nasogastric tube insertion can occur at anytime point along the palliative and end of life care journey. Consent from the AYA is paramount; benefits and risks should be explored, including risk of aspiration, balanced against the pleasure of eating. Rationalisation of medications in an AYA with difficulty in swallowing and utilising alternative routes of administration may reduce the oral intake burden for the AYA.

9.10 Corticosteroids

One of the mainstays of treatment in reducing neurological symptoms is corticosteroids. They are often part of the AYA's chemotherapy and radiotherapy regime, supportive care management for various symptoms and used in emergencies, for example, spinal cord compression. Corticosteroids have a well-known side effect profile with both short and long term sequelae. Effects on mood and sleep disturbance are particularly an issue in AYA population. Dexamethasone is often the corticosteroid of choice in the setting of neurological decline in the brain tumour population, used with limited published data to indicate best approach to dosing and weaning. Some centres give 5-day pulsed courses whereas others taper over a longer period, balanced against clinical effect. A practical approach should consider the lowest effective dose for the least possible time with clear objectives for determining clinical benefit. Prior steroid use, effectiveness and side effects, may support decision making on an individualised risk-benefit ratio. Notwithstanding the experience of the clinical team, often the AYA will have a clear view of the use of steroids due to previous clinical benefit and the effects it has had on their mood, appetite and physical appearance.

9.11 Gastrointestinal Issues

9.11.1 Nausea and Vomiting

Nausea and vomiting are common issues in cancer care. In palliation, the approach is similar to on treatment, where often the cause is multifactorial. Anxiety, pain, gastrointestinal upset, raised intracranial pressure and side effects of medication, in particular opiates, are common causes. Simple measures including avoiding strong smells and having small frequent meals may help. Select an anti-emetic medication based on their site of action in the emesis pathway considered to be the dominant cause in the AYA. If combining medication, ideally prescribe from different groups but many will overlap in their site of action. Beyond the standard antiemetics 5HT3, cyclizine and Hyoscine, Metaclopramide can be used but has an increased risk of extrapyramidal side effects in adolescents. Other prokinetic agents may be used in the palliative care setting including Domperidone and erthyromycin. Levomepromazine is an effective antiemetic, with dose related sedation properties. Haloperidol is an alternative antiemetic and Lorazepam is often tried in anticipatory nausea. Often non-enteral routes are needed initially to gain control of symptoms before converting to enteral formulations. In opiate induced nausea, the symptoms often resolve after a few weeks and discontinuation of the antiemetic can be trialled. Non-pharmacological approaches including seabands and acupuncture may provide benefit.

9.11.2 Bowel Obstruction

AYAs presenting with bowel obstruction are often highly symptomatic. Often the obstruction is recurrent and can become refractory to treatment. The gastro-intestinal symptoms and bowel function may improve with a combination of anti-inflammatory (for example, dexamethasone), anti-secretory (for example, Octreotide) and a prokinetic (for example, Metaclopramide) [50]. If the bowel obstruction is complete, a prokinetic is not recommended. A wide-bore nasogastric tube may be useful in decompressing the stomach and enabling rapid relief of symptoms. The aim is to enable some oral intake (for pleasure and satis), pain control and reduction in nausea. Intravenous fluids or TPN may be useful as a short-term measure until oral intake has returned. In patients with severe pain, patient controlled anaglesia (PCA) can be of benefit since analgesia can be given parenterally. Alternatively buccal, sublingual and transdermal routes are indicated.

9.11.3 Secretions

Drooling and secretions are particularly challenging in the AYA with a brain tumour. The balance between very loose secretions, which without an effective swallow can spill into the airway, and thick secretions that the AYA cannot cough and clear, requires constant reassessment. Medication including Hyoscine and Glycopyrronium can be used to thicken secretions and saline nebulisers at various concentrations can loosen secretions.

Many dying patients develop noisy breathing from excessive secretions sitting on the vocal cords and upper airway; often referred to as the 'death rattle'. Oral suctioning of secretions may give comfort but will not reach the secretions sitting beyond the oral cavity. Deep suctioning of these secretions may induce bradycardia and cause distress if a gag is present. Management of the other end of life symptoms and drying of the secretions with medication may reduce but not completely eliminate the noisy breathing. An awareness is needed, that excessive respiratory secretions are a dose-related side effect of the benzodiazepines, which are often administered in the dying setting. Families should be reassured that this symptom, though distressing to the listener, is unlikely to be causing any distress to the patient.

9.12 Experimental Therapy

Many AYA and their families continue to search for cure. They may engage in clinical drug trials and/or look at non-traditional approaches, including diets and herbal remedies. Phase I and II trials are available for AYA patients but some may have to wait until they are 18 years to enter relevant adult trials. Until then the patient may have access to Paediatric trials. Palliative care support alongside on-going experimental therapy is important in controlling symptoms and facilitating care, especially when coming off trial. The enrolment on a early phase trial does not effect end of life care characteristics, suggesting that quality end of life can be delivered regardless of early phase trial participation [51].

Open communication on the types of non-traditional therapies being tried is needed to monitor drug interactions and side effects with conventional therapies. The MDT can provide the AYA and their families with support in navigating the choices in trialling non-traditional approaches to cancer-directed therapy.

9.13 Recreational Drugs

"I took my MST (Morphine sulphate tablets) this afternoon when I woke up and also had some Sevredol (Morphine IR) 'cos my pain was really bad. I'm not sleeping 'cos I'm short of cash to buy my weed." (patient, 18 years)

"I know Ketamine, my mate took some at the back of science class." (patient, 17 years)

Availability, exposure, experimentation and use of recreational drugs are prevalent in the AYA population. Awareness and acknowledgement of the presence of recreational drugs with the AYA may support an open discussion on personal use and experience and perceptions of effect and impact. AYAs will generally not raise the topic independently and, therefore, it should be introduced by health professionals in an unjudgemental manner and away from parents. Awareness of the role of social drug taking is an important part of assessing and managing an AYA's pain and other symptoms and should be explored with all AYAs. Education about the difference and safety between prescribed medication and similar drugs available on the street should be explored. Impact on the interaction of alcohol with prescribed medication and recreational drugs should be explained.

Prescribed medication is also potentially open for abuse and clinicians should be aware how each medication formulation could be abused. Intraveneous Cyclizine (antiemetic) when given as a fast intravenous push gives a 'rush to the head' enjoyed by some. Oxycodone tablets can be crushed and snorted and Fentanyl patches can be rolled and smoked or give a rapid increase in dose in a very hot bath. This should not prevent prescribing of these medications to manage symptoms but enables the prescriber to be alert to telltale signs of abuse.

9.13.1 Driving with Opiates

Check the country's driving regulations since they vary. In the UK the AYA must be on a stable dose of opiates to drive. Caution is required about recreational sports involving machinery, for example, jetski and motor-cross, which are not always included in the regulations.

9.14 Social Media and the Internet

#DNR or #resus (patient, 19 years)

Internet and social media are the social hub and life of most AYAs. Their use, and lack thereof, can often inform professionals about the AYA's current psychological and physical wellbeing.

Social media enables AYAs to keep in touch with friends and family and update them on their progress and care. Vblogging and other diary type formats are widely used to share their experiences, offering help to others, and find meaning for themselves. Themes of adolescent bloggers include 'normalizing the news, facing treatment failure, and reconciling 'chronos'-the finite concept of time' [52]. The balance between sharing and over exposure is a constant issue requiring support and guidance. Trolling can happen to anyone and even in bereavement. As the AYA becomes more unwell they may start to cut themselves off and reduce the forums and platforms they use. Every missed party or social event pinged to their phone can be keenly felt. Discussions with AYA about the use of social media sites and passwords to electronic devices should be had with the AYA prior to end of life. Some AYA families use their social media sites as memorials and maintain them including notifying friends of funerals and memorial events. For some families this can be very precious in the initial period after an AYA dies.

AYA and their families use the internet to search for better understanding of their condition, treatments and prognosis. When the prognosis is poor, alternative therapies, experimental therapies and sharing of information and experiences abound. It can provide a wealth of helpful information and support but it can also be the conveyor of inaccurate information peppered with unsubstantiated reports of miraculous cures bought at house re-mortgaging prices. Navigating this information overload and sense of unproven possibilities can be overwhelming and require support from both oncology and palliative care teams.

9.15 End of Life

Once the end of life phase is recognised, discussions and decisions around level of intervention, monitoring, goals and place of care should take place. Review of appropriate medication and completion of Emergency Health Care Plans (DNR orders) should take place. Currently AYAs still receive chemotherapy (11%) within 14 days of death with 22% admitted to intensive care in the last month of life; 68% of AYAs receive at least 1 medically intensive end of life care measure [53].

When planning end of life care, the preferred place of death should be identified. Despite most stating a preference to be at home if they were dying [11] most AYA actually die in hospital [53]. When making decisions about place of care at end of life, a realistic and achievable picture should be presented, since the preferred place of care may not be possible due service provision or impractical in meeting the health needs of the AYA. Services and professionals should flex and accommodate the AYA and their family wishes as much as possible whilst continuing to balance the needs of their other patients. A community team may be able to offer end of life care 24/7, but only for short periods of time, or, hospitals may not be able to promise a bed, specific staff or additional accommodation if the AYA is entering their end of life phase.

Stopping the routines of ward life can be beneficial through reducing personal intrusion and anxiety around changing observations, or, results that require no positive action or intervention by the professional to improve the wellbeing of the AYA. The continuation of some routines, however, can bring comfort and reassurance. Therefore an agreed plan with initial removal of interventions that the AYA dislikes or dreads, eg, blood pressure readings, especially at night, is a good first step.

Levels of intervention and monitoring should be agreed based on the perceived benefit to the AYA. The rationale for stopping of routine investigations and rationalization of antibiotic and antifungal therapy should be explained. Simple checklists can be useful to ensure all aspects of care are considered. When referring to a hospice at end of life, clarify the level of intervention and monitoring a hospice can provide prior to offering the service, for example, most children's hospice, cannot take a patient on Total parental nutrition (TPN) who is not on an established community TPN program.

AYA usually have few or no comorbid conditions prior to their cancer diagnosis. Their bodies are young and vital. End of life care in the AYA with cancer can in some cases be protracted. Managing a prolonged end of life phase can be physically, emotionally and practically challenging for the AYA, their loved ones and professionals. AYAs often have a keen awareness of their changing condition and often recognize when death is close.

When preparing the AYA, their family and professionals for end of life care, consider the possible modes of death and prepare for these circumstances. Explaining the possible modes in simple terms enables the AYA and their family to plan, be prepared and act on manifesting symptoms quickly to alleviate these symptoms and minimise suffering. As part of the process of dying, controlling of symptoms through effective symptom management may enable a short period of stability. Professionals call this 'the window' (or the 'rally'). Families may be keen to reduce medication or reconsider curative options. AYAs and their loved ones should be encouraged to make the most of this brief period, if it occurs.

9.15.1 End of Life Care Symptom Management

The end of life phase in the AYA can occur rapidly over a few hours, or be prolonged, lasting several weeks. Distinct issues around symptom management arise that may be challenging to manage. AYA experience both physical symptoms, commonest being pain and dyspnoea, and psychological symptoms, including sadness, anxiety, fear and guilt in the end of life phase [3]. End-of-life care can include transfusions, artificial nutrition, corticosteroids, pain control, sedation but also palliative chemotherapy [3].

The fears around medication speeding up the dying process should be explored and assurances given. The clinician should explain the role of each medication at end of life, to alleviate suffering and allowing a good death and that the lack of medication will not stop death. Professionals should be aware that all treatment has inherent risk and be familiar with the concept of the doctrine of double effect: 'A single act having two possible seen effects, one good and one harmful, is not always morally prohibited if the harmful effect is not intended'. Professionals should improve their knowledge of medication used at end of life so they are confident and assured in the right approach to managing the AYA's end of life phase.

Blood and platelet transfusions, which may have provided symptomatic relief in palliation, for example, symptomatic anaemia, provide no clinical benefit in this phase of illness.

Nutrition and hydration can be maintained with the insertion of a nasogastric tube. Guidance is available on if and how various medications can be given down a nasogastric tube [54]. However, at end of life, gastric absorption curtails and often a significant reduction in feed volume is required, conversion to rehydration fluid or stop/starting small volumes of feeds may need to be considered. Mouth care should be maintained. Some AYAs refuse nasogastric tubes and their wishes should be respected. If end of life is prolonged, hydration in the form of intraveneous or subcutaneous fluids can be explored if the AYA is not able to take some oral sips of fluids. In practice this is uncommon.

Route of administration may alter, if an AYA has a nasogastric tube insitu, some deaths may be managed with transdermal, buccal and nasogastric routes. Vigilance of continued gastric absorption during end of life care is imperative with conversion of medication to intraveneous (if central venous access is present) or subcutaneous infusions, if necessary.

Infusions, either intravenously or subcutaneously, over a 24 h period can be commenced with up to five [55] compatible drugs being mixed in one driver. These may include a benzodiazepine (to manage agitation and seizures), opiate (to manage pain and breathlessness), antiemetic and an antisecretory as the mainstays of end of life care. Not all are required and should only be added if clinically indicated, or, a high clinical concern of occurrence. Initial infusion doses should be based on conversion from current oral dosing. Bolus doses of appropriate medications can continue to be given, as needed, to control breakthrough symptoms. Bolus volumes of up to 3 mL may be tolerated subcutaneously. The infusion dose can then be increased based on the breakthrough doses needed in the preceding 24 h. Caution should be exhibited if breakthrough doses total more than a 30–50% increase in the resultant background infusion. Review of the clinical effect of the current medications may be needed; the addition of Haloperidol or switch to Levomepromazine may be required, for example, if escalation of the benzodiazepine for agitation is not providing adequate effect. Compatibilities [55] and the infusion site should be checked regularly. Dexamethasone has been added to infusions to maintain the subcutaneous site.

9.16 Parents and Caregivers

> *'When I die I want my ashes to be spread outside my favourite shop so I can shop there every day, what about you?'(mother to her 17 year old)*

Parenting the AYA brings its own challenges, as the AYA matures they move from a family centred/parent led view to a friend centred/independent view. With illness comes a temporary reverse or brake on this transition. With palliative care and the natural protective instincts of a parent, conflict around decision-making and information sharing can occur between the AYA and their parents. The death of one's child brings unimaginable loss and professionals often have a difficult task in navigating and supporting parents whilst ensuring the AYA are centre to the discussions and decision-making process. There is not always consensus between AYA and their parents on the importance of dying a natural death, dying at home and "wanting to know if I were dying."

Many AYAs report feeling comfortable discussing end of life, and the majority preferred to talk about end of life issues before they are facing end of life [11]. The AYA's family communication and decision-making culture may have a significant impact on how information is shared and decisions reached. Some AYA may, and some may not, wish to be part of the discussion. Check out with the AYA how they would like to hear news, especially difficult news; it may be they choose to hear news by themselves, with their parents or want their parents to hear some news first. Respecting the AYA's decision is imperative. Encouraging families to initiate conversations with AYAs away from the consultation room is part of the support that an MDT can offer. Professionals should never lie, or collude with families, in withholding information from the AYA, on the perception of causing too much distress. However, professionals can support the AYA and family in maintaining hope and a planned approach in how to communicate difficult news.

9.17 Siblings and Friends

I'm going to tell my brother and sister first and then invite my friends over on Friday night and tell them....so hopefully they are ok to go to school on Monday. My friends want to book a holiday next July for when I've finished treatment and I'm better; they don't understand why I won't put down a deposit. (patient 18 years)

AYAs have the right to control how information is shared with friends, school, siblings and the wider family and community. The opportunity to say previously unsaid words, make further memories, and say goodbye is an important aspect of end of life care for the AYA, their siblings and the friends they leave behind. Siblings should have information shared openly and honestly [24] be given the opportunity, if they wish, to be involved in the palliative care process and be actively engaged in funeral and memorials. 'Bereaved siblings of adolescents with cancer who died report anxiety, depression, and illicit substance use increased during the first year after their sibling's death. Siblings who reported dissatisfaction with communication, poor preparation for death, missed opportunities to say goodbye, and/or a perceived negative impact of the cancer experience on relationships tended to have higher distress and lower social support scores. Almost all siblings reported that their loss still affected them.' [56].

AYAs may decide to share their news with their friends, some may choose to do this directly or some through their parents or one close friend. Up until end of life the AYA may have welcomed frequent visitors but towards end of life AYAs may be more reluctant for friends to visit. This is in part due to their physical changes and encroaching illness, which may manifest increasing distressing symptoms. This lack of desire for visitors should not be seen as a reflection on their friendships, more on the impact of their disease.

9.18 Bereavement

Bereavement support should be part of the palliative care process. Bereavement work can start at diagnosis, through palliation, and end of life. On-going access to spiritual and psychological support is important with the level of engagement and support needed varying on the stage of illness and the individuals involved. For some specific support groups for parents, grandparents and siblings may be beneficial, while for others, one to one work or specific therapies (eg music or art) is more effective. Maladaptive grief requires psychological and sometimes psychiatric input. Identification of risk factors (for example a history of depression, anxiety disorders or drug and alcohol abuse) may be useful in enabling early referral to appropriate services.

Conclusion

A palliative care ethos should be embedded within an oncology service with the concepts of maintaining hope whilst offering choice, planning and effective symptom management. Palliative care should be, where possible, uniquely tailored to the individual AYA patient. For the professional, the challenge is, as far as possible, to ensure the AYA, at the pace of their choosing, to be well informed, their decisions respected and their choices realized.

Early referral to palliative care, should be seen as providing benefit with the aim to improve the AYA's well being and it may, in some cases, be life prolonging and be offered hand in hand with on-going cancer directed therapy. Services should provide a MDT approach to care, death and bereavement, tailored to the AYA's needs but considering also the AYA's family and friends. It should always seek to improve symptom burden with effective symptom management, enable choice and decision-making through advance care planning and support the AYA in living and dying well. AYAs are astute and visceral in their views and wishes; listening to their voice will, not only, benefit them but it will enhance the care and service delivery for all AYAs receiving palliative care.

References

1. Eurostat http://ec.europa.eu/eurostat/statistics-explained/index.php/File:Causes_of_death,_by_age_group,_EU-28,_2011.png.
2. Keim-Malpass J, Erickson JM, Malpass HC. End-of-life care characteristics for young adults with cancer who die in the hospital. J Palliat Med. 2014;17(12):1359–64.
3. Cohen-Gogo S, Marioni G, Laurent S, Gaspar N, Semeraro M, Gabolde M, Dufour C, Valteau-Couanet D, Brugières L. End of life care in adolescents and young adults with cancer: experience of the adolescent unit of the Institut Gustave Roussy. Eur J Cancer. 2011;47(18):2735–41.
4. Temel J, Greer J, Muzikansky A, Gallagher E, Admane S, Jackson V, Dahlin C, Blinderman C, Jacobsen J, Pril W, Billings J, Lynch T. Early palliative care for patients with metastatic no-small cell lung cancer. N Engl J Med. 2010;363:733–42.

5. Jalmsell L, Lövgren M, Kreicbergs U, Henter JI, Frost BM. Children with cancer share their views: tell the truth but leave room for hope. Acta Paediatr. 2016;105(9):1094–9.
6. George R, Hutton S. Palliative care in adolescents. Euro J Cancer. 2003;39(18):2662–8.
7. Grinyer A, Barabarachild Z. Teenage and young adult palliative and end of life care service evaluation. London: Teenage Cancer Trust; 2011.
8. Valdez-Marinez E, Noyes J, Bedolla M. When to stop ? Decision-making when children's cancer treatment is no longer curative : a mixed-method systematic review. BMC Ped. 2014;14:124.
9. Masso M, Allingham SF, Banfield M, Johnson CE, Pidgeon T, Yates P, Eagar K. Palliative care phase: inter-rater reliability and acceptability in a national study. Palliat Med. 2014;29(1):22–30.
10. Montel S, Laurence V, Copel L, Paquement H, Flahault C. Place of death in adolescents and young adults with cancer: first study in a French population. Palliative and supportive care. 2009;7:27–35.
11. Jacobs S, Perez J, Cheng YI, Sill A, Wang J, Lyon ME. Adolescent end of life preferences and congruence with their parents' preferences: results of a survey of adolescents with cancer. Pediatr Blood Cancer. 2015;62(4):710.
12. Bluebond-Langnar M, Belasco J, Goldman A, Belasco C. Understanding parents' approaches to care and treatment of children with cancer when standard therapy has failed. J Clin Onco. 2007;25(17):2414–9.
13. Hammes BJ, Klevan J, Kempf M, Williams MS. Pediatric advance care planning. J Palliat Med. 2005;8:766–73.
14. Gold standards frame work. www.goldstandardsframework.org.uk/advance-care-planning
15. Lyon ME, Jacobs S, Briggs L, Cheng YI, Wang J. Family-centered advance care planning for teens with cancer. JAMA Pediatr. 2013;167(5):460–7.
16. Lyon ME, Jacobs S, Briggs L, Cheng YI, Wang J. A longitudinal, randomised, controlled trial of advance planning for teens with cancer: anxiety, depression, quality of life, advance directive, spiruality. J Adolesc Health. 2014;54(6):710–7.
17. Zadeh S, Pao M, Weiner L. Opening end of life discussion: how to introduce voicing my CHOiCES, an advance care planning guide of adolescents and young adults. 2014 1478. ACP for AYA. Pediatr Blood Cancer. 2013;60(5):715–8.
18. westmidlands. https://wmppcn.wordpress.com/wm-toolkit/.
19. Weaver MS, Heinze KE, Bell CJ, Wiener L, Garee AM, Kelly KP, Casey RL, Watson A. Hinds PS; establishing psychosocial palliative care standards for children and adolescents with cancer and their families: an integrative review. Palliat Med. 2016;30(3):212–23.
20. Bates AT, Kearney JA. Understanding death with limited experience in life: dying children's and adolescents' understanding of their own terminal illness and death. Curr Opin Support Palliat Care. 2015;9(1):40–5.
21. Harding R, Simms V, Calanzani N, Higginson IJ, Hall S, Gysels M, Meñaca A, Bausewein C, Deliens L, Ferreira P, Toscani F, Daveson BA, Ceulemans L, Gomes B. If you had less than a year to live, would you want to know? A seven-country European population survey of public preferences for disclosure of poor prognosis. Psychooncology. 2013 Oct;22(10):2298–305.
22. Wiener L, Zadeh S, Battles H, Baird K, Ballard E, Osherow J, Pao M. Allowing adolescents and young adults to plan their end of life care. Ped. 2012;130(5):897–905.
23. Fraser J, Harris N, Berringer AJ, Prescott H, Finlay F. Advanced care planning in children with life-limiting conditions—the wishes document. Arch Dis Child. 2010;95(2):7982.
24. Warnick AL. Supporting youth grieving the dying or death of a sibling or parent: considerations for parents, professionals, and communities. Curr Opin Support Palliat Care. 2015;9(1):58–63.
25. Wolff A, Browne J, Whitehouse W. Personal resuscitation plans and end of life planning for children with diasability and life-limiting/life threatening conditions. Arch Dis Child Educ Prac Ed. 2011;96:42–8.
26. Breault J. DNR, DNAR or AND? Is language important? Ochsner J. 2011;Winter 11(4):302–6.
27. Sokol D. The death of DNR. BMJ. 2009;338:b1723.
28. Wiener L, Zadeh S, Wexler LH, Pao M. When silence is not golden: engaging adolescents and young adults in discussions around end-of-life care choices. Pediatr Blood Cancer. care. 2013;60(5):715–8.

29. Kondryn H, Edmondson C, Hill J, Eden T. Treatment non-adherence to teenage and young patients with cancer. Lancet Oncol. 2011;12(1):100–8.
30. Kamperidis N, Goodhand J, Chowdhury F, Koodun Y, Direzke N, Naik S, Sanderson I, Croft N, Langmead F, Irving P, Rampton D, Lindsay J. Factors associated with nonadherence to Thiopurines in adolescents and adult patients with inflammatory bowel disease. J Ped Gastro Nutrition. 2012;54(5):685–9.
31. Landier W. Adherence to oral chemotherapy in childhood acute lymphoblastic leukaemia : an evolutionary concept analysis. Onco Nursing Forum. 2011;38(3):343–52.
32. Anghelescu DL, Zhang K, Faughnan LG, Pei D. The safety and effectiveness of patient-controlled analgesia in outpatient children and young adults with cancer: a retrospective study. J Pediatr Hematol Oncol. 2015 Jul;37(5):378–82.
33. Othman A, Mohamad M, Sayed H. Transdermal fentanyl for cancer pain management in opioid-naïve pediatric cancer patients. Pain Med. 2016;17(7):1329–36.
34. Likar R. Transdermal buprenorphine in the management of persisting pain-safety aspects. Ther Clin Risk Manage. 2006;2(1):115–25.
35. Seyfried O, Hester J. Opioids and endocrine dysfunction. Br J Pain. 2012;6(1):17–24.
36. Anghlescu D, Patel R, Mahoney D, Trujillo L, Faughnan L, Steen B, Baker J, Pei D. Methadone prolongs cardiac conduction in young patients with cancer-realted pain. J Opioid Manag. 2016;12(2):131–8.
37. Rasmussen V, Lundberg V. Extreme doses of intravenous methadone for severe pain in two children with cancer. Pediatr Blood Cancer. 2015;62:1087–90.
38. Bredlau A, McDermott M, Adams H, Dworkin R, Venuto C, Fisher S, Dolan J, Korones D. Oral ketamine for children with chronic pain: a pilot phase 1 study. J Pediatr. 2013;163(1):194–2000.
39. Bredlau A, Thakur R, Korones D, Dworkin R. Ketamine for pain in adults and children with cancer: a systematic review and synthesis of the literature. Pain Med. 2013;14(10):1505–17.
40. WHO Guidelines on the pharmacological treatment of persisting pain in children with medical illness 2012.
41. Paulsen Ø, Aass N, Kaasa S, Dale O. Do corticosteroids provide analgesic effects in cancer patients? A systematic literature review. J Pain Symptom Manag. 2013 Jul;46(1):96–105.
42. Butkovic D, Tljan S, Mihovilovic-Novak B. Experience with gabapentin for neuropathic pain in adolescents: report of five cases. Paediatr Anaesth. 2006;16(3):325–9.
43. Vondracek P, Oslejskova H, Kepak T, Mazanek P, Sterba J, Rysava M, Gal P. Efficayc of pregablin in neuropathic pain in paediatric oncological patients. Eur J Paediatr Neurol. 2009;13(4):332–6.
44. Nayak S, Cunliffe M. Lidocaine 5% patch for localized chronic neuropathic pain in adolescents: report of five cases. Paediatr Anaesth. 2008;18(6):554–8.
45. Valrie C, Bromberg M, Palermo T, Schanberg L. A systematic review of sleep in pediatric pain populations. J Dev Behav Pediatr. 2013 Feb;34(2):120–8.
46. Walter L, Nixon G, Davey M, Downie P, Horne R. Sleep and fatigue in pediatric oncology : a review of the literature. Sleep Med Rev. 2015;24:71–81.
47. Yennurajalingam S, Bruera E. Role of corticosteroids for fatigue in advanced incurable cancer: is it a 'wonder drug' or 'deal with the devil'. Curr Opin Support Palliat Care. 2014;8(4):346–51.
48. Miller S, McNutt L, McCann MA, McCorry N. Anorexia in palliative medicine: a systematic review. J Palliat Med. 2014;17(4):482–5.
49. Sizoo EM, Grisold W, Taphoorn MJ. Neurologic aspects of palliative care: the end of life setting. Handb Clin Neurol. 2014;121:1219–25.
50. Berger J, Lester P, Rodrigues L. Medical therapy of malignant bowel obstruction with Octreotide, dexamethasone, and metoclopramide. Am J Hosp Palliat Care. 2016;33(4):407–10.
51. Levine DR, Johnson LM, Mandrell BN, Yang J, West NK, Hinds PS, Baker JN. Does phase 1 trial enrollment preclude quality end-of-life care? Phase 1 trial enrollment and end-of-life care characteristics in children with cancer. Cancer. 2015;121(9):1508–12.
52. Keim-Malpass J, Stegenga K, Loudin B, Kennedy C, Kools S. "It's back! My remission is over": online communication of disease progression among adolescents with cancer. J Pediatr Oncol Nurs. 2016;33(3):209–17.

53. Mack JW, Chen LH, Cannavale K, Sattayapiwat O, Cooper RM, Chao CR. End-of-life care intensity among adolescent and young adult patients with cancer in Kaiser Permanente Southern California. JAMA Oncol. 2015;1(5):592–600.
54. White R, Bradnam V. Handbook of drug administration via enteral feeding tubes. 3rd ed; 2015.
55. Dickman A, Schneider J, Varga J. The syringe driver: continuous subcutaneous infusions in a palliative care. 2005.
56. Rosenberg AR, Postier A, Osenga K, Kreicbergs U, Neville B, Dussel V, Wolfe J. Long-term psychosocial outcomes among bereaved siblings of children with cancer. J pain symptom manage. 2015;49(1):55–65.

10 What Adolescents and Young Adults Want Health Professionals to Know

Jeanette Hawkins

10.1 This Is What I Want to Tell You About Being Diagnosed with Cancer

10.1.1 Listening to AYAs Talking About the Time of Diagnosis

It is a privilege to hear a group of young people talking openly about their lives. Often such discussions are not held in the presence of older adults. Discussion amongst peers with cancer can be vibrant, provide incredible insight into the complexities of human life, funny, sad, flamboyant, shocking and demonstrate great wisdom and experience. Developing this chapter offered a glimpse into the nature of today's youth in a modern, economically developed country in an era of beautiful diversity, intelligence and technology. The high potential they exude is a devastating mirror image of the risk that their diagnosis may snatch it all away from them with very little warning. Yet, you quickly get the feeling that while they want empathy and understanding they certainly do not want sympathy and platitudes. They want life; to live it as fully as they can, to understand how the diagnosis will impact on their lives and how they can minimise that impact. They want real and honest approaches, delivered with kindness and consideration. The structure of this chapter puts the AYA voice first to focus on their actual views of what health professionals need to know rather than presumed views [1, 2].

The first point of contact with health professionals is often with the Family Doctor/General Practitioner (GP). Several young people talked about their GP not picking up the signs of cancer with consequent delays in diagnosis. One young person related how she got to the point where she felt no-one was helping or listening to her, which resulted in depression and a desire to end her own life. This wasn't an isolated scenario and young people frequently felt they were not listened to when visiting the GP. They were sometimes treated like novices and patronised when they

J. Hawkins, RGN, RSCN, DPSN, MSc
CLIC SARGENT, London, UK
e-mail: Jeanette.Hawkins@clicsargent.org.uk

J. Chisholm et al. (eds.), *A Practical Approach to the Care of Adolescents and Young Adults with Cancer*, https://doi.org/10.1007/978-3-319-66173-5_10

explained signs and symptoms, being made to feel silly if they stated they felt there was something seriously wrong.

For young people who are moving away from dependence on their parents, to even make an appointment and visit a GP takes courage. They may find it difficult to explain what their symptoms are, or focus on what they feel is important for the GP to know and perhaps miss stating something important that they assume to be irrelevant [3, 4].

Once AYAs are in hospital the strongest message from around the time of diagnosis was "*we have no idea what you're going on about. It's all just jargon.*" This was a top point made by almost every young person I had contact with in researching this chapter. "*We haven't got science degrees (yet!), so expect our science knowledge to be low unless we tell you otherwise.*" It was evident that what appears as common language in most haematology or oncology services is a foreign language to the young. Thrown into this alien landscape, why would they know what bone marrow does, what a stool is, or have a clue why health professionals would want to examine and measure their "*body rubbish*"? In amongst the fear, brain-fog and time standing still that occurs at diagnosis, young people understand little of what is said to them and are often too scared or bewildered to ask before they have built any relationships with health professionals. One young person said they made notes of words and acronyms on their phone while health professionals talked, asking "*what did anyone do before google*?" [5–7].

An excellent example of language that is common to health professionals and a mystery to AYA is the Multi-Disciplinary Team (MDT); the team of professionals who work together to diagnose, treat and care for the AYA with cancer. "*Everyone talks about the MDT. What the hell is an MDT? I thought it was the Managing Director of the Trust to start with. I'm still not sure what it is.*" Other young people explained it was a meeting of the team of professionals taking care of them, which prompted a conversation that some young people felt their team didn't meet or speak to each other or to other departments. "*People have no idea what's going on with me, do they really meet?*" We return to this point later in the section on living with cancer.

AYAs recognised that cancer still feels like a taboo subject to say out loud. Young people felt that cancer needs to be spoken about more so that it becomes more acceptable to talk about in everyday lives. There was a clear message that young people felt health professionals should be leading the way with this. It was unhelpful if the word was skirted around at diagnosis by using words like lump or tumour. At worst it makes the young person unclear whether it's cancer or not and at best it perpetuates a culture that inhibits open conversations about cancer.

The second foremost question that sits in young people's minds once diagnosis is shared and inhibits further understanding is "*Am I going to die?*" This terrible possibility occupies their mind to the extent that it drowns out almost everything else that is said, the world stops and lives are put on hold [6, 8]. The acknowledgement of the possibility of death or relapse stays with young people to a greater or lesser extent for a long time depending on their individual circumstances. For many this becomes part of what contributes to their eventual changed outlook, greater enjoyment of life, nothing worse to face, and learning early in life what is truly important [9–13].

The impact on family was expressed by AYAs as "*total shock.*" Family members were recognised to be deeply upset and yet hid their emotions, in the recognised family ritual of mutual pretence [14]. Amongst families, the AYAs recognised that there were very complex emotions going on that they did not always understand.

Many young people said that healthcare professionals didn't explain that it might be like this, let them know that this might be normal or help them learn how to manage it. For some the diagnosis brought them closer to family or friends and they often found themselves worrying about family members [13, 15]. Brassil et al., describing AYA cancer experience in the context of stem cell transplant in the USA included a closer relationship with God in their findings, but this did not come up in conversation with AYAs in the UK, which may be a cultural difference [9] (Fig. 10.1).

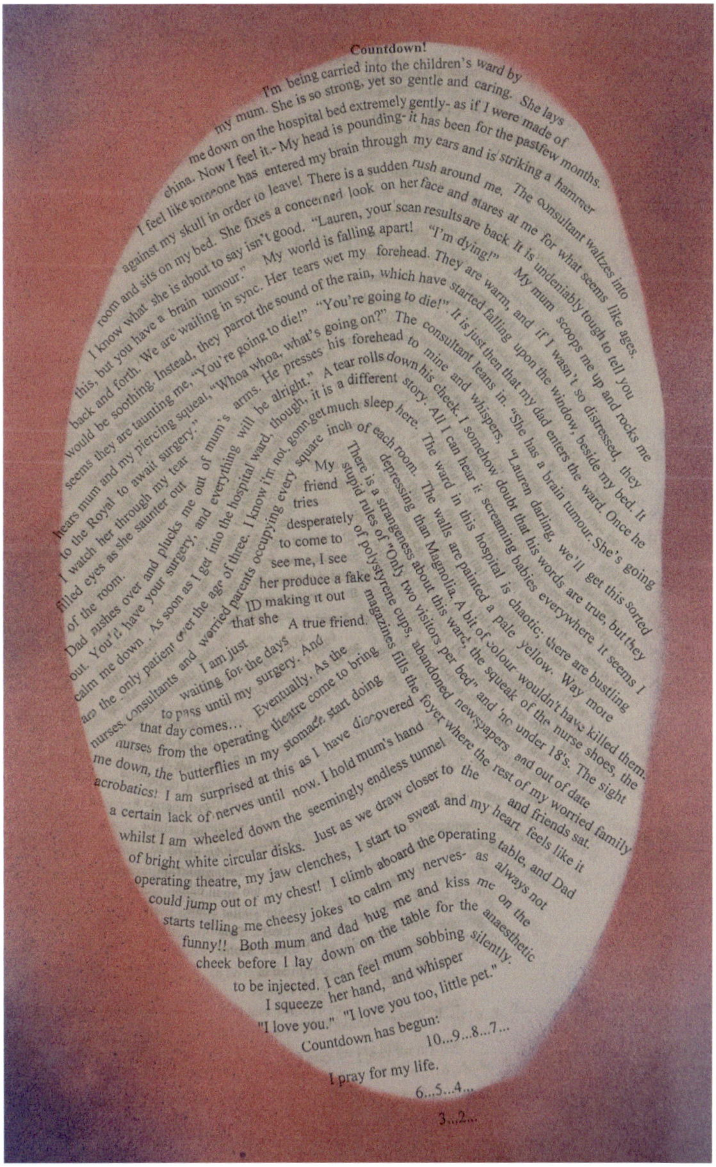

Fig. 10.1 Lauren Thumbprint Art "The Countdown" from the Northern Ireland Arts project 'Hello, my name is not cancer'

After receiving the initial diagnosis, AYAs attention rapidly moves on to considering the potential impact this will have on their lives. Older adolescents and young adults are often at university or in first jobs or training posts. They may have achieved some independence from parents and have new friendship groups who were not necessarily connected to their original home and family. For some this was what they described as "*having my own life for the first time*," so when the diagnosis was made (and temporarily bypassing the panic of the potential risk to life) it wasn't the diagnosis that was scary, it was the loss of their new found independence, friends, career, opportunities that scared them most. Davies, Kelly and Hannigan discuss this strong desire to be aligned to their peer group in their discussion paper on decision-making [15, 16].

The young people talked about their responses and coping mechanisms at diagnosis. They felt it was important for health professionals to understand that even adolescents and young adults may have already acquired "*emotional baggage*" in their short lives, just like most of the adult population. "*At diagnosis I ended up repressing a lot of memories and kept it quiet that these had returned, because I had no idea how to deal with it and no-one explained this might happen.*" They described having 'normal problems' but not yet acquiring years of adult experience, thus not knowing how to deal with things. They felt that health, social care and education professionals needed to offer guidance on how to deal with diagnosis, and treatment and what to expect in their own emotional responses, so that they didn't "*stress over little things.*" Belpame describes this as anticipatory guidance and believes that regaining control is key to recovery [17]. "*I was offered emotional support within the phone call [to Redkite]. I also received a follow up call which was very thoughtful.*"

Lots of young people talked about neutropenia and getting infections being scary. "*As soon as I walk out the door, I don't know what I'm going to be exposed to.*" The young people consulted said they were always worrying about becoming ill. One young man's job brought him into frequent contact with the public and children, and he related how he became scared of contact with them, and being very wary of customers with colds. "*It's awful when previously I enjoyed the interaction with kids in the shop and now, basically ..... thinking ..... you could kill me.*" When talking about living with fear, another young person said, *"I'm not sure you ever get over the 'germ obsession' thing."* [2].

A picture emerged of AYAs trying to navigate through life-changing events and manage normal everyday AYA life simultaneously; feeling inexperienced in how to integrate the two. This has been described as a duel crisis [13, 18]. Some young people talked about the support they got from charity Social Workers such as CLIC Sargent or Redkite or activity coordinators from Teenage Cancer Trust who helped in ways that general healthcare did not reach [19]. "*CLIC Sargent mops up what the NHS fails to do. The NHS tells you lots of stuff you're not really interested in or can't understand at the start. What I needed to know was practical stuff like, 'when can I start driving again,' 'can I take my exams'.*" "*I mean there were very specific questions, like for me it was how long can I get back into sports, contact sports and stuff because my doctor kind of set this off hand."*

Quite quickly after diagnosis AYAs began to build relationships with health professionals (and where available, with social care professionals.) In stark contrast to young people's concerns about their interaction with the family GP, their confidence in the hospital consultant (usually the treating oncologist) was high. Young people recognised their Consultant's knowledge and expertise and it gave them confidence in how their cancer was managed. This confidence did not translate to all health professionals and AYAs were astute at recognising when a health professional lacked competence, confidence or knowledge [20]. AYAs struggled with more than just medical jargon; they expressed limited understanding of clinical procedures, tests and investigations. They were able to discern staff they trusted and those they didn't by their ability to fully explain procedures or reasons for treatment in a way they could understand. They were wary and felt insecure when staff just left a medication cup with tablets in by their bedside without explaining what it was for. Several young people mentioned being given inadequate explanation about what medicines were for [21]. A particular problem in UK hospitals was the impact of staff shortages and agency staff which left AYAs in some situations feeling less safe when their healthcare providers did not seem to be as confident or knowledgeable as the permanent staff [1].

Young people found it difficult when health care professionals gave inconsistent messages. They gave examples of doctors giving differing contraceptive advice and mixed messages about what contraception they should use. There was lack of clarity around contraception and its purpose: preventing pregnancy, preventing infection or protecting partner from chemotherapy exposure? In other examples, a young person was told by one doctor it was advisable to have sperm frozen for fertility risk, while another said it wasn't necessary.

10.1.1.1 Section 1 Summary

In this section AYAs wanted health and social care professionals to know about their experiences getting to diagnosis in primary care, unfamiliar language barriers at diagnosis, immediate concerns about death and how difficult it is to ask important questions in front of close family or partners. They discussed their initial responses to the impact on their life and some of the things they found useful or difficult. The published literature reviewed matches much of what was said in the conversations, but little appears to have been written so far about the presence of parents at diagnosis specifically. One study examined the shared experience of AYA cancer and included caregivers in their analysis of perceptions of illness severity and posttraumatic stress symptoms, describing cancer as a "dyadic illness" [22]. Place of care and the hospital environment did not feature in the UK conversations, but research from Canada, where AYA specific services are not yet established, reports AYAs requesting suitable age appropriate environments (not with very young children or older adults) with access to health and supportive care professionals who have an understanding of the needs of young people [2, 10, 23].

The overwhelming nature of diagnosis is well documented with much recognition of the shock, time freezing, feeling numb, not being able to process information, and yet despite this recognition AYAs still experience health professionals delivering diagnosis in one long session using phrases they don't understand [1, 6].

This is what I want health professionals to know when you tell me I have or might have cancer

GPs/family doctor When I visit the surgery on a few occasions with the same or similar symptoms, it helps me to know you are listening to me if you ask how worried I am. It helps if you ask how many times I've been in with this before. It helps if you ask to see me again, in a short timeframe, to review what is happening. It helps if you ask me to write down things that are unexplained, severe, worsening, don't go away or keep returning [7].

Information Needs I need simple explanations about my diagnosis and proposed treatments in plain everyday language, and in short episodes [5, 21]. I need time to understand it and will need things repeating. It helps when you try to find out how much I have understood. At diagnosis information needs to be face to face, although age appropriate written and digital material to back up the verbal information is also helpful.

Personal Communication It helps when you make sure I have had some time without parents or partners to talk about very personal things, like relationships and contraception. It helps if you give me time between giving information and offering private opportunities to ask questions about the diagnosis and treatment away from close family and friends.

Team work and communication It helps build confidence in my care and safety if the team helping me give consistent, simple information and have communicated well with each other. It helps if professionals have specific training in the care of AYAs with cancer.

Facing mortality and living with fear I have no idea how to manage this yet, but I will. Give me time; there is nothing I want more than to feel normal again. Be honest and kind. Give me anticipatory guidance. Explain things to me including what my medicines are for [11, 15] (Fig. 10.2).

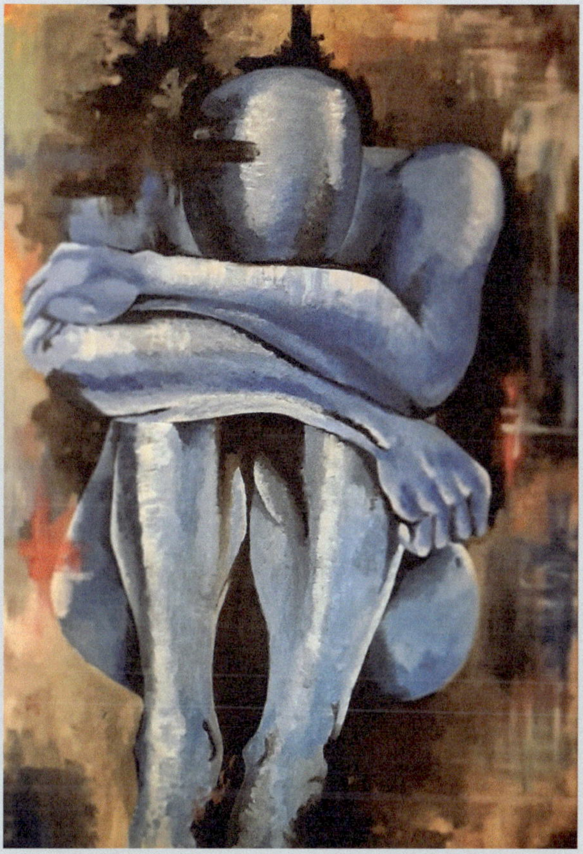

Fig. 10.2 Shock of diagnosis by Holly Hamer

10.2 This Is What I Want to Tell You About Day to Day Living with and Beyond Cancer

10.2.1 Listening to AYAs Talking About Day to Day Living with and Beyond Cancer

The theme of living day-to-day with and beyond cancer provides the best illustration of how developmental stage and the goals of adolescence and young adulthood impact the cancer experience and are impacted by the cancer experience [13, 24]. Age, cognitive, social, emotional, physical, sexual, cultural development and competence are recognised to play a major part in the AYAs experience of cancer [16, 25]. In published literature these developmental stages usually encompass increasing autonomy (moving from dependence to independence), making decisions about education and work, intimacy and sexuality, child rearing, developing an identity of self and body image, and establishing a personal set of values and standards [1, 9,

16, 26]. In their study on adolescence and identity, Stegenga & Macpherson, note that at in no other life period except infancy is there so much development occurring [13]. They found that over time adolescents with cancer must integrate their adolescent identity with their cancer identity [18]. Lee et al., propose that with good support from professionals and security of close family and friends, adolescents were able to integrate body image changes into a positive self identity and develop protective strategies [27]. Similarly, in a stunning account of what it is to be human after years of cancer relapses, Speraw describes that sheer determination to be normal helps the development of self-concept for AYA cancer survivors [20].

The members of the Young People's Reference Group at CLIC Sargent described themselves as a spontaneous age group and felt the ability to be spontaneous must be factored into care to help them get through treatment. Too many restrictions were not helpful, and they rebelled against being given long instructions about things they could not do. They needed to know what was not advisable, as well as what was OK, so they could be spontaneous when the situation allowed. This was demonstrated in their discussions about relationships and sex. While they had been told some things they shouldn't do, they were not told what they could do. One young man amusingly related how he was left "Googling" 'oral sex' [AND] 'neutropenia' [AND] cancer [AND] chemotherapy [AND] 'multiple partners' [AND] 'kissing too much' and laughing about how much trouble that can get you into on the internet. He said, "*Either that stuff just isn't there on the internet or it's well hidden, so people need to tell us.*" Young people also found confusing and contradictory information on the internet, like don't kiss as much when you're having chemo, leading to questions about how much is "much" and is a lot with your regular partner different from a little with lots of partners? The people they were comfortable talking about sex with varied. Some were very comfortable talking with doctors while others felt it would be weird to talk to their doctor about sex and preferred to have these discussions with a nurse or a social worker. Health and social care professionals need to be comfortable and confident leading conversations about sex and relationships as AYA felt there was a lack of information given [28]. This also included being offered the opportunity to talk about the strain on romantic relationships, the treatment effect on their sex life and loss of libido. Young people often didn't realise what they needed to ask until they found themselves in a "*spontaneous*" situation; so forewarned is forearmed.

It was not surprising that AYAs wanted professionals to know they had information needs about relationships and sex, and separately about long term effects on fertility and reproduction [8, 29]. Developmentally this is a period of sexual and relationships exploration and for some young adults moving into longer term relationships and longer term life plans. Decisions relating to this become so much more difficult when the future may be unpredictable [16, 24]. An interesting study by Quinn GP et al. notes that historical health-related quality of life (HRQoL) tools have been used for AYA in some studies but were validated for use with adults and may lack specificity to the needs of AYA with cancer leading to under-reporting the prevalence of certain factors affecting them as survivors [30]. These under-reported HRQoL factors from their study were relationship problems, self and identity problems, and feelings about parenthood.

Whilst some young adults did not want parents around for sensitive or personal conversations, sometimes they did [8]. One young person said, "*I remember thinking, where's my mom, I need my mom*." This was different for younger adolescents who were much more used to having parents around in medical consultations, but this was not the case for every younger adolescent either. Older teens and young adults collectively felt that when health professionals asked personal questions with parents present, it was really uncomfortable and lacked respect. There were also messages for health professionals around privacy in relation to breaking bad news and other private situations. AYAs stated it was a bad experience for them when health professionals just pulled a curtain across and assumed that gave them dignity and confidentiality. They may internalise emotions because they feel unable to scream, shout, cry loudly or even just speak at all if they think someone the other side of the curtain is listening.

Similarly asking a young person if they have any questions about diagnosis, treatment or any aspect of care with parents in the room is considered pointless because young people say they are inhibited to ask what they really want to know in front of them, or will give incomplete answers to questions. The issues around parents or partners presence came from a range of perspectives for AYAs. Some of their questions may be around things they don't want their parent or partner to know about, like relationships and sex. Often, it was their respect for the feelings and emotional needs of parents or other family members present that inhibited communication, such as really wanting to know if this diagnosis or relapse meant they were going to die. There was a big plea from all young people to be offered at least 5 min of every appointment or in-patient interaction without parents. Crawshaw et al. offer sound advice on how to give choice about fertility conversations, but also noted the value of mothers' support for both sexes, demonstrating that parental support can be valuable as well as inhibitory [8]. Even worse than not being given time alone without parents to talk about their own needs, AYAs also experienced being in the room with parents, and health professionals turning direct to parents and saying "*so, how has he been?*" as though they were invisible. The AYA is left thinking "*hello, I'm here, can anybody see me*." Davies et al., describes how paternalistic instinct by both parents and professionals can isolate the AYA with cancer in medical communications [16].

Parents were described by some as part of the problem for AYAs managing their illness and self-care recovery, while at the same time being a major part of their support and return to daily life. Family were described as extending the recovery period by being "*too helpful*" like making the young person use a wheelchair for convenience or speed. However, AYAs were quick to defend their 'over helpful' parents, as this young lady from Australia explains, "*I had one lady tell my mum to stop helping and that I'm 21 and that I should do this by my self. This was hard as my mum and been there for me through everything and I thought that was just rude.*" Similarly health professionals can be too helpful and override self-care in attempts to get the job done quickly and easily [20].

During day-to-day living with and beyond cancer AYAs need to make multiple health-related decisions. The burden of these decisions, multiple factors and consequences to be taken into account are far beyond the normal experiences of their AYA peers. Davies, Kelly & Hannigan provide a valuable discussion paper which reviews decision making against the backdrop of altered autonomy and dependence [16]. A normal AYA pattern of development in decision-making involves shifting responsibilities from parents over time in parallel to transition through legal, ethical, social and developmental stages. There is strong evidence that the cancer diagnosis and treatment period "suspends" and in some cases "regresses" progress through this normal pathway. Parents frequently become more involved in decision-making, and in some cases may "take over" the responsibility entirely. This may impact on the young person losing control of the majority of their daily life choices, leaving them feeling powerless, frustrated and restricted [6, 20, 25].

> "You can't avoid it, you are a child again [1]."

However, while dependence on parents is greater than that of peers, AYAs with cancer also report feeling more mature than their peers due to wider a scope of experiences for personal development [13]. In some other aspects however, AYA survivors felt their development was 'stunted' or lagged behind peers due to the effect of "life on hold" during treatment [13]. In addition control over cancer-related decisions may also be given away to health professionals. For adolescents under the age of consent (which can vary by country) the degree of choice they are permitted in decision-making can also be affected by whether the parent and health professionals feel the young person is making the 'right' choice [16]. AYAs looked to health professionals to help parents understand when the young person should be regaining their independence. Davies et al., pick up the question of how nurses can work effectively when there is tension between parents and AYAs in regard to decision-making, offering a reminder to employ

> "…non-judgemental approaches to care and 'keep in check' …personal values and belief systems [16]."

Sometimes young people found it hard to be with people who got upset, especially when they needed to make big decisions. In research by Belpame et al., AYAs described avoiding negativity and being unable to share negative thoughts with close relatives [1]. Avoiding confrontation was seen as a way to hold on to normal life. AYAs expressed frustration at being made into a hero or heroine, constantly being told "*You're being so brave,*" "*You're being really positive,*" when this wasn't a choice; they had no option but to get on with things. In some literature AYA's did talk about making a choice to stay positive and this aligned with the power of optimism to help coping strategies [9, 17]. This applied to professionals as well as friends and family. Over time young people with cancer found it easier to be around their peers with cancer [24]. They felt they were able to relax and be themselves more around people who "*got it,*" "s*taff who helped me keep normality.*" AYAs felt it was crucial that health professionals understood that spending time at home and being independent was very important and needed to be prioritised more in care planning, alongside creating opportunities to connect with non-cancer friends and cancer friends [2, 13]. The hopefulness of life returning to "normal" has been identified as being motivational for helping to get through treatment, and professionals have a role to play in maintaining that hope, alongside balancing honesty and interpretation of what the "new normal" will likely be in life with and after cancer [6, 13, 15, 27, 31].

Young people talked a lot about friends not knowing how to cope. Some experienced the painful loss of very close friends who just didn't know how to deal with the situation and became distant from them. They related how friends didn't know what to say so they stayed away [13, 32, 33]. Young people had very strong feelings about social isolation, describing it as being "*horrendous*." They said that no-one mentioned this at all and they felt nurses needed to be able to talk to young people about it. Brassil et al., propose that professionals need to help support AYAs with sustaining relationships [9, 11, 24]. Some found friends a distraction, a space where they didn't have to talk about cancer. Some encountered people who only wanted to be friends now they had cancer [13]. Others felt friends didn't understand the full severity of what they were going through. Impacting significantly on social isolation was the loss of confidence and self-esteem with changing body image and reduced independence [24, 27, 33, 34] (Fig. 10.3).

Over time it became increasingly difficult having to explain things constantly to friends. AYAs recognised that not only did friends move away from them, they also moved away from some friends [9]. Social media is a choice method through which

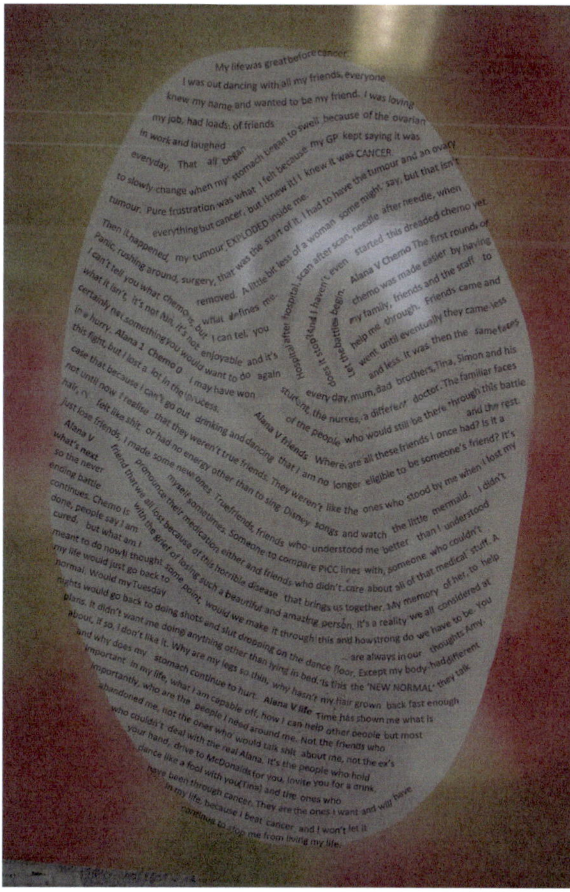

Fig. 10.3 Alana Thumbprint Art "My life was great before cancer" from the Northern Ireland Arts project, "Hello, my name is not cancer."

many AYAs communicate and this became another aspect of managing social isolation. While it could be a source of support and connection, there was also the dilemma of whether to post things about their diagnosis or treatment on social media [6, 12, 24, 34]. In addition some faced the distress of people making negative comments about how their appearance had changed, both innocently and maliciously [27]. Keim-Melpass et al. , propose that patient led narratives help AYA make sense of their world and normalise their experience, and while studying blogs for truly patient centred research is valuable, it is also potentially limited by the characteristics of AYA who chose blogging as a form of expression and have access to the internet [12].

The fact that AYAs need help and support to both understand and manage isolation, loneliness, changes in the way others interact with them, both short and longer term, is evident in much of the literature [17]. There is juxtaposition between never being alone (parents at the bedside, multiple professionals around constantly, friends and family more in touch than normal) and at the same time feeling alone, missing friends and family who have stepped away from contact [20]. What is less clear in published literature is who is best placed to undertake this support. Hospital based health professionals have a significant role to play in preparing AYAs for these challenges but their focus on treatment and physical restriction within the boundaries of the hospital, may mean this is a better focus for charities[1,2,3,4,5], support groups, education and social care professionals [31, 35] (Fig. 10.4).

"*People's demeanour instantly changes when you say I have, or have had cancer.*" This change in attitude filtered into almost every aspect of their lives from their Mum's over-protection to the encounter with a stranger in the street. It impacted greatly on job seeking. "*Do you put the cancer diagnosis on the CV or not when you know this will change their attitude towards you, but if you don't you won't get understanding for any ongoing limitations you have.*" Tied in with the challenge of looking for jobs were also issues around muscle wasting, self-esteem and appearance for the young people. They described the very real challenges faced either after treatment when hair has grown back or if you have a cancer treatment that doesn't result in hair-loss such as less advanced thyroid cancer [36]. They found it hard when they looked normal but actually had a lot of muscle wasting and fatigue. A recent study in Norway suggests fatigue is a long term problem for some [34, 37]. AYAs talked about sometimes struggling with everyday activities that would be considered

[1] http://www.clicsargent.org.uk/ CLIC Sargent is the UK's leading charity for children and young people with cancer, and their families. When cancer strikes young lives CLIC Sargent helps limit the damage cancer causes beyond their health.

[2] http://www.redkite.org.au/ Redkite is an Australian cancer charity providing essential support to children & young people (0–24 years) with cancer, and the family and support network who care for them.

[3] https://www.teenagecancertrust.org/ Around seven young people aged between 13 and 24 are diagnosed with cancer every day in the UK. They need expert treatment and support from the moment they hear the word 'cancer.'

[4] https://www.teencanceramerica.org/ Teen Cancer America partners with hospitals throughout the United States to develop specialized facilities and services for teens and young adults with cancer.

[5] https://www.canteen.org.au/ CanTeen helps young people deal with the challenges cancer brings.

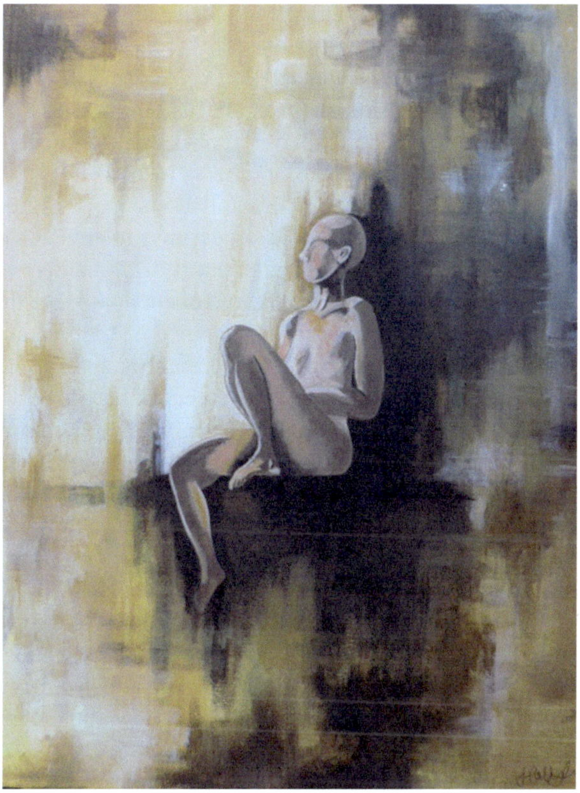

Fig. 10.4 "Watching from the side-lines" by Holly Hamer

easy for someone their age. *"I can't do that like I used to, just isn't possible any more. But sometimes people look at you like you're putting it on, the cancers' behind you now, get on with it."* Sometimes there were self-acknowledged contradictions in how the young people felt about their ongoing limitations. While they didn't want to be the one always having to say, *"I've had cancer treatment, I can't do that now,"* they also didn't want to be restricted by other people telling them what they couldn't do or shouldn't do, preferring to always try to see if they can [20].

In the conversations with AYAs they recognised the sometimes contradictory nature of their feelings, needing others to acknowledge their cancer limitations but not wanting to be reminded and restricted by others about their cancer, needing gentleness and needing a push. Social Workers have particular skills in helping young people manage this and can act as a bridge between the AYA and health professionals. Belpame et al., identified that healthcare professionals often experience AYAs as a mass of contradictions.

> They can be perceived as compliant and noncompliant, independent and vulnerable, or demanding as well as acquiescent.

They propose that to understand this behaviour health professionals need to understand the origins of adolescent behaviour. Belpame et al., identified that a cancer diagnosis for AYAs created a very self conscious and self-centred perspective, but following the same contradictory behaviours described above, AYAs at the same time did not want to "lose themselves to the cancer experience." They identified that the cancer experience was so intense and exhausting that AYAs may have "no spare energy" to be considerate to the needs of others at times [1, 6]. Other researchers found that the cancer experience also had the capacity for survivors to be more compassionate to the needs of others [1, 15, 18].

Young people wanted information to be made available for friends and employers about ongoing restrictions on exercise tolerance and the longer term impact of cancer treatment. They talked about it being harder when treatment completed or when they were past the intense treatment phase and "looked normal again." In this situation an obvious cancer appearance had an advantage in harnessing support, while at the same time looking different is a risky situation for adolescents [13]. Employers, friends and flatmates expected them to be able to return to pre-diagnosis levels of energy, fitness and strength rapidly on completing treatment [38]. AYAs didn't want to have to keep playing the "cancer card" and explain about their ongoing limitations, having to say "*I have cancer.*" Acknowledging the cancer identity but not being defined by it was strong factor in these conversations and recognised in published literature [13, 27]. The request for information for flatmates extended to information to help them understand about infection risks, the need to keep bathrooms and kitchen areas clean, and the urgency in responding to temperatures when unwell. AYAs faced a real dilemma in communicating what employers needed to know about how the cancer and treatment affected them and what help they needed, with increased risk involved in an interview situation, "*I wanted the job on merit, and couldn't take the risk they would pass me over because of it.*"

The need for understandable age-appropriate information is well recognised in research literature and there is evidence that quality of life and sense of control can be improved when information needs are met [2]. Furthermore, it is recognised that AYA have a greater need for information than older adult cancer patients but also that too much information about things that are not imminent can be overwhelming [1, 26]. Information can also be part of seeking control but also rejecting information can be a sign of avoidance to maintain control and cope with uncertainty [9, 17]. The AYAs conversations in this chapter parallel the findings in the DeRouen et al. study, that information needs to include recurrence risk and handling concerns about this, late effects, fertility and reproduction, alongside information about how the cancer experience is likely to impact on daily life including financial support, healthy lifestyles, how to talk about cancer, how to manage friends and family reactions, and impact on self-image and mental health, to improve AYAs sense of control. Unmet information needs were associated with lower levels of overall mental and physical health [26].

Chapter 4 covers the psychosocial aspects of the cancer experience in more detail but it would be remiss not to acknowledge here, that in conversations with AYAs about what they wanted health professionals to know, they talked about their changed perspective on their life, changing priorities and life goals, living each day like it was their last, constant worry about their health and mortality, worry the cancer might return or that they would develop secondary cancers [6, 9, 11]. All of this caused sleep problems, permanent anxiety and overthinking. They expressed the need for more emotional and psychosocial support than most of them were able to access, but they wanted psychological support that was constructive and purposeful. They did not appear to be fans of psychological approaches where they were constantly asked "so how does that make you feel?" or "what do you think about that?" They felt they were too engrossed in the energy of trying to get well and make any sense of anything to respond to this approach. They were looking for coping strategies, ideas to help build resilience, ideas on how to stay connected to friends, ideas on how to manage everyday life, or ways to adjust their life or life goals in the reality of living with or beyond cancer. Conversely they also wanted health professionals to recognise that they may not appear to have taken in the severity of their situation, but just because they weren't crying or planning their funeral it didn't mean they hadn't taken it in. It has been noted that many health professionals believe that it is normal for AYAs to experience anxiety and depression as a result of the cancer diagnosis and not recognise problems that need intervention [25]. If left unsupported, these emotional side effects can manifest as physical effects, non-compliance, and withdrawal from their social network [24].

AYAs talked about experiencing mental health issues as a result of the diagnosis, which were encountered at different times for different individuals; (diagnosis, during treatment, or when treatment finished) when the realisation and effort of rebuilding their life became apparent [6]. Taylor et al. found that survivors who had signs of post traumatic stress could also jeopardise their future health because they lacked confidence to raise concerns [15, 39]. AYAs felt that health professionals didn't explain that they could experience depression or anxiety. AYAs assumed this would be more expected or 'normal' if you reached a point of facing death, thus experiencing a degree of guilt or embarrassment about their mental health if they were not imminently in that situation. They were not aware that this might be "normal or predicted" simply as an effect of the life changes they were experiencing and were therefore afraid to tell anyone. Some described the cancer experience as being like post traumatic distress disorder (PTSD), with lots of the impact kicking in after the experience, something that has become more recognised as a potential consequence of treatment for around 13% of patients based on studies in the UK, USA and Europe [39–41]. People think that if you look ok, you are ok [11] "*I looked happy on the outside but I didn't feel it on the inside; I felt lost and now I'm trying to find a job and feel like I don't know my self.*" Conversely, some young people offered the view that if the Consultant was really open and honest they didn't feel like they experienced PTSD. They knew what was going on. One young person explained how the Consultant was kind and candid saying, "*you could die during this surgery.*" AYAs felt that if nothing was hidden, it helped them to cope in the here and now, instead of storing up distress that would emerge later. This insight from the AYA reflects the view offered by Hobbie et al., that contrary to what might be expected, focusing on real issues and honest information helps survivors to learn to accept the uncontrollable aspects of life with cancer. One study in the USA distinguishes between PTSD and posttraumatic growth, stating that "re-experiencing" and "intrusive thoughts" can be an adaptive process and does not need to be pathologised, unless it becomes overwhelming. Health professionals can support this adaptive growth [12, 42].

Research from Belgium identified that AYAs may initially perceive the diagnosis as a temporary state after which they will get better and return to normal, and therefore it can be later that the reality and longer term consequences of treatment are realised [1]. This may explain the pressures on mental health further down the line. This is highlighted by McDonnell et al., who report that,

> literature to date has typically found adolescent cancer survivors to be psychologically resilient; however, there is a subset of individuals who experience psychological difficulties following their transition into survivorship.

McDonnell and colleagues report that anxiety in AYA survivors is as yet understudied, and that uncertainty about the future, the possibility of recurrence and troubling memories could give rise to specific anxiety disorders, but that prevalence reduced over time if they remained disease free [34]. Survivors report both negative and positive consequences of the cancer experience. Negatives include bodily concerns and health worries, thoughts about loss and life, psychological problems, difficulty interacting with others, fertility, frustrations with ongoing health care. Positive consequences include positive view of self or life, compassion for others, closer relationships, increased knowledge, financial gain (health insurance). Consequences can change over time and researchers suggest that helping AYA to see a longer term view can be helpful [15, 18, 34].

A factor that impacted greatly on AYAs mental health was the grief they experienced if another young person with cancer died. Some had no experience of death or only in elderly relatives, but certainly few had experience of the death of a young person or friend. They found it very difficult if health, social care or education professionals did not acknowledge their grief or even mention the person who died. Few professionals offered them support afterwards. A big source of trauma was experienced if, on a subsequent admission, they were admitted to the bed where a friend had died.

Some young people talked about how their emotions were affected by significant changes, such as the disease becoming resistant to treatment, needing to progress to bone marrow transplant or finishing treatment. There was a big resurgence of 'diagnosis' emotions at these times, but also a sense of feeling quite alone and not being able to talk to anyone. They tried to turn to family but realised that family were too entangled themselves. Friends had people in their own families who were fighting cancer and talking to them felt too negative for their circumstances. The healthcare team were very focused on getting through the next part of treatment or moving to follow-up. This was a time point where AYAs were thankful for the support of their social worker who became the less emotionally invested person they could talk openly to, and who they used for support more than anyone at that time, as this quote from Australia shows. *"At that time, a lot of the doctors were saying, "You can go see a counsellor. It's okay to go see a counsellor," but I was kind of more comfortable around my social worker because she had been there for me from the beginning to the end."*

In the first section, AYAs discussed their impression that professionals within teams and across departments did not talk to each other nor hand over important information. They experienced multiple healthcare workers, often not seeing the same hospital staff during repeat admissions or clinic visits. Access to case files, not reading case files, or not being able to locate up-to-date information in case files contributed to poor communication. AYAs expressed the feeling that many of the people looking after them didn't know what's going on. Other challenges that AYAs faced was a lack of forward planning. During treatment AYAs felt confident that when they returned to the hospital with a problem, it was largely managed well on the day, but many experienced a lack of foresight from health professionals to plan ahead and try to minimise problems for them in the future. "*They don't think about tomorrow, they just think about what they have to do with you today. They treat you on the day and if something happens they deal with it. There's no forward planning or preventative measures. Their reactions are slow – as good as me catching a ball!*" (Young man post Brain Tumour who struggled with lack of physical coordination). They also felt it took too long to get referrals to other services when they needed other services, an example being over 3 months to get a physio appointment after the referral was sent for someone with immediate post surgical needs.

Scans were another aspect of care that heightened anxiety and stress when waiting for results, especially when they got the feeling that there was no rush on the side of the hospital to get the results to them, or going to clinic for results and medical staff not knowing that's what they had come for. AYAs describe intense emotions with loss of sleep leading up to scans, but felt health professionals saw scans as routine and something they got used to. Waiting for scans was stagnating time [6]. Young people experienced lots of failed communication. They described turning up for consultations and the doctor asking what they had come for. Conversations repeatedly transpired like this. "*What have you come for today?*" "*I don't know, you sent me an appointment letter.*" "*Have you had an MRI today?*" "*No.*" Poor communication between teams was one of the biggest causes of bad experiences for AYA cancer patients. The effects ranged from anger, distress, anxiety, frustration, fear that no-one knew what was going on, loss of confidence in the treating team, time wasted, increased risk, loss of control and isolation.

Time wasted was another bugbear. So much precious time wasted sitting around in hospitals waiting [1, 12, 15]. Keim-Melpass et al. identify how discussing "time" has become a contemporary proxy for discussing "death," employing phrases such as "buying time" and "not enough time" which health and social care professionals should be tuned in to an awareness of [12].

> But remember as you waste your time,
> That for people like me,
> Time is life,
> And should be wasted with thought,
> Not wasted by the hour.
> Tracy Wollington 1980 [43]

There was huge frustration if medical staff were very late for clinic appointments. "*If I'm late for an appointment, I get the third degree and they threaten to discharge me. If he's late for the appointment, I just have to wait, sometimes for hours. I lose money, earnings, tutor time.*" If medical staff were late for appointments and apologised and still gave the person the time they needed, the AYA could accommodate this sad failing of the UK NHS to stick to appointment times. When there was no apology and their appointment was clearly rushed and only partially focused on the task, the AYA felt faceless and unimportant [20].

During treatment the daily struggles that accompanied medication was discussed alongside lack of clarity from health professionals about what some of the treatment was and it's importance, especially oral medications [21]. "*I had terrible weight gain. Half a year later they told me it was the steroids. So I didn't take the steroids. They made me feel horrible. But no-one told me how important they were until ages afterwards. Then there was this big conversation where my Dad said something about the steroids, and that I don't take them because they don't help, and then they said, "They're like chemo, as important as chemo." I felt so bad for not taking them, I didn't know.*" Another young person said, "*I didn't take my home meds for a while, like for a whole month. My memory was affected by the tumour and I just forgot about them. My endocrinology consultant told me to set an alarm on my phone every day – easy as that, simple tip, and I never forgot them again.*"

For the AYAs who had moved past treatment the reality or risk of late effects was discussed. Their message for health professionals in relation to late effects was that they needed to be told more about these earlier on and they needed the information repeated in short episodes [8, 29, 40, 44]. "*I'd had chemo already. If they'd thought of it earlier I'd have been able to have fertility preservation.*" For one young person the discussion about fertility was nothing more than a single sentence. "*This drug might affect your fertility.*" "*When? How? I've never even considered having children before. I was too shocked to even think what to ask, and then that was it, …the conversation was over, subject over …..before it even began.*"

More sensitivity is needed to consider giving advanced warning about hard questions or hard hitting information that might otherwise take a young person unawares. This was illustrated during a conversation on sperm banking. A young person recalled being faced with a form that asks "Do you want someone to be able to use your sperm if you die?" Firstly, this is a shocking question if you haven't been prepared for it, and secondly it is a very difficult question to answer at their age if they haven't been given some time to think about it and discuss it with important people in their lives. This also usually occurs at a time when they are still in the shock and brain fog of having just been diagnosed [8, 24].

AYAs with cancer experience many social problems as a result of their cancer or treatment and those who had access to a social worker usually found this extremely helpful unless the worker was overly sympathetic without giving much in the way of practical support. It is also noted that some AYAs have pre existing social issues exacerbated by diagnosis and, if they had been managing these, the diagnosis and longer term effects can tip them into not coping. UK young people wanted social care providers and agencies to know that they find the welfare benefits system very hard to understand. Many had had negative experiences with the system experiencing delayed payments, leaving them without funds or owing money on accommodation contracts if they had to leave university. Some AYAs had only just become financially independent from parents, and described guilt about taking benefits or that taking benefits made them feel as if they had lost control of their financial independence.

Those young people who were diagnosed while away from home at university found this especially tough. Most found the university unsupportive. There was considerable complexity around organising what needed to change as a result of the diagnosis and negotiate on contracts made – this included accommodation, funding and student finance and deferring places. Young people found this hugely complex to navigate at a time when they were feeling unwell and they were coping with the shock of diagnosis [33, 35]. When they deferred their course, the student finance stopped but benefits did not kick in until about 6 months after diagnosis for some, leaving them with no income for several months. The financial impact of a cancer diagnosis will certainly be an issue for almost all AYAs but the issues involved and degree of impact will also be affected by the healthcare system of their country [24, 26, 45]. DeRouen et al., when writing about the USA, states that [26],

> AYAs diagnosed with cancer between 15 and 39 years of age have the lowest rates of insurance coverage

AYAs wanted healthcare professionals to know that they needed preparing for life past chemo [11, 39]. They expected that once chemo finished, life would pretty much get back to where it was after a period of recovery [1]. In reality they find that friends and family haven't had the same "pause" button pressed on their lives and they have moved forward while the AYA lived in their "*bubble world*." Life after cancer was referred to as having a "*hidden disability*." Hair grows back and to most people everything looks pretty normal again. "*I even forget sometimes when I look in the mirror.*" After cancer young people are often still managing short or long-term effects of treatment discussed earlier.

Preparation for transition was vital. "*Don't just tell me I'm not going to be your doctor anymore, it's time you moved over to the adult service. I was really shocked. I trusted him.*" Those young people who were given transition planning in a staged way over time were able to cope better with the move. "*It didn't happen straight away then, so I had time to get used to it and that helped.*" This also applied to other professionals involved in their care such as social workers, whose practice in the UK is to help the young person towards managing their own life independently (not necessarily waiting for life to be perfect; it rarely is) but having helped the young person to manage the normal ups and downs of life. If the young person was suddenly faced with the social worker saying that they were closing the case now, the AYA was left feeling let down and stranded. A more positive experience was had when the worker had a transition plan for gradually handing back control to the young person.

Some had negative experiences after transition. "*After I transitioned a lot of appointments stopped or were not as frequent. They don't monitor my bloods the same or do scans. Things could be going wrong for all anyone knows; I've hardly seen anyone in ages.*" In situations like this it appeared that no-one had explained how follow-up care might be different in the adult service or that it may be part of a planned reduction in surveillance over time. Lehmann et al. explain that frustration with health care can result from survivors feeling their late effects problems are viewed as less important [18].

Another example of a lack of forward planning or poor coordination of follow-up services was being required to attend the treating hospital near the family home for routine follow-up endocrine bloods. "*Why do I have to drive all the way back to my treating hospital for that? Why can't I get these bloods done where I'm at university? There's a big cancer centre there, why can't they do it and send the results over?*" Davies, Kelly and Hannigan explore the need for health professionals to assist AYAs with decision-making about place of care, but this is often focused on place of treatment and should expand to consider place of follow-up [16, 44].

When discussing with one UK team how they managed the long term follow-up and late effects service and whether or not young people were given time in late effects clinics without parents or partners, they explained that they had a dedicated 'Long Term Follow-up email address.' This email inbox was reviewed daily on week days and was advertised to young people as a place where they could email private questions that they didn't want to discuss in front of parents or partners, or if they had questions ahead of their appointment or thought of questions after their consultation.

10.2.1.1 Section 2 Summary

In this section AYAs wanted health, social care and education professionals to know about striving for normality, information needs, privacy, contradiction and individuality, dependence and frustration, the power of positive, anxiety and mental health, death of a peer, the construct of time, social challenges and preparation for transition.

In synthesizing the conversations of AYAs with cancer and reviewing the literature on this topic there are clear messages. Exploring thoughts and feelings and expressing them in some form is helpful in normalising the cancer experience. Managing posttraumatic growth, and integrating their normal AYA identity with a cancer identity, while maintaining a sense of personhood that is not exclusively defined by the cancer is possible. Health, social care and education professionals alongside charities and support groups can help AYAs explore and express their world in the most meaningful way for them [15][6,7,8,9,10,11].

[6] https://www.mskcc.org/experience/patient-support/activities

[7] https://jtvcancersupport.com/

[8] http://www.clicsargent.org.uk/content/join-clic-sargents-online-community

[9] http://www.clicsargent.org.uk/news/11-11-2015-kaiser-chief-and-x-factor-star-help-cancer-patients-follow-their-musical-dreams

[10] https://www.youtube.com/watch?v=uZfjCTSuuRU&app=desktop

[11] http://www.lillyoncology.com/support-resources/lilly-oncology-on-canvas.html

This is what I want all health, social care and education professionals to know about how to support me living with and beyond cancer

AYA age appropriate care We need to be supported by people who understand our age group and the ways in which we are biologically, developmentally, psychologically, socially and culturally different from young children and older adults [25].

Building strategies for developing a positive self image and identity It helps if you try to understand the impact of treatment on my body image and help my family and I to develop ways to accept theses changes. Discussing how to manage social interactions and cope with relationships that are affected by my self image will enable me to stay connected to education and work and may help with treatment compliance particularly in relation to steroids [27, 32, 33].

Private time When you offer me discreet opportunities to have a private or sensitive conversation with you away from my parents or partner, I feel more respected, more able to express my true needs and I have a better experience.

Talk to me not my parents, or talk to me and my parents, but ask me first.

Sex It helps if you explain what is ok with regard to sex when on treatment, as well as what should be avoided. How much kissing when I'm neutropenic? Can I enjoy multiple partners as long as I use barrier contraception? Is oral sex OK?

Help with decision making It helps me if you are confident with knowledge of the legal framework in my country for consent and refusal of treatment and care. I might need you to be brave in helping me to be a part of informed decision-making [46].

Anxiety, depression, grief At some point during my treatment or life after cancer I will get this. I may still put a brave face on. I may say I'm fine. I'm not. I need you to tell me what to expect and how to manage it.

Contradiction and adaptation What I want and need each time we meet may ebb and flow. I am constantly moving between regression, development and evolution, but I am rarely still and always looking to the future.

Time has new meaning for me Time freezes, moves slowly, speeds up, stagnates, becomes a measure of risk, frightens me, heals, becomes precious. Consider my view of time when you plan my care [6, 20].

10.3 This Is What I Want to Tell You About Your Interactions with Me

10.3.1 Listening to AYAs Talk About Their Interactions with Health Professionals

Young people wanted health professionals involved in their care to get to know them as a person and find out how they want to be treated. Being so much more than their diagnosis was an important message. They asked that health, social care and education professionals remembered what they themselves were doing at a similar age.

"I know they don't know what we're going through, but try and get on our level; cancer isn't the only thing in our lives" AYAs wanted health professionals to treat them as an individual, "more than a number," and to give them;

"a voice in the care and support they receive [2]."

There was clear recognition and respect for the fact that individuals have to be "*professional,*" but at the same time they wanted them to "*act normal,*" *have a laugh sometimes and show they are human.*" "*That's always important…just having positive people around you. I didn't like people feeling sorry for me. I didn't like that. I like people that would walk in and just be funny and just have jokes and just be comfortable.*" Young people were clear that they wanted professionals to be able to relate to them and build relationships, which included emotional engagement, but that the professionals also had to have clear professional boundaries [1, 6, 12, 20]. AYAs do not want health, social care or education professionals to be unbounded and over-familiar with them.

In terms of qualities or characteristics for health professionals, the young people felt that health professionals in this field needed to be "*people persons.*" "*I love how they listen to what you have to say and try and convince you that you're not alone.*" They wanted to be talked to as if they were a friend, have their name remembered and have a chat. Generally they felt they had this with many nurses but not always. A positive attitude and the importance of humour was cited in published literature as supporting a positive attitude and being essential in helping AYAs to cope [1, 6, 12].

Being honest was highly valued by AYAs. In discussions, two young people shared how they felt their Consultant pitied them and wasn't being 'straight' in terms of prognosis, trying to give them false hope. Young people described that some days you need a soft, gentle and comforting approach and some days you need the push. Overall they preferred a direct and honest approach; "*say it how it is, but deliver it gently.*" It's difficult for healthcare professionals to pitch this right every time, and being a good interpreter of adolescent body language is a must. One young man was talking about his oncologist and said "*She was really hard on me at diagnosis. I was really upset and she said, come on now, you need to be strong and get on with this thing. It felt hard and callous and from then on, every time I had an appointment I felt I had to put a brave face on.*" This of course, highlights the need to try to get to know the young person individually and be flexible with the approach [1, 20].

Poorer experiences were described where the professionals approach was seen as inflexible, such as strict adherence to rules and procedures, especially around set wake up times on the ward [2]. Conversely good experiences were cited as professionals who were friendly and bubbly, willing to help, had their own personality, introduced themselves and made the AYA feel comfortable asking for help [2, 32]. They valued staff who made them feel equal, asked permission, always involved them in decision making, spoke directly to them and remembered their names. Like each AYA is individual and has their own unique personality, AYAs appreciated it when healthcare, social care and education professionals showed something of their own personality rather than standing behind a particular persona as a nurse, or a doctor. In the UK, they did not want health professionals to be too formal; "*no shaking hands and stuff.*" This professional individuality is beautifully illustrated in the following set of photographs.

> Lying in a hospital bed far from feeling 100%; with a thousand thoughts floating around my head accompanied by the ominous beep-beep-beep of the pumps, trolleys rattling up and down the ward and countless nursing footsteps moving busily to and fro, I was understandably unable to focus. Sometimes I found it difficult to remember the simplest things such as the names of the amazing professionals caring for me, ensuring my chemotherapy was running smoothly. Something that stood out throughout my treatment was the individuality of each medical person by my bedside; more specifically their personalised pockets which were constantly at eye level as I lay there. Having something routinely familiar helped a lot during chemo treatment and these unique and often quirky pockets helped me feel secure, comforted and served as a reminder to whom each one belonged. These personal pockets are from some of the nurses who I thank for me being here today, they broke up the monotony and sterility of the clinical environment and they brightened up my days.
>
> Aimee Mary Jordan 2016 (Fig. 10.5).

When discussing communication style and approach young people recognised that different people have very different needs at different times during their diagnosis, treatment and life beyond cancer. Tough talk works for some, sometimes, but it is not right for everyone on every occasion. But interestingly AYAs recognised that they definitely needed a tough talking to at some point along the way. All of them needed lots of comfort too. Not too harsh and callous. Not too soft, wishy-washy and unclear. I am reminded of a phrase heard at a conference many years ago "*a firm hand in kid gloves*" [47].

In one scenario a young man talked about what he called "*Ostrich Syndrome*" and explained how he came to recognise he had been burying his head in the sand. He had moved away to a new job and stopped taking his oral medication for several months. When parents called he would say he was doing fine. This links back to the work of Belpame et al., which identified how AYAs can employ avoidance to hold on to normality and manage coping, becoming a "director" to master and manage their environment [1]. Other researchers also identify a higher level of wishful thinking and avoidance/ignoring problems in survivors compared to health peers [41]. It wasn't until meeting with this young man's Consultant that she challenged him on the fact he wasn't taking his treatment. He say's the Consultant's approach was absolutely what he needed to shock him back to reality. She was really firm and said "*you cannot do this, this is life and death stuff. Then she went on to explain why.*" Despite how direct she was it was also said with kindness and understanding.

Parents were also mentioned in this discussion. When parents were too gentle and sympathetic, young people found this stifling and came to realise that it wasn't helping them to learn to manage their situation or get past some of the challenges they were facing. They were very respectful of parents who employed "*tough love*"; kind and caring but retaining some firmness and the odd push. "*I can't thank my Dad enough for making me get out of bed every day. Really at the start, all you're thinking is 'am I going to die,' nothing else goes in. He got me going again.*"

Young people said they didn't always have the same perception of when they were OK, ill or seriously ill as the professionals. This can manifest in positive ways as in this scenario, "*Sometimes I needed reminding that it's OK to find it hard to get up in the night and make a cup of tea.*" Or it can be a source of conflict as this scenario describes. "*He was really pleased that the cancer was shrinking but I was*

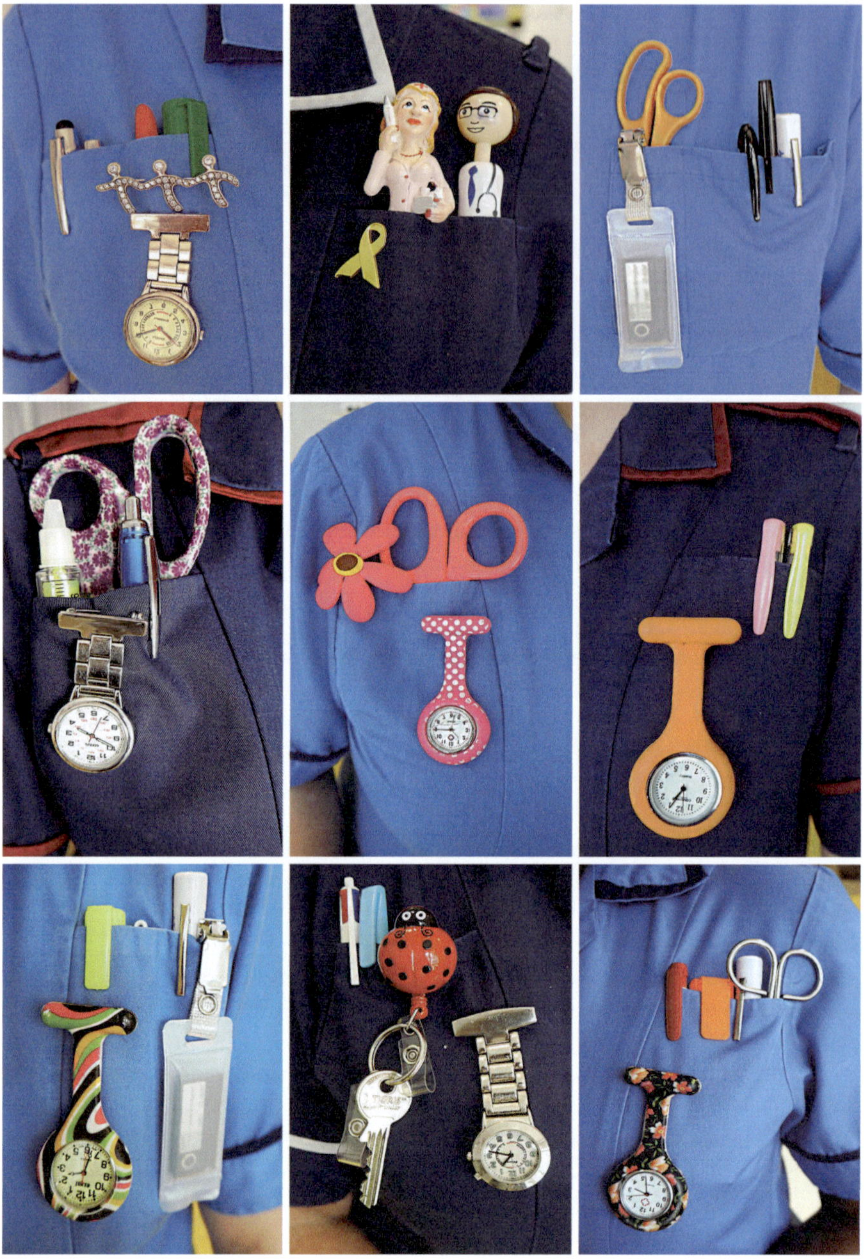

Fig. 10.5 "Personal Pockets" by Aimee Jordan

really angry about it all. I had bad side effects, the steroids made me really spotty, I had a lot of weight gain and he wanted me to be happy. He couldn't get his head round why I wasn't. For me it was the worst message in the world that the chemo was working and he wanted me to have more. I couldn't see beyond to the positive."

When it's not possible or necessary to be face to face, support and communication via telephone seemed to work for most young people in the conversations, although one young lady expressed not liking to talk on the phone. The phone call offered a personal touch and gave them an opportunity to ask questions. Text was considered a useful tool but mainly for reminders before appointments, and potentially less satisfactory as a medium for dialog. "*I email my oncologist and it's the best thing ever*" explained one young person. The oncologist emailed blood results and always stated "*email back if you have any questions*." She felt this approach saved the oncologist time and saved her from worrying, waiting for calls or appointments, and dealt with problems quickly at low cost. Letters were less satisfactory as a medium for communication. Letters can appear cold, often made assumptions that the young people felt were not correct, and there was no opportunity to ask questions. Letters were useful to confirm information shared verbally. In countries with vast land mass and sparse populations the needs for communication via digital technologies are likely to be different and emerging. For AYAs born since the 1980s their comfort with digital communication is usually way in advance of the health, social and education professionals supporting them [6, 12].

10.3.1.1 Section 3 Summary

In this section AYAs wanted health and social care professionals to know about individuality and personal connections, professional behaviour with a human touch and good humour. They talked about style and approach and methods of communication.

This is what I want health, social care and education professionals to know about how to interact with me

Trust I have entrusted my life to you, because I have nowhere else to turn [20]. Communicate with me and with other people in the team so that I feel safe and that you all know what's going on with me.

I am not my cancer Support my efforts to grow, believe in me. "Being different does not equate to being less." Discover my strengths and help me use them to overcome my challenges [20]. Sometimes I will need you to be brave for me or to help me find the courage I need [46].

Humanity Show me the person you are, and get to know the person I am. Be kind and friendly but retain your professional boundaries. Every interaction counts.

Tough Love I may have cancer, but sometimes I need a push in the right direction.

Acknowledgments All the young people supported by CLIC Sargent or Redkite who offered their thoughts and experiences freely to inform this chapter. In particular the Young People's Reference Group, the Participation Team & Rachel Blackford. http://www.clicsargent.org.uk/

Simon Darby (social worker) who introduced me to the Arts Project in Northern Ireland "Hello, my name is not cancer."

Laura Monaghan for contributing her thumbprint "Countdown" from the Northern Ireland Arts Project

Alana McCrea for contributing her thumbprint “My life was great before cancer.” from the Northern Ireland Arts Project

Shona McDowell (social worker) who introduced me to Holly’s art.

Holly Hamer for contributing her art work ‘Shock of diagnosis’ and ‘Watching from the sidelines.’

Sam Collins (social worker) who supported two focus groups and introduced me to Aimee’s photography.

Aimee Jordan for contributing her Photography ‘Individuality’

Kailly Woodroffe at http://www.redkite.org.au/ who linked the themes of the chapter with practice in Australia and Redkite research

The CLIC Sargent Research and Policy Team for support with research.

The literature search strategy was developed by Royal College of Nursing Library and Heritage Centre (UK), with grateful thanks to the RCN Library staff for their support. The Royal College of Nursing Library and Heritage Centre

References

1. Belpame N, Kars MC, Beekman D, et al. The AYA director: a synthesized concept to understand psychosocial experiences of adolescents and young adults with cancer. Cancer Nurs. 2016;39(4):292–302.
2. Hedström M, Skolin I, von Essen L. Distressing and positive experiences and important aspects of care for adolescents treated for cancer. Eur J Oncol Nurs. 2004;8:6–17.
3. CLIC Sargent. Best chance from the start: improving support to identify cancer in children and young people. 2016. http://www.clicsargent.org.uk/content/better-care-diagnosis. Accessed 15 Jan 2017.
4. Gibson F, Pearce S. Eden T et al. Young people describe their prediagnosis cancer experience Psycho-oncology. 2013;22:2585–92.
5. CLIC Sargent. Coping with cancer: supporting young people’s resilience. 2014. http://www.clicsargent.org.uk/sites/files/clicsargent/Coping%20with%20cancer%20report.pdf. Accessed 15 Jan 2017.
6. Keim-Malpass J, Steeves RH. Talking with death at a diner Young women’s online narratives of cancer. Oncol Nurs Forum. 2012;39(4):373–406.
7. Teenage Cancer Trust 2014 Cancer Warning Signs. https://www.teenagecancertrust.org/get-help/i-think-i-might-have-cancer/cancer-warning-signs Accessed 15 Jan 2017.
8. Crawshaw MA, Glaser AW, Hale JP, Sloper P. Male and female experiences of having fertility matters raised alongside a cancer diagnosis during the teenage and young adult years. Eur J Cancer Care. 2009;18:381–90.
9. Brassil KJ, et al. Exploring the cancer experiences of young adults in the context of stem cell transplant. Cancer Nurs. 2015;38(4):260–9.
10. Coelho P. Veronika Decides to Die. 2000th ed. London: Harper Collins; 1998.
11. Hauken M, Larsen T, Holsen I. Meeting Reality: Young adult cancer survivors’ Experiences of re-entering everyday life after cancer treatment. Cancer Nurs. 2013;36(5):17–26.
12. Keim-Melpass J, Stegenga K, Loudin B, Kennedy C, Kools S. “It’s back! My remission is over”: Online communication of disease progression among adolescents with cancer. J Pediatr Oncol Nurs. 2016;33(3):209–17.
13. Stegenga K, Macpherson CF. I’m a survivor, go study that word and you’ll see my name. Cancer Nurs. 2014;37(6):418–28.
14. Bluebond-Langner M. The private worlds of dying children. In: Hanks G, Cherney N, Christakis N, Fallon M, Kaasa S, Portenoy R, editors. Oxford textbook of palliative medicine. 4th ed. Oxford: Oxford University Press; 1978. p. 1355.
15. Woodgate R, West C, Tailor K. Existential anxiety and growth: an exploration of computerized drawings and perspectives of children and adolescents with cancer. Cancer Nurs. 2014;37(2):146–59.

16. Davies J, Kelly D, Hannigan N. Autonomy and dependence: a discussion paper on decision-making in teenagers and young adults undergoing cancer treatment. J Adv Nurs. 2015;71(9):2031–40.
17. Anderzén-Carlsson A, Sörlie V, Kihlgres A. Dealing with fear – from the perspective of adolescent girls with cancer. Eur J Oncol Nurs. 2012;16:286–92.
18. Lehmann V, Grönqvist H, Engvall G, Ander M, Tuinman M, Hagedoorn M, Sanderman ME, von Essen L. Negative and positive consequences of adolescent cancer 10 years after diagnosis: an interview-based longitudinal study in Sweden. Psycho-Oncology. 2014;23:1129–235.
19. Redkite. Redkite music therapists. 2015. http://www.redkite.org.au/support/music-therapists Accessed 15 Jan 2017.
20. Speraw S. "Talk to me –I'm human": The story of a girl, her personhood, and the failures of healthcare. Qual Health Res. 2009;19(6):732–43.
21. Sposito A, Silva-Rodrigues F, Sparapani V, et al. Coping strategies used by hospitalized children with cancer undergoing chemotherapy. Journal of Nursing Scholarship Brazil. 2015;47(2):143–51.
22. Juth V, Cohen-Silver R, Sender L. The shared experience of adolescent an young adult cancer patients and their caregivers. Psycho-Oncology. 2015;24:1746–53.
23. Tsangaris E, Johnson J, Taylor R, Fern L, Bryant-Lukosius D, Barr R, Fraser G, Klassen A. Identifying the supportive care needs of adolescent and young adult survivors of cancer: a qualitative analysis and systematic review. Support Care Cancer. 2014;22:947–59.
24. Docherty SL, Kayle M, Maslow GR, Santacroce SJ. The adolescent and young adult with cancer. A developmental life course perspective. Seminars in :Oncology Nursing. 2015;31(3):186–96.
25. Lauer AL. Treatment of anxiety and depression in adolescents and young adults with cancer. Journal of Paediatrics Oncology Nursing. 2015;32(5):278–83.
26. DeRouen MC, Smith AW, Tao L, et al. Cancer-related information needs and cancer's impact on control over life influence health-related quality of life among adolescents and young adults with cancer. Psycho-Oncology. 2015;24:1104–15.
27. Lee M-Y, Mu P-F, Tsay S-F, Chou S-S, Chen Y-C, Wong T-T. Body image of children and adolescents with cancer: a metasynthesis on qualitative research findings. Nurs Health Sci. 2012;14:381–90.
28. CLIC Sargent. Relationships and sex. 2015. http://www.clicsargent.org.uk/content/relationships-and-sex Accessed 15 Jan 2017.
29. CLIC Sargent. Cancer and fertility. 2016. http://www.clicsargent.org.uk/content/cancer-and-fertility Accessed 15 Jan 2017.
30. Quinn GP, Huang IC, Murphy D, Zidonik-Eddelton K, Krull KR. Missing content from health-related quality of life instruments: interviews with young adult survivors of childhood cancer. Qual Life Res. 2013;22:111–8.
31. Insley E, Streich L. The new normal (executive summary) In: The new normal; evaluation of the social care service for young people. 2015. http://www.clicsargent.org.uk/content/new-normal-evaluation-our-social-care-enhanced-service-young-people. Accessed Aug 2016.
32. CLIC Sargent. Impact of cancer on a child's world. 2010. http://www.clicsargent.org.uk/content/impact-cancer-childs-world. Last accessed 15 Jan 17.
33. CLIC Sargent. No young person with cancer left out. 2013. http://www.clicsargent.org.uk/content/no-young-person-cancer-left-out. Last accessed 15 Jan 17.
34. Kim B, Gillham D. The experience of young adult cancer patients described through online narratives. Cancer Nurs. 2013;36(5):377–84.
35. Wakefield C, McLoone J, Butow P, et al. Support after the completion of cancer treatment: perspectives of Australian adolescents and their families. Eur J Cancer Care. 2013;22:530–9.
36. Easley J, Miedema B, Robinson L. It's the "good" cancer, so who cares? Perceived lack of support among young thyroid cancer survivors. Oncol Nurs Forum. 2013;40(6):596–600.
37. Hamre H, Zeller B, Kanellopolous A, Kiserud CE, Aakhus S, Lund M, Loge JH, Fossa SD, Ruud E. High prevalence of chronic fatigue in adult long-term survivors of acute lymphoblastic leukaemia and lymphoma during childhood and adolescence. Journal of adolescent and young adult oncology. 2013;2(1):2–9.

38. Scott K. Give me time to heal. Nurs Stand. 2008;23(9):61.
39. Taylor N, Absolom K, Snowden J, Eiser C. Need for psychological follow-up among young adult survivors of childhood cancer European. J Cancer. 2012;21:52–8.
40. Hobbie WL, Stuber M, Meeske K, Wissler K, Rourke MT, Ruccione K, Hinkle A, Kazak AE. Symptoms of posttraumatic stress in young adult survivors of childhood cancer. J Clin Oncol. 2000;18(24):4060–6.
41. McDonnell G, Baily C, Schuler T, Verdeli H. Anxiety among adolescent survivors of paediatric cancer: a missing link in the survivorship literature. Palliat Support Care. 2015;13:345–9.
42. Zebrack B, Kwak M, Salsman J, Cousino M, Meeske K, Aguilar C, Embry L, Block R, Hayes-Lattin B, Cole S. The relationship between posttraumatic stress and posttraumatic growth amongst adolescent and young adult (AYA) cancer. Psycho-Oncology. 2015;24:162–8.
43. Wollington T. "Time" in I'm still running: selected poems by adolescent with cancer. Privately Published. 1980.
44. McClellan W, Klemp J, Krebill H, et al. Understanding the functional late effects and information needs of adult survivors of childhood cancer. Oncol Nurs Forum. 2013;40(3):254–61.
45. CLIC Sargent. What about money. 2016. http://www.clicsargent.org.uk/content/what-about-money-2 Accessed 15 January 2017.
46. Kippen R. Stand up for me and be brave: what young people want from social workers the Guardian social care network: social life blog. 2016. https://www.theguardian.com/social-care-network/social-life-blog/2016/jul/06/stand-up-for-me-and-be-brave-what-young-people-want-from-social-workers. Accessed 9 July 2016.
47. Spinetta J. Conference lectures. Psychological late effects: the myths of surviving childhood cancer. Late effects conference. Manchester, UK. May 1993. 1993.

11 Caring for the Carers

Lesley Edwards and Laura Beek

11.1 Introduction Who Are the Carers?

Cancer is inherently a family disease, reverberating through the family and impacting all facets of the world of the child, young person and his or her family or partner and doing so over an extended period of time [1, 2]. In addition to coping with the diagnosis and treatment, the young person (term used throughout to represent Adolescent/Young Adult/AYA) is also in a developmental phase of discovery with psychosocial and identity changes and is also developing new types of relationships with peers and families and with a new set of hospital and community professionals [3]. For AYA, cancer diagnosis, treatment and subsequent late effects can be particularly disruptive to their social maturation, their development of social cognition and relationships awareness, and emotional regulation that guide them throughout the remainder of their lives [4, 5]. The impact of the diagnosis, prognosis, proposed treatment and potential long term effects are felt not only by the young person but also by their family including parents, siblings, children, peers and partners. For young people who are married or in committed relationships when they are diagnosed, they can be forced into dependence on a spouse or partner in a way they never conceived imaginable [6]. The TCT Blueprint of care [7] sets out advice about recognising the importance of support for the young person, the importance of

L. Edwards (✉)
Consultant Clinical Psychologist Royal Marsden Hospital, Sutton, Surrey, UK
e-mail: lesley.edwards@rmh.nhs.uk

L. Beek
Clinic Psychologist, Prinses Máxima Centrum voor Kinderoncologie, Utrecht, The Netherlands

J. Chisholm et al. (eds.), *A Practical Approach to the Care of Adolescents and Young Adults with Cancer*, https://doi.org/10.1007/978-3-319-66173-5_11

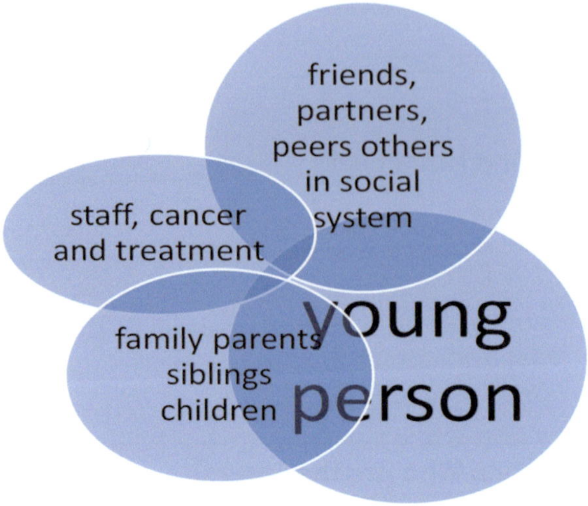

Fig. 11.1 Support system of the young person with cancer

discovering through dialogue which the important support networks are and the importance of maintaining relevant and appropriate boundaries for staff whilst understanding that communication with this developmental age group may be different than for other age groups. Staff expertise and training is crucial in developing good working practices.

It is of note that the wider social system is also likely to include the important roles of school, college, work, spiritual or religious support. It is therefore imperative to understand the multiple influences on the young person, taking into consideration the roles of the sub-systems in their social world, which all play prominent roles in adjustment and outcomes. Co-incidentally the patient's cancer, medical world and treatments become part of their social ecology because they are important factors that enter into the lives of children and young people [2] (Fig. 11.1)

11.2 Developmental and Disease Trajectory Issues

The role of parent, partners and family can be complex in a social unit where the independence of the young person is the aim. Many young people do regress and many parents are faced with a grown up child who is behaving like a much younger child and has retreated to needing to be 'mothered'. This can be in contrast to their behaviour when with peers, friends or partners. There is a need to recognise that a young person can hold conflicting views when faced with challenges and may need to be treated in different ways by different carers.

The young person and their carers are facing potential loss of future, loss of their dreams which may lead to both feeling out of control and have detrimental effect on their self-esteem. Staff working with young people need to have an in depth understanding of these impending developmental issues, recognising that independence

Table 11.1 Important developmental information for staff to know [7]

• Parents may re-evaluate their relationship with the young person when a cancer diagnosis is made. How the relationship changes is dependent on the relationship before their diagnosis. Some young people rely on their parent/carers to be there with them, others find it embarrassing and stifling. In addition, regressive or childlike behaviour may be observed. Changes in the parental relationship are often a source of family conflict that will need careful management and support from the young person's healthcare team
• Some patients may be parents themselves. Young parents in some circumstances may resume an adolescent role thus affecting their behaviour as a parent. Conflicts of interest can occur regarding the care of a child between the patient, their parents or partners where a child of the young person is involved. If their cancer cannot be cured, they will have the added burden of choosing who will look after their child/children after their death. In some situations legal issues may arise. If this is likely the young person should be supported to discuss and document their wishes where possible
• Young people may be diagnosed during a time when they are beginning to establish an important personal or sexual relationship. A cancer diagnosis is challenging even in strong relationships, as it can test partners' perseverance and care. New relationships can be very vulnerable to existing parental relationships. Conflict may occur in establishing who the significant carers are for that young person. Patients may revert to parental care at this time and new partners can feel isolated

and identity are fragile. They must also recognise the importance of education or lack of it, the complexity of relationships and that the development of sexuality and fertility can be in a state of crisis [8].

The Teenage Cancer Trust TCT [7] outlined the importance of staff understanding the complex interaction of adolescent development with cancer diagnosis and family dynamics (Table 11.1):

11.2.1 Stage of Diagnosis and Treatment and Impact on Carers

Adams and Deveau [9] outlined that as doctors forewarn patients and family members about possible physical side effects, so must the carers be warned about the different psychological issues which may emerge as the young person and their carers go through treatment, the stress both the carers and patient may be under and what to expect. The carers must be able to to think carefully through what may or may not help.

At diagnosis carers and family may question "why my child?", "why my girlfriend?", "why my mummy?" It is normal to search for meaning and explanations, trying to achieve some degree of control over the situation. Immediately following a life-threatening diagnosis like cancer, the adolescent or young adult and his carers can experience acute medically related traumatic stress. Although most families are resilient and access their natural coping resources to adjust in time, it is important to talk through with the carers and patient the stress they may be under, and what to expect [10]. Feelings faced can be similar to those illustrated in a loss and grief model (Table 11.2):

In order to offer the best care the importance of good psychosocial screening from diagnosis onwards is the first step in identifying risks (and competencies) and

Table 11.2 Diagnosis—Loss and grief feelings and what can help

Loss and grief feeling	What can help carers
Shock, denial and confusion	Understand the need to repeat information, acknowledge how to negotiate relationships with hospital staff, especially when the young person is an adult themselves. This is particularly resonant when the young person has regressed and their parent has been drawn back into being the responsible adult.
Sadness and depression	Acknowledging feelings and then consideration of whether it is better for carers to show or not to show feelings, acknowledging that all are affected, but not wanting to be a burden upon others.
Anger	Recognising it is common to blame others for what is happening, blaming God, and blaming self. Therefore to think creatively how to express feelings, what works for each individual and encouraging them to do what helps.
Guilt: feeling that somehow it was their fault, carer can feel helpless	Sometimes this leads to a parent or sibling spoiling the young person. It is useful to recognise that guilt is a common and normal reaction to cancer, most parents want to protect their children and feel they have failed as a parent in some way; in this case it is important to get an outside perspective. Children of the young person, can also show very strong feelings of wanting to protect their parent and want to make everything better; or conflictingly display vulnerable out of control behaviour if all they feel is chaos. Creating a safe place to talk and be listened to is important and creative ways of working with children of the patient or siblings can be explored from psychological support or play therapy team.
Understanding and acceptance	Thinking about how much should the young person know, in whose interest is the carer or staff member acting? How to negotiate a shared and safe understanding of what is happening.
	Remember that for most people information is learned in stages, what the illness is called, what this means, understanding it is serious, specifics of diagnosis and prognosis. Specific knowledge depends on age and understanding of the young person.

determining need for further evaluation and support. Some of the young people diagnosed with cancer and their families have pre-existing vulnerabilities/deficits that may complicate treatment and that would benefit from psychological intervention.

11.2.2 During and After Treatment

Cancer can be seen as a barrier to normality by the young person making them feel that the treatment or follow up goes on forever, making them different and isolating them from friends and peers, at a time when they would normally be identifying more with them. This can result in conflict and a separation from or rejection of the young person's peers or partners. This sense of isolation can lead to overcompensation, including increased risk taking, outdoing their peers, resisting treatment or non-compliance. Carers can feel increasingly tense and fatigued as treatment continues, roles within the family can become blurred and the cancer continues to be the major focus of everyone's life, taking its toll on all in the family. Parents can struggle with balance between over protecting and overindulging. What is important is that carers are as consistent as possible and an understanding of their needs must be shown by the supporting staff.

Some young people who present as defiant or refusing treatment or follow up feel unsupported, angry, not listened to or feel that that parents are being talked to without them. Having an open dialogue and noting that most families do remain together and that families do need to work on strengths as well as recognising weaknesses helps families to pull together rather than pulling apart. Siblings can feel very left out and rejected, and if they feel unnoticed can present with attention seeking behaviour or problems at school. A parent's role for the young person undergoing treatment is to help the young person to learn and grow despite their illness, for all to recognise they are a young person first and a cancer patient second.

11.2.3 Palliative Care

If the young person can no longer be cured, carers have an important role to play, to help the young person feel safe and contained, to enable them to ask questions and discuss feelings if they need to and learn to balance the needs of all in the family, whilst having the devastating need to grieve themselves [9, 11, 12]. Carers need to be able to take care of themselves in order to be able to meet the needs of others. It is recommended to seek support, whether practical, psychological, financial or spiritual. It is helpful to consider and anticipate questions the young person or siblings might ask, what kind of answers to give and work out who to go to for advice.

Parents and at times partners can experience suicidal ideation and even suicidal intent when faced with the potential death of the young person. If this is the case, a risk assessment needs to be undertaken and an appropriate safety plan drawn up with the carer, placed in the young person's notes and their family doctor must be informed so that all parties know which emergency numbers to call.

11.3 Carers, Family and Partners

11.3.1 Family (Including Parents, Siblings, Children and Important Other Members of the Family)

Being a family caregiver can have positive altruistic benefit but may also have an impact which is burdensome, placing the caregiver at risk of physical and psychological morbidity and financial disadvantage [13, 14]. The primary care giver chosen by the young person may vary over time and may include their partner, a friend or a parent. For parents, it can feel impossible to cope, feeling at times overwhelmed by emotions, with signs of depression, anxiety, panic, or at times post traumatic disorder (PTSD) or suicidal ideation. Therapeutic support can help to provide the parent carer with coping strategies and non-judgemental listening. It is not always the most obvious person that the young person turns to: the role of important others including teachers, mentors and other adults can never be underestimated, and the close family may feel rejected. It is notable that there are many examples of resilience but a substantial minority struggle to cope; it is always important to note that families and social systems are complex, and there are many ways in which family functioning may be either a hindrance or an asset in the context of child and young adult's cancer [2].

Good clinical practise is to identify a key staff member who can either provide support for the caregivers or sign post them to available face to face or online support. Most cancer centres use a key worker system and the carers need to feel part of the system, valued and know who to go to for their advice or support. It is important to consider both culturally appropriate resources and where appropriate spiritual resources. The support worker needs access to a database of local support networks whether locally or online and/or to be able to signpost the carer to the hospital patient support Team. Given the varying needs of young people, a variety of informal and formal support is usually offered.

Family involvement should always be on the terms laid down by the young person (this will be influenced to some degree, by the age and psychological state of the individual) and a flexible approach should be adopted. Treating teams should consider the following:

- Information needs of the young person's support networks [15]. Do they have any questions? Do they feel fully informed about the treatment and have all resources that they can access been highlighted to them? This is an important issue as it has been suggested that information needs can be unmet [6]
- Practical needs of support networks—for example, do carers need assistance with travel to and from the hospital? Has general financial or employment or support advice been given. Do they have other dependents?
- Support needs of significant others—are they given time and opportunity to talk about the young person's situation? Would the support of other parents or guidance to online parent/carer networks be beneficial?

There is a special requirement to address the information and psychological needs of the children of young people themselves. Cancer Research UK recognised that talking to children about cancer can be very difficult and upsetting [16]. Adults sometimes try to protect children from such a situation by not discussing it with them. But even if adults don't tell them openly about what is happening, children will inevitably know when something is seriously wrong. It is recommended that children need to be told what is happening, in an age appropriate way. There is good guidance available in the Cancer Research UK website and Macmillan Cancer Support websites [17]. They recommend letting children know what is happening, as this generally helps them cope better with a parent's illness. There are booklets with some useful information about what to tell children when an adult has cancer and how children cope. For example "Talking to children when an adult has cancer"' and "Talking to children about cancer" [17]. Cancernet [18] also has excellent information and links to other useful websites in the United States.

11.3.2 Partners and Peers

Partners and peers of the young person may find themselves in a very vulnerable position, where their relationship has changed, but they are still are an important part of the young person's life. They can find a much higher requirement to co-exist with the young person's family than would be usual. In the same way that parents, siblings and children of the young person need available support, so do the partner and friends who also play a vital role in role in helping the young person feel contained [7]. The relationship with the patient's partner can change immensely throughout treatment, therefore sensitive handling of issues involving their changing relationship, including sexual relationships, fertility and physical changes coupled with an experienced approach will help the partner to feel an important part of what is happening to the AYA [19].

Young people who do have partners can be forced by medical circumstances into dependence on their partner in a way they never conceived imaginable. This can be a source of distress and ultimately have a major impact on the relationship affecting how both people view the other. They can often discover that they have quite different coping strategies [6].

Interestingly, Zebrack et al. [20] found that only 50% of young people ranked having support from family, partner and friends as a top five need at diagnosis and in treatment whilst meeting other survivors was identified as a top five need for all patients. Developmentally, social connections with same age peers who have a cancer history may be more beneficial or at least different from the support of family or friends. The caring aspect of the peer support role cannot be underestimated, but could potentially pose the risk of potentially having to deal with the raw emotions of another peer whilst being in the same position yourself: ideally some supervision or guidance for peer support groups would be beneficial. Clinicians and community-based agencies running peer-support programs for teens are now recognizing a growing need for extending peer support to a substantial subset of young adult patients and survivors [21].

11.3.2.1 Good Practice Guidelines for Family, Partner and Peers Support

It is necessary to offer psychological care for the young person and their carers as part of the overall medical and clinical care of the patient [22]. Applying standards of psychological care to identify both the families, and partners who are resilient and those who are vulnerable to match screening and interventions to levels of risk, would ensure that young person and their carers are offered targeted interventions within the context of their social, clinical and medical systems, taking into account their individual needs as well (Table 11.3 and Fig. 11.2). Using this checklist can help the caregiver recognise emerging stress.

Alongside the recognition of stress, there are risk factors which may help to identify those families in need of increased support. Based on Kazak's [2] work these may include:

- Single parent
- Poor social support system
- History of prior mental illness in patient or caregiver
- No confiding relationship (patient or carer)
- History of poor family functioning or prior involvement with social care system
- Financial difficulties
- Behaviour problems in childhood (young person)

Table 11.3 Best support provision of family members, peers and partners support (based on [7] with additions)

• Best practice is delivered through a combination of expert medical management and expert age-appropriate psychosocial management. Treating teams should access services/support or liaison offered by AYA Principal Treatment Centres
• Screen all patients and family members using a psychosocial assessment tool such as holistic needs assessment [23] or family assessment tool PAT 2.0 [2] which was initially developed for use in the paediatric population, but potentially could be proposed for use in the AYA population. Then refer on to support services as appropriate (e.g. psychology, psychiatry, counselling, occupational or physio- therapy, pain and symptom control team)
• Ensure psychosocial assessment and screening is continued throughout treatment, and into survivorship recognising that individual circumstances will change during the care pathway
• Ensure early referrals for risk issues including safeguarding and mental health risk, self harm or suicidal ideation. Remind staff that we are all responsible for referring and contacting safeguarding and psychiatric liaison teams; do not wait for someone else to do it
• Consider the use and creation of peer support and contact groups which can be seen as crucial to identity and coping [20] alongside appropriate guidance
• Ensure robust referral pathways for psychology, psychiatric services and counselling are in place to refer patients or carers when necessary
• Ensure a portfolio of support services and local resources are available for wider family members and carers
• Consider use of checklist to identify increased stress in caregivers (Fig. 11.2)

11.3.3 Spiritual and Cultural Support

Spiritual and cultural support are considered to be important care needs both in treatment and into palliative care, However, some studies indicate that health professionals express discomfort or lack of knowledge or skill in addressing these issues. Studies of minority and cultural groups suggest patients and families need healthcare professionals to understand and ask about socio-cultural traditions and norms, including gaining an understanding of a belief that God or an alternative is the determination of outcome for some patients. It is important to note patients and their families who receive a cancer diagnosis often begin to think about the meaning and purpose of life. They ask questions like 'Why me?' and 'Why now?' This kind of existential philosophical questioning is common both to people of no faith and to people of faith. Evidence suggests that addressing spiritual concerns and receiving good spiritual care contributes to patients' and family members' sense of wellbeing and quality of life, A robust referral pathway to chaplaincy and spiritual support will enhance good practise [7].

11.3.4 Research on Support Provision for Family Members

Hudson et al. undertook a systematic review in order to identify developments in family carer support that have occurred over the last decade. The focus of the review was interventions that targeted improvements in the psychosocial support of family carers of palliative care patients. The review found that having a variety of support to choose from enhances coping in carers [24]. The authors conclude that

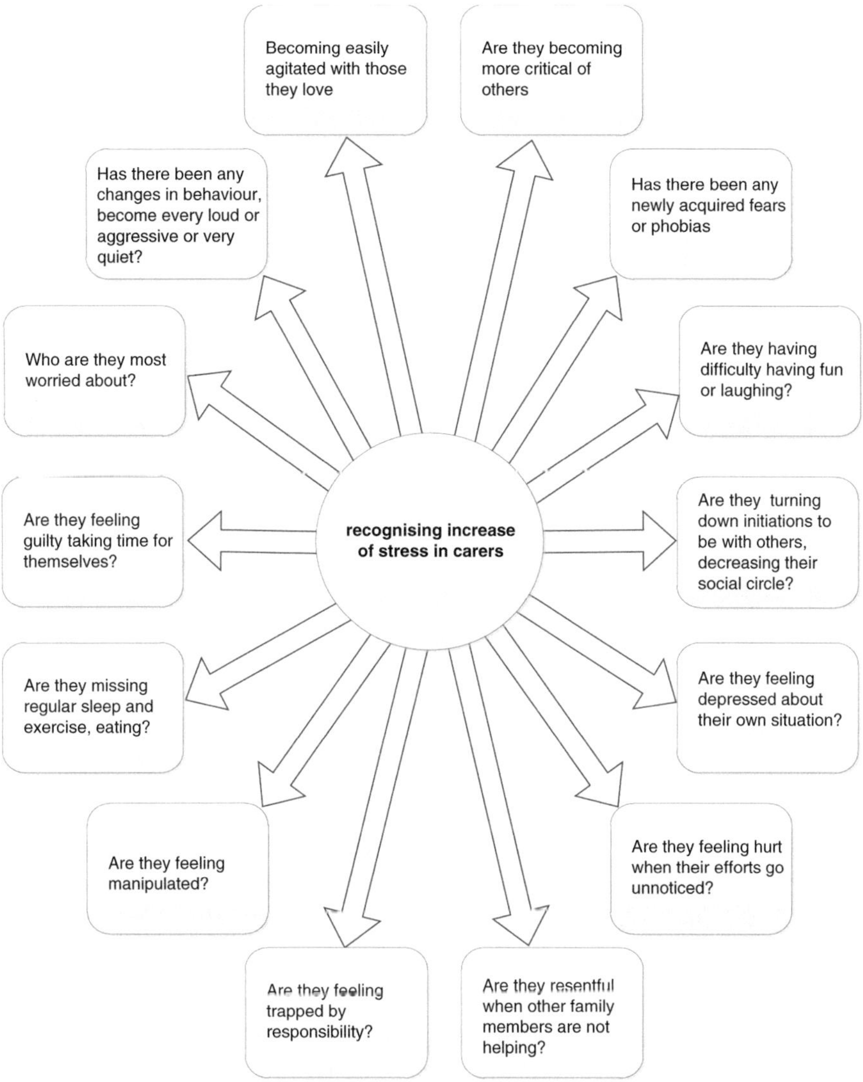

Fig. 11.2 Checklist of how to recognise increase of stress in family or peer/partner caregivers, are carers

interventions are needed: some of these can be generic, but that there will always be a need for individual variation. There remained however some excellent key questions which arose from the review.

- First, how can psychosocial interventions be designed to be effective given the typically short or variable period of time available to intervene?
- Second, what is the most useful way to determine which family or partner carers need significant psychosocial support, what assessment/identification methods should be used?

- Third, how can health services meet the support needs of the entire family and partners when many services may only be resourced to support the primary family carer?
- Finally what are the priority interventions and methods of delivery that are required for development and testing in the family carer population?

Group, individual, family or couple therapy have all been advocated as potential models that could be offered, but this does depend on funding of the support services and skills of the available team. Again it is crucial that there is a readily available and well known referral pathway to access psychological and counselling support both within and outside the primary treatment centre.

It is well known that being a carer can have devastating consequences and systematic review demonstrated the considerable challenges faced by carers [25]. These included adverse psychological, social, and financial consequences which can present somatically and can be exacerbated by the longevity both of treatment but also of long term effects and impacts which reverberate through the family [25]. There is widespread agreement that a more comprehensive model of psychosocial support, alongside protected funding is needed throughout the disease trajectory for patients, their partners and family members [7, 13, 26].

11.3.5 Types of Support Available

11.3.5.1 Online Support and Forums

Given this is a digital age and social media and the use of the internet is prevalent, ideally different types of support could be introduced so the young person and their carers have a choice of where to access such support. In the UK, the Children's Cancer and Leukaemia Group provides a useful leaflet giving guidance both to young people and carers about good websites [27], but also signposts to social media chat rooms and forums which can be accessed for support. Of note a report on the relatively low use of age-appropriate, internet-based resources among teenagers in their study (15.5%) surmised that, although teenagers may be heavy users of computers and social media in general, perhaps only a minority of these recently diagnosed patients use the internet for cancer-related information and support; in contrast, nearly half of young people aged 20–39 years who were treated in adult care institutions wanted but did not use age-appropriate internet resources for information and support, despite the existence of emergent social media and resources designed specifically by and for AYAs (eg, Planet Cancer, mAssKickers, StupidCancer.com [21]).

11.3.5.2 Face to Face Support for Family Members, Partners and Friends?

A wide variety of support groups and individual supports have been described. Information needs to be available from appropriately trained staff who can either offer the support, refer on or signpost to local or online services. These services include (Table 11.4):

Table 11.4 Face to face support

Drop in parent meetings
Couple therapy
Family therapy
Individual support for partners
Peer group informal and formal support/social groups
One off targeted days for children of adult patients
Breakfast brunches for all family members
End of treatment days
Coping with treatment days
Art therapy, music therapy
Games and film clubs
Mindfulness sessions for parents/young people and family members
Activity based support activities both in and away from hospital
TCT sponsored well being events, Find Your Sense of Tumour conferences or equivalent
Bereavement groups for parents/siblings and partners (separate groups)

11.4 Carers: Staff Members

To be able to effectively look after the young person and their families, staff need to be aware of the particular needs and developmental tasks of this group. Good education and training as well as a genuine desire to work with this age group is crucial to be able to form caring relationships and to anticipate what may happen and how to approach situations in a creative yet containing manner [28]. The 2012 TCT blueprint of care stresses the importance of having specialised staff who are not afraid of frank discussions, who can cope with open criticism and challenges and who can negotiate both with the young person and their family. Caring for a young person generates both negative and positive reactions, and the mood of both the young person and their carer can change in an instant. Knowing how to react in situations which can easily become volatile is a challenge [29]. The importance of specific adolescent and young people training is important. TCT wards or community teams tend to be made up of either paediatric or adult trained teams, who may not have had the experience of working with this fascinating, but at times challenging age group.

11.4.1 Training Needs of Staff

(See Table 11.5)

Table 11.5 A rolling training programme including

• *Learning opportunities*
• A variety of learning experiences including didactic learning, experiential learning, observation, shared learning with other disciplines and the opportunity when possible to learn from young people and their carers directly
• Staff need access to attend AYA specific courses and conferences
• Staff should be encouraged to utilise and join existing national AYA professional networks which offer expertise, peer support and mentorship (eg in UK TYAC/TYAC MDT)
• Staff need to attend advanced communication courses
• Staff support and supervision is essential, transparent support mechanisms need to be established
• Importance of promoting staff support either in an individual or group format
• *Specific teaching areas*
• Developmental awareness; what developmental tasks the young person faces, how these are interrupted or challenged by cancer
• The adolescent, how they think, the uniqueness of the adolescent brain, how they challenge and make sense of the world
• Understanding their psychosocial needs
• Young people may demand more time from staff than other groups. Spending time is crucial in developing therapeutic relationships, and staff need to be supportive in meeting this need
• Confidentiality issues are paramount for this population including limits of confidentiality and importance of boundaries
• Recognition that non adherence and noncompliance is common: There is a need for negotiating skills, listening to what the reason was for noncompliance and creative ways to approach within an MDT framework
• Creativity in how to balance needs of the young person, their partners, peers and family members who all may have important roles to play
• Understanding the role of school/college/university further education
• Communicating with young person: both facilitators and what to avoid
• Mental health needs and role of risk assessment and management and development of liaison networks for access to mental health services
• Clinical practice guidelines including in UK mental health act and mental capacity act, risk assessments
• Instruction in how to use holistic needs assessments and guidelines as communication tool, and incorporating into good practise
• Ongoing awareness of boundaries, self care and risk of compassion fatigue and burnout

11.4.2 Boundaries

The development of a solid therapeutic relationship with firm boundaries means staff can apply their professional knowledge and experience towards meeting health and psychosocial needs of their patients. This needs to be tempered with recognition that boundaries exist to protect the needs of the patients and needs of the staff member [30]. Boundaries can further be complicated if the majority of the staff are of a similar age to the patient, or if the patients are the same age as staff members own children, which can bring up issues of over identification and awkwardness. Working as a member of an MDT with young people affects staff on many levels; there are always some patients and families who affect us deeply. There may be many reasons why this can happen including identifying with them in some way, triggers or reminders of important relationships, or having formed a bond with the family and then treatment not going as expected can feel unbearable. There must be recognition that there need to be boundaries to protect staff from getting hurt, getting too close to a family or stopping staff from burning out.

11.4.3 Boundary Challenges Specific to Working with AYA Patients and Their Carers

The informal setting of the AYA ward, means informal approach and informal language may be used which promotes more time with patients and family and promotes some self disclosure.

The longer the stay, the more involved the team become with the patient and carers lives; and thus the potential for the carer and young person to see staff more as friends then as members of staff because of the huge amount of time spent together.

The use of modern technology and the potential shared interests with staff, relaxed communication style, an emotionally demanding group, and the need to think in the moment, on your feet can all lead to potential for breaking of boundaries.

Managing relationships and boundaries with young people can be challenging to healthcare professionals, particularly for inexperienced and younger members of the team. Staff are expected to foster a friendly and age-appropriate approach. These factors can introduce unique challenges to maintaining appropriate professional boundaries with the young person (Fig. 11.3).

11.4.3.1 *What are Professional Boundaries?* (Based on Santa Cruz [31] with Additions)

- Professional boundaries are clearly established limits that allow for safe connections between service providers and their clients
- "Being with" the client, not becoming the client
- Being friendly, not friends
- The ability to know where you end and the client begins
- A clear understanding of the limits and responsibilities of your role as a service provider

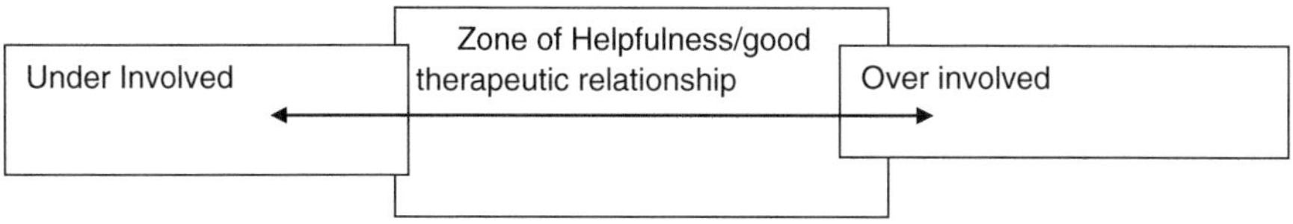

Fig. 11.3 A continuum of professional behaviour based on Santa Cruz [31]

Boundary violations occur when there is confusion between the needs of the staff member and that of the patient and mayinclude excessive personal disclosure, secrecy, feelings the staff member is the only one that can care for the patient properly and inappropriate use of social media. Social media is part of most people's lives but can blur lines between professional and personal lives and it is strongly recommended to have a clear policy discouraging use of personal social media with patients or their carers (see Table 11.6 for red flag behaviours of staff).

Table 11.6 Red Flag behaviours of staff with regards to professional boundaries which need to be addressed promptly (based on NCSBN [30] with additions)

• Discussing intimate or personal issues with a patient
• Patient and staff member refer to each other as friends
• Staff member receives or gives gifts to patient
• Patient asks for personal information about staff member including telephone number, facebook etc
• Staff member reveals excessive personal information or personal problems to patient
• Staff member unable to sleep because of worrying about patient
• Discussion about patient or work dominates staff social interactions with friends and family
• Staff member offers assistance outside their role eg babysitting, driving to appointments
• Engaging in behaviours that could be interpreted as flirting, or starting a sexual or intimate relationship with a patient
• Keeping secrets with a patient or for a patient
• Believing you are the only one who truly understands or can help the patient, taking on the. 'rescuer/hero role'
• Having favourites to work with, stopping others from working with the patient or refusing to work with other patients.
• Spending more time than is necessary with a particular patient
• Speaking disrespectfully about colleagues/managers to patient or their family
• Meeting patients in settings beside those used to provide direct patient care or meeting when you are not at work
Consequences of having loose or poor boundaries (from Santa Cruz with additions):
• Compassion fatigue, feeling your role is unsustainable
• Splitting in teams (cannot all agree, exhausting, disagreeing with colleagues)
• Client may miss out on appropriate or helpful services
• Client may feel betrayed or abandoned by other staff
• Staff member may not trust other team members to fulfil their responsibilities, as they believe only he/she can provide a good service
Techniques for creating and maintaining healthy professional boundaries
• Establish clear agreements regarding role of staff, what your availability is, how to communicate with your staff/management system
• If boundary issues appear, address them promptly, be sensitive to feelings
• If you do self disclose, ensure any information is minimal and related only to patients goals, too much self disclosure can shift focus from patient to staff
• Remember that how someone interprets your words may not be what you were trying to get across, must get them to repeat back, check they understood
• Use supervisor/peers as sounding board, to ensure still providing objective compassionate care

11.4.4 Stress and Burnout

The impact of working with this population can put staff members as well as family members under huge stress, and at risk of stress, burnout and compassion fatigue' The stress comes in part from burnout, the chronic psychological syndrome of perceived demands from work outweighing perceived resources in the work ([32]):

Burnout is a cumulative process marked by emotional exhaustion and withdrawal associated with increased workload and underlined by institutional/managerial stress [33]. Burnout results from prolonged high levels of stress at work [34] and, if not addressed, contributes to staff leaving the workplace [32] Burnout can be experienced both by family members, and members of staff looking after the patient and family.

Compassion fatigue [33] is the emotional reaction created by the trauma of helping others in distress, which leads to a reduced capacity for empathy towards suffering in the future, associated with the kind of work you do; it is a consequence of the strain of exposure to working with those who are vulnerable suffering or undergoing trauma. Compassion fatigue develops over time, and the ability to feel and care for others becomes eroded with emotional blunting. It has been described by Potter [32] as the cost a caregiver may experience as a result of caring for others; resulting from giving high levels of energy and compassion over a prolonged period to those who are suffering, often without experiencing the positive outcomes of seeing patients improve.

Mukerjee et al. [35], have developed specific tools acknowledging that working in paediatric and young adult oncology means there may be specific aspects of this work which increase the risk of burnout and also of mental health difficulties. These may include: administering and managing complex treatment regimes which have a significant impact on the child's or young person's health and well-being; the untimeliness of the death of a child; supporting and managing demands from families; and recognition that many staff work over their allocated hours; and may have children themselves which can be an extra potential identification of stress. Staff working within the specialism may need ongoing and specialised support if they are to avoid burnout and mental health difficulties.

Three sources of stress were associated with burnout and psychiatric morbidity: feeling overloaded, and its impact on home life; feeling poorly managed and resourced; and dealing with patients' suffering. Burnout was also associated with low satisfaction in relationships with patients, relatives, and staff, professional status/esteem and intellectual stimulation. In addition, being younger and being single were independent risk factors for burnout. Burnout was more prevalent among consultants who felt insufficiently trained in communication and management skills [36]. Burnout is usually reported more for junior doctors aged below 30 or 40 [37], but there is a debate that this may present in a U shaped curve, both peaking at junior level, but with a second peak aged 50–60 [38]. Ramirez's study also reported prevalence of burnout up until ages of 55 (Table 11.7) [36].

11.4.4.1 Stress and Resilience Assessment

Mukerjee et al. have developed two new robust stress and resilience measures for staff working in paediatric and young adult oncology:

60 item WSS_PO (Work Stressors scale-paediatric oncology) measuring total intensity of work related stressors, including sub scaled scores for ill patient (caring

Table 11.7 Key messages for staff training in oncology on burnout: (ECEPO undated)

1.	Key manifestationss of burnout are exhaustion, cynicism, and a sense of personal ineffectiveness
2.	Burnout often presents as a feeling that you "don't care anymore"
3.	Burnout is more related to the situation and perception of poor management than the individual
4.	Burnout is more prevalent among women than men and those in earlier stages of their careers
5.	Long work hours and work-home interference are strongly associated with burnout
6.	Burnout arises from chronic mismatches between people and their work settings
7.	Job engagement (energy, involvement, and efficacy) is conceptualized as the opposite of burnout
8.	Burnout, in contrast with depression, is specific to the work context
9.	Lifestyle management techniques (exercise, meditation, humour, etc.) may decrease vulnerability to burnout
10.	Burnout may be prevented by changes in management and guidance combined with educational interventions and improved communication
11.	Burnout is common; expect it and prevent it. The working conditions and often institutional poor management practice, not the patients, are the most common cause of burnout
12.	Trying to simply pretend it is not happening and soldiering on regardless doesn't work. Burnout needs to come out into the open with opportunities to change working conditions and have a frank discussion with the management system to effect change

for an ill or dying patient), parent (dealing with parents and families) and organisation (team conflict, workload and work environment source of stress).

The 35 item WRS-PO (Work Rewards Scale-paediatric oncology) provides a total score of the perceived intensity of rewards/what helps staff to cope.

11.4.5 What Can Help Staff?

A number of factors can help staff: knowing who to go to if support is needed; creating a supportive atmosphere; not dismissing early signs of stress and burnout; creating a culture of working together with colleagues to problem solve; recognising staff need to feel valued and listened to; being able to all play some part in organisational change when needed [39]. Beresford surveyed children's and young people's specialist cancer treatment centres in the UK found a wide variability about the types of support on offer [39]. Doctors were the professionals least likely to access support. The authors also concluded that there is a need to recognise that the organisational culture both at an institutional and departmental level plays a role in workforce well-being.

11.4.5.1 What Helps Staff to Cope

A realistic understanding of the demands faced by staff both in workplace and to an extent at home, and an understanding of the impact that work is having on coping, work–life balance and mental health all facilitate coping. Access to appropriate support is crucial, and needs to be available for all levels of staff throughout the hierarchy, either provided in house or externally. Not only will this help the individual staff members concerned, and patients in their care, but it will also be beneficial to the rest of the MDT, who have to deal with the consequences of a colleague experiencing burnout.

Some people prefer to seek support on an individual basis, in or away from the hospital, others are happy in a group format. Access to support needs to be transparent, encouraged by managers and available if staff are to remain in a job which both challenging and rewarding. Working in austere times in underresourced teams contributes to the problem and should be recognised. Transparent management and knowledge of who to go to if a staff member feels stressed, can see boundaries being breached or is aware of bad practise is important. Accessing support needs to be seen as an acceptable way of coping, not as a failure, and this means gentle encouragement from management downwards that it is acceptable and encouraged to seek support.

It is however crucial to note that support services alone cannot prevent stress, burnout and staff turnover; there needs to be a top down approach from the management teams to recognise that at times changes in practice are needed.

11.4.5.2 Offer Clinical Supervision

The purpose of clinical/reflective/professional supervision is to provide a safe and confidential environment for staff to reflect on and discuss their work, usually using case study discussion and personal and professional responses to their work, usually by a monthly closed group. Clinical supervision can also be offered on an individual or peer group format. It can help staff to manage the personal and professional demands created by the nature of their work; this is particularly important for those who work with people who have complex and challenging needs. Clinical supervision provides an environment in which they can explore their own personal and emotional reactions to their work. Clinical supervision has been associated with higher levels of job satisfaction, improved retention, reduced turnover and staff effectiveness. Effective clinical supervision may increase employees' perceptions of organisational support and improve their commitment to an organisation's vision and goals [40].

11.4.5.3 Offer Confidential Individual Support

Confidential support can be offered through though a staff support service, occupational health or through individual consultation with psychology/wellbeing teams or external referral. If this is offered, support and recognition that this is acceptable needs to be given from the management teams, and early referral is recommended if staff feel stressed or are showing early signs of burnout. Working together with occupational health teams will enable staff to feel supported and find a safe place to work through any issues and put in place strategies or changes to work with support arranged as needed.

11.4.5.4 Group Support

Many members of staff request and take part in regular group support sessions with their peers. A variety of group types are on offer, including general drop ins, theme led support, regular complex decision making meetings or de-briefs following the death of a patient. The formats are variable and creativity is needed when working out what suits the majority as it will be very difficult to accommodate all individual needs. Regular consultation with staff and managers is needed to ensure that a variety of support is offered.

Balanced with formal support, the encouragement of team away days, social outings and social time away from the hospital is also encouraged to enhance team working and to understand and get to know the individual team members. No one works in isolation and sharing of the challenges and successes of the job is needed.

11.4.5.5 Debriefs/reflective space after death or critical incident/complex decision making

There are times when a critical incident has occurred and the staff need space and time to reflect, think through what worked and did not work, talk through how this made them feel and consider any learning or action points. The staff facilitating such meetings, ideally with 2 co-facilitators, aim to ensure it is not seen as a blaming and shaming exercise and that the purpose of such a meeting is clear to all, that everyone does have a chance to contribute, and that agreed documentation or action points are carried out.

11.4.5.6 Schwartz Rounds [41]

A structured forum where all staff, clinical and non clinical, come together regularly to discuss the emotional and social aspects of working in healthcare, has been introduced in many hospitals over the last few years. The purpose is to understand the challenges and rewards that are intrinsic to providing care. Evidence shows staff who attend feel less stressed and isolated. The underlying premise is that compassion shown by staff can make all the difference to a patient's experience of care, but that in order to provide compassionate care, staff must feel in turn supported in their work (Table 11.8).

Table 11.8 Different types of staff support

Traditional Staff Forums	Schwartz Rounds
Grand Rounds aim to help medical staff learn about recent developments in medicine and focus on the clinical details of a case	*Schwartz Rounds* do not focus on the clinical aspects of patient care; instead learning is focused on understanding staff experience from a social and emotional point of view
Balint groups follow a similar format to rounds in terms of their reflective nature and focus on emotional impact, but they are only open to certain members of clinical staff	*Schwartz Rounds* are open to all staff members including non-clinical staff. Three or four stories are told at each round, which are used as a springboard for a wider discussion beyond the case itself
Supervision/clinical supervision involves expertise and advice; is generally aimed at a specific staff group; focuses on technical aspects of care, clinical outcomes or personal development, unlike rounds	*Schwartz Rounds* are not designed as a form of peer supervision and do not fit the traditional model of clinical supervision
Debriefings are usually structured meetings that aim to help staff following stressful or traumatic clinical events, through education, normalising and support	*Schwartz Rounds* should not be used as a form of debriefing. If there is a case that has been particularly troubling for staff and the organisation, a certain amount of time will need to pass before it is addressed in a round

11.4.5.7 Praise and Rewards for Staff

Underlying all the different support mechanisms around for staff, is the need for all staff to feel what they do is worthwhile, that their views are important and that they are valued and have a voice. The appraisal system, is a mechanism which can be seen as an opportunity for reward and recognition, but is more often seen as a necessary exercise to get through every year and for some staff groups contributes to revalidation. Every institution, if really paying attention to their staff, needs to think how to really engage with their staff and how to address the hierarchy that always exists, but which can make it difficult for some members of the team to ever feel important or heard. NHS institutions often call themselves a family, but often this is a family that does not function very well, communication issues exist, roles may not be clear, and some members of the family feel invisible. If we are truly to care for the carers, whether family members or staff, the carers need to be noticed, time taken to understand their views and to work together to meet the needs both of patient, carer and staff.

11.5 Carers: Support Staff Who Look After Other Carers

The final group of carers are those whose work primarily is to look after all the other carers, those offering the clinical supervision, running the staff groups, offering individual support, giving expert advice, chairing debriefs offering consultation on complex decisions or risk issues.

Clinical psychologists, staff support workers (often counsellors) and social workers as part of their clinical practice guidelines have ongoing supervision to reflect upon practice and the complex issues that arise. In terms of a team working to support other carers, peer supervision and case study discussions about complex families, safeguarding or risk issues are held regularly to ensure any burden is shared. Support needs to be in conjunction with team leaders, managers, and the management executive as an entity.

11.6 Final Words on Self Care

Carers play a crucial role in the wellbeing and social system of any young person going through treatment and they need ongoing support at all levels to facilitate coping and understanding when faced with such a complex situation. The better informed and supported a carer is, the better they can find ways to cope, or find ways of finding someone to help. The importance of self-care is crucial: at all levels we need to be able to look after ourselves in order to be able to meet needs of others. The capacity for compassion and empathy, and understanding of our own strengths and limitations seem to be at the core of our ability to do the work and at the core of our ability to be wounded by the work [42] (Table 11.9)."

Table 11.9 Care for the caregiver

For family member, staff or carer of any type: Tips adapted from words shared by Marilyn Goodhew, play specialist
• Be gentle with yourself
• Work - life balance, make sure there is one
• Remind yourself you are an enabler not a magician, we cannot change anyone else, just change how we relate to them
• Say I choose rather than I should, I have to...
• Remember your sense of humour
• If you never say no, what is your yes worth?
• Aloofness and indifference are far more harmful than admitting an inability to do more
• Change your routine often and your tasks when you can
• Create a calm safe spot, use it daily, we all need a man cave or a woman cave...
• Schedule withdrawal time, time away, limit any encroachments
• Be your own resource, get creative, try new approach, try something new
• Use supervision, mentoring, coaching, counselling as a source of support and strength
• Learn to recognise the difference between complaining that relieves and complaining that reinforces negative stress
• Remember that in the light of all the pain that we see, we are allowed to feel helpless sometimes and admit it without shame
• Caring and being there sometimes is more important than doing
• Give support and encouragement and praise to peers and management when things are done well, learn to accept it in return
• On the way home focus on a good thing that occurred during the day, jot it down so you can remind yourself in the gloom there is something good to focus on
• Remind yourself what you really enjoy
• Laugh, play have fun
• If we care for ourselves we can care for others

References

1. Burton M, Watson M. Counselling people with cancer. West Sussex: Chichester; 1988.
2. Kazak A, Noll R (2015) The integration of psychology in pediatric oncology research and practice. American Oncologist 70(2):146-158. https://doi.org/10.1037/a0035695
3. Whiteson A, Whiteson M. Foreward. In: Selby P, Bailey C, editors. Cancer and the adolescent. London: BMJ; 1996.
4. Quinn P, Goncalves V, Sehovic I, Bowman M, Reed D. Quality of life in adolescent and young adult cancer patients: a systematic review of the literature. Patient relat Outcome Meas. 2015;6:19–51.
5. Warner E, Kent E, Trevino K, Parsons H, Zebrack B, Kirchhoff A. Social well-being among adolescents and young adults with cancer: a systematic review. Cancer. 2016;122:1029–37.
6. Zebrack B, Isaacson S. Psychosocial Care of Adolescent and Young Adult Patients with Cancer and survivors. J Clin Oncol. 2012;30:1221–6.
7. Teenage Cancer trust (TCT)2012 Blueprint of care.
8. Grinyer A. The biographical impact of teenage and adolescent cancer. Chronic Illn. 2007;3:265–77.
9. Adams D, Deveau E. Coping with childhood cancer: where do we go from here? Canada: Kindridge Publications Ontario; 1989.

10. Patiño-Fernández AM, Pai ALH, Alderfer M, Hwang WT, Reilly M, Kazak AE. Acute stress in parents of children newly diagnosed with cancer. Pedatric Blood Cancer. 2008;50(2):289–92.
11. Children's Cancer and Leukaemia Group. In: Edwards L, editor. Facing the death of your child; suggestions and help for families, before and afterwards. CCLG Leicester. 2015.
12. Proot I, Abu-Saad H, Crebolder H, Goldsteen M, Widdershovn K. Vulnerability of family caregivers in terminal palliative care at home: balancing between burden and capacity. Scand J Caring Sci. 2003;17:113–21.
13. Hudson P, Aranda S. The Melbourne family support programme: evidence based strategies that prepare the family caregiver for supporting palliative care patients. BMJ Support Palliat Care. 2016;4(3):231–7.
14. Northouse L, Williams A, Given B, McCorkle R. Psychosical care for family caregivers of patients with cancer. Journal of Clnicial Oncology. 2012;30(11):1227–34. https://doi.org/10.1200/JCO.2011.395798.
15. Macmillan Cancer Support. A Practical guide to living with and after cancer, a sort guide to make sure no one faces cancer alone. 2015.
16. Cancer Research UK (CRUK undated) Support for children whose parents have cancer. Read more at http://www.cancerresearchuk.org/about-cancer/cancers-in-general/cancer-questions/support-for-children-whose-parents-have-cancer#4QCItbA9ghKUh0a1.99 Accessed 10 Sep 2016.
17. Macmillan Cancer Support. Talking to children when an adult has cancer. 2016. http://www.macmillan.org.uk/information-and-support/coping/talking-about-cancer/talking-to-children Accessed 1 Jul 2016.
18. Cancernet. http://www.cancer.net/coping-with-cancer/talking-with-family-and-friends/talking-about-cancer/talking-with-your-children. Accessed 10 Sep 2016.
19. Fossa S, Dahl A. Fertility and sexuality in young cancer survivors who have adult onset malignancies. Hematol Oncol Clin North Am. 2008;22(2):291–303.
20. Zebrack B, Bleyer A, Albritton K, Medearis S, Tang J. Assessing the health care needs of adolescent and young adult cancer patients and survivors. Cancer. 2006;107(12):2915–23.
21. Zebrack B, Block R, Hayes-Lattin B, Embry L, Aguikar C, Meeske K, Li Y, Butler M, Cole S (2013) Psychosocial use and unmet need among recently diagnosed adolescent and young adult cancer patients. Cancer. 119(1):201-214. https://doi.org/10.1002/cncr.27713.
22. World Health Organisation (WHO) 2002 National Cancer control programmes: policies and managerial guidelines 2nd Edition geneva WHO 11.1.
23. Macmillan Cancer Support. A Practical guide to living with and after cancer, having a holistic needs assessment. Macmillan Cancer Support. 2015.
24. Hudson P, Remedios C, Thomas K. A systematic review of psychosocial interventions for family carers of palliative care patients Biomedcentral (BMC). BMC Palliat Care. 2010;9:17. https://doi.org/10.1186/1472-684X-9-17.
25. Michels C, Boulton M, Adams A, Wee B, Peters M (2016) Psychometric properties of carer reported outcome measures in palliative care a systematic review30(1):23–44.
26. Surbonne A, Baider L, Weitzman T, Brames J, Rittenberg C, Johnson J. Psychosocial care for patients and their families is integral to supportive care in cancer: MASCC position statement. Support Care Cancer. 2010;18:255–63.
27. Children's Cancer and Leukaemia Group. How can the internet help us? A guide for parents and families using online childhood cancer information. 2014. http://www.cclg.org.uk/write/MediaUploads/Publications/PDFs/How_can_the_internet_help_us_(May_14).pdf. Accessed 10 Jul 2016.
28. Wiener L, Weaver M, Bell C, Sansom-Daly U. Threading the cloak palliative care education for care providers of adolescents and young adults with cancer. Clini Oncol Adolsec Young Adults. 2015; https://doi.org/10.2147/COAYA.S49176.
29. Nijboer C, Treimstra M, Tempelaar R, Sanderman R, Van den Bos GA. Measuring both negative and positive reactions to giving care to cancer patients: psychometric qualities of the caregiver reaction assessment (CRA). Soc Sci Med. 1999;48:1259–69.

30. National Council Of State Boards of Nursing (NCSBN). A Nurse's guide to professional Boundaries. 2014. https://www.ncsbn.org/ProfessionalBoundaries_Complete.pdf. Accessed 25 Jul 2016.
31. Santa Cruz County Service Integration. Maintain professional boundaries in interpersonal work. 2008. https://www.ualberta.ca/medicine/departments/anesthesiology-pain-medicine/staff-wellbeing/-/media/275648b805574c9cb6b19f6b4fce950c.ashx. Accessed 25 Jun 2016.
32. Potter P, Deshields T, Divanbeigi J, Berger J, Cipriano D, Norris L, Olsen S. Compassion fatigue and burnout: prevalence among oncology nurses. Clin J Oncol Nurs. 2010;14(5):E56–62. https://doi.org/10.1188/10.CJON.E56-E62.
33. American Institute of Stress. Is it burnout or compassion fatigue? 2011. http://www.stress.org/military/for-practitionersleaders/compassion-fatigue/. Accessed 20 Aug 2016.
34. Maslach C, Leiter M. The truth about burnout: how organizations cause personal stress and what to do about it. San Francisco, CA. 1998.
35. Mukherjee S, Beresford B, Tennant A. Staff burnout in paediatric oncology: new tools to facilitate the development and evaluation of effective interventions. Eur J Cancer Care. 2014; https://doi.org/10.1111/ecc.12176.
36. Ramirez AJ, Graham J, Richards MA, et al. Mental health of hospital consultants: the effect of stress and satisfaction at work. Lancet. 1996;347:724–8. PMID: 8602002
37. EPEC™-O. Education In Palliative And End-Of-Life Care For Oncology, Self-Study Module 15: Cancer Doctors and Burnout. https://www.cancer.gov/resources-for/hp/education/epeco/self-study/module-15/module-15.pdf.
38. Skovholt T, Trotter-Mathison M. The resilient Practioner: burnout and compassion, fatigue prevention and self care strategies for the caring professions. Abingdon: Routledge; 2016.
39. Beresford B, Gibson F, Bayliss J, Mukherjee S. Preventing work related stress among staff working in children's cancer principal treatment Centres in the UK: a brief survey of staff support systems and practices. Eur J Cancer Care. 2016; https://doi.org/10.1111/ecc.12535.
40. Care Quality Commission. Supporting information and guidance: supporting effective clinical supervision. 2013. https://www.cqc.org.uk/sites/default/files/documents/20130625_800734_v1_00_supporting_information-effective_clinical_supervision_for_publication.pdf. Accessed 20 Aug 2016.
41. Point of Care Foundation. Scwartz Rounds. 2015. https://www.pointofcarefoundation.org.uk/our-work/schwartz-rounds. Accessed 21 June 2016.
42. Good Therapy.org. Who's taking care of the caretaker/A Guided Self-Care Assessment for Helping Professionals. 2014. http://www.goodtherapy.org/blog/whos-taking-care-of=the-caretaker-1022144 Accessed 19 May 2016.

MIX
Papier aus verantwortungsvollen Quellen
Paper from responsible sources
FSC® C105338

If you have any concerns about our products,
you can contact us on
ProductSafety@springernature.com

In case Publisher is established outside the EU,
the EU authorized representative is:
Springer Nature Customer Service Center GmbH
Europaplatz 3, 69115 Heidelberg, Germany

Printed by Libri Plureos GmbH
in Hamburg, Germany